DEDICATIONS

Dedicated to Steve, with love and thanks for many wonderful years together; to our children, who enrich my life; and to my students, who keep the job interesting.

Kate Baldwin

I would like to dedicate this to my wonderful wife Paula and my two fine sons, Michael and Matthew, whose companionship makes it all worthwhile.

John Young

Dedicated to Seb and Adey who fill my life and to my students who inspire me to do my best.

Lekidelu Taddesse-Heath, MD

I dedicate this book to my wife Fran, my children, and my students.

Ray Hakim

Preface

This book is designed to aid students who want a comprehensive review of histology, cell biology, and basic pathology. It consists of a set of multiple choice exam questions, written in the style of the USMLE exams. As is the case with USMLE questions, some answer choices are partially correct, but the single best answer is indicated. Each question has an explanation of why the correct answer should be chosen and a reference to one or both of the companion texts: *Wheater's Functional Histology, 5th Edition* by Young, Lowe, Stevens, and Heath or *Wheater's Basic Histopathology, 5th Edition* by Young, O'Dowd, and Stewart. Where possible, histology and cell biology are presented as applications of the core basic subjects. Many questions are written as introductory level clinical scenarios in order to give students practice in problem solving.

Since histology, cell biology, and pathology are disciplines that depend heavily on images, we have included many questions based on images. The illustrations come from one or the other of the two companion texts and are in full color.

Many of the questions can be answered using a knowledge of histology and cell biology and will be appropriate for students beginning their second year of medical school. These questions will be useful in reinforcing understanding of these subjects and providing practice in applying information mastered. Other questions require some knowledge of pathology and will serve as an introduction to this discipline. More advanced students who are preparing for the USMLE exams may use these questions to review and to test their retention of histology, cell biology, and pathology.

It is our expectation that this review book will encourage remediation where needed and will act as a guide for students by revealing any areas of weakness. By closely tying the questions to material in the companion textbooks, we have attempted to make this remediation/review process as efficient as possible.

Kate M. Baldwin
John K. Young
Lekidelu Taddesse-Heath
Raziel S. Hakim

Acknowledgments

The authors are indebted to Barbara Young, James S. Lowe, Alan Stevens, and John W. Heath, authors of *Wheater's Functional Histology, 5th Edition,* and to Barbara Young, Geraldine O'Dowd, and William Stewart, authors of *Wheater's Basic Pathology, 5th Edition.* These two texts served as the reference texts for this review book, and it is our expectation that readers of this book will seek out further information from these companion texts as they discover a need to supplement or correct their knowledge of cell biology, histology, and pathology.

We would also like to thank Elsevier staff members Kate Dimock, Senior Acquisitions Editor; Christine Abshire, Developmental Editor; and Sharon Lee, Project Manager for their help and support during the preparation of this book.

Contents

The Cell

FH5 Chapter 1: Cell Structure and Function
FH5 Chapter 7: Nervous Tissues
FH5 Chapter 14: Gastrointestinal Tract
FH5 Chapter 16: Urinary System
FH5 Chapter 17: Endocrine System
BH5 Chapter 1: Introduction

1

Cell Structure and Function

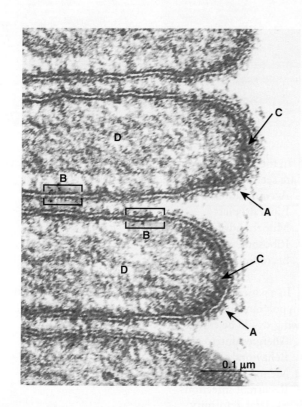

0.1 µm

1 Which of the labeled structures in the figure above contain the most sugar groups?

2 What occupies most of the light region in the middle of the plasma membrane shown in the figure?
☐ A. Cholesterol and glycolipid
☐ B. Choline and serine
☐ C. Fatty acids and cholesterol
☐ D. Fatty acids and ethanolamine
☐ E. Serine and ethanolamine

3 A group of plasma proteins called *complement inhibitors* protect cells from complement-mediated cell damage and require an anchoring protein to attach them to the cell membrane. Which of the following would be a direct consequence of an absence of the anchoring protein on red blood cells?
☐ A. Denaturation of hemoglobin
☐ B. Hemolysis
☐ C. Inability to carry oxygen
☐ D. Increased DNA transcription
☐ E. Rapid protein synthesis

4 In a female patient born with Turner syndrome, a genetic disorder that results in only one X chromosome, how many Barr bodies would be present?
☐ A. 0
☐ B. 1
☐ C. 2
☐ D. 3
☐ E. 4

5 Which cytoplasmic organelle would be most abundant in plasma cells?
☐ A. Lysosomes
☐ B. Microtubules
☐ C. Peroxisomes
☐ D. Rough endoplasmic reticulum
☐ E. Secretion granules

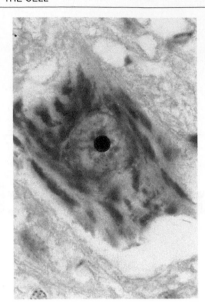

6 In the figure above, a neuron with an unusually prominent, dark-staining nuclear structure is shown. This structure is specifically linked to which cellular process?
☐ A. Exocytosis of neurotransmitter
☐ B. Mitosis
☐ C. Production of ribosomal subunits
☐ D. Reuptake of dopamine through dopamine transporters
☐ E. Synthesis of glycogen

7 Hepatocytes detoxify barbiturates using cytochrome P-450 enzymes. Where are these enzymes mainly found?
☐ A. Golgi apparatus
☐ B. Lysosomes
☐ C. Peroxisomes
☐ D. Proteasomes
☐ E. Smooth endoplasmic reticulum

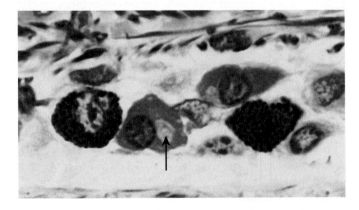

8 In a cell shown in the figure above, there is a clearly circumscribed, pale-staining region in the cytoplasm (*arrow*). What occupies this region?
☐ A. Golgi complex
☐ B. Lysosomes
☐ C. Mitochondria
☐ D. Rough endoplasmic reticulum
☐ E. Zymogen granules

9 Binding specificity between a vesicle and the membrane of its target is established by having what vesicle- and target-specific proteins?
☐ A. GTPases
☐ B. Lectins
☐ C. Pore proteins
☐ D. SNARE proteins

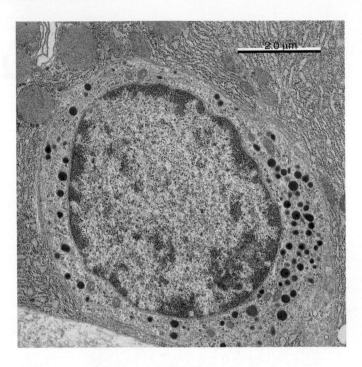

10 In the figure above, what numerous dark-staining structures are seen within the cytoplasm of the cell?
☐ A. Accumulations of glycogen
☐ B. Lipid droplets
☐ C. Mitochondria
☐ D. Ribosomes
☐ E. Secretion granules

11 In a patient with an inherited defect of phagocytic function in polymorphonuclear neutrophils (PMNs), which of the following would be expected?
☐ A. Allergies due to mast cell degranulation
☐ B. Behavioral abnormality
☐ C. Mental retardation
☐ D. Recurrent infections
☐ E. Skeletal deformity

13 The cell in the figure at the bottom left is enriched in organelles to carry out which cellular process?

☐ A. Apoptosis
☐ B. Mitosis
☐ C. Phagocytosis
☐ D. Protein synthesis
☐ E. Storage of secretory proteins in vesicles

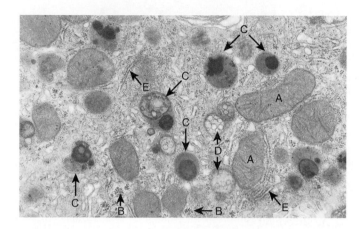

14 Which structures in the cell shown in the figure above would be expected to accumulate in a patient with Hurler syndrome?

Receptor-mediated endocytosis

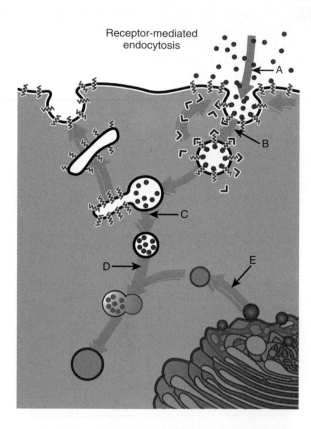

12 A patient has been diagnosed with *familial hypercholesterolemia*, and a lab test shows severely elevated low-density lipoprotein (LDL) in her blood. The diagram above shows the mechanism of cellular uptake of LDL. Which stage is likely deficient in this patient?

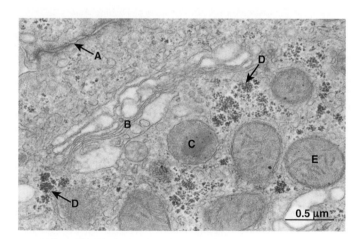

15 Which labeled structure in the figure above would be expected to stain most intensely with antibodies to catalase?

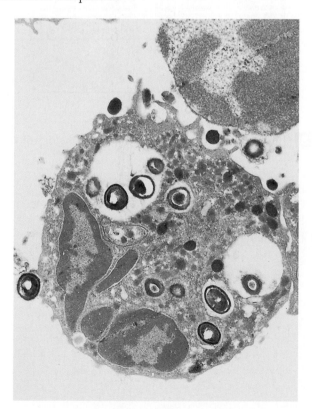

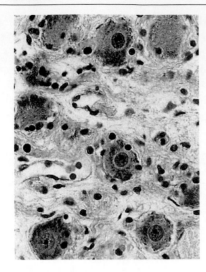

16 Brown granules of lipofuscin are detected in a tissue section from an elderly patient (see above figure). In which cell type is lipofuscin a normal, rather than a pathologic, constituent?

☐ A. Brown fat cell
☐ B. Ganglion cell
☐ C. Keratinocyte of the stratum basale of the skin
☐ D. Keratinocyte of the stratum granulosum of the skin
☐ E. Macrophage

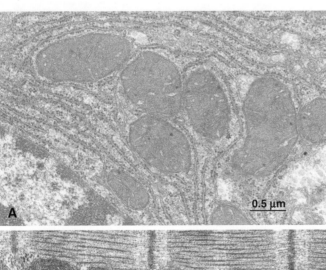

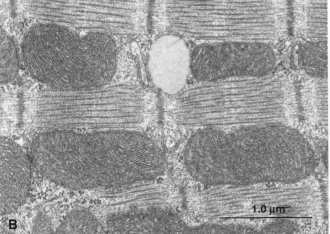

17 Compare the two images at the bottom left and determine which shows the cell with the highest energy requirements. How do you know this?

☐ A. The cell in A because of the large amount of matrix in the mitochondria
☐ B. The cell in A because of the larger size of the mitochondria
☐ C. The cell in A because of the prominent matrix granules in the mitochondria
☐ D. The cell in B because of the densely packed cristae in the mitochondria
☐ E. The cell in B because of the regular orientation of the mitochondria

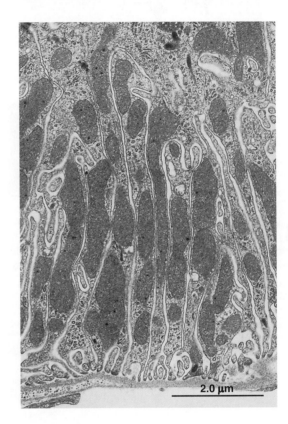

18 The cell in the figure above has the morphology of a cell specialized for what?

☐ A. Absorption and digestion
☐ B. Antibody secretion
☐ C. Glycogen synthesis and detoxification of drugs
☐ D. Ion transport
☐ E. Protein synthesis

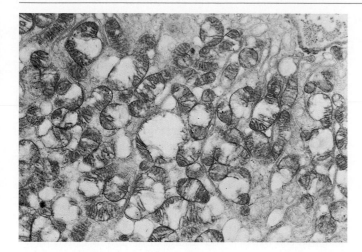

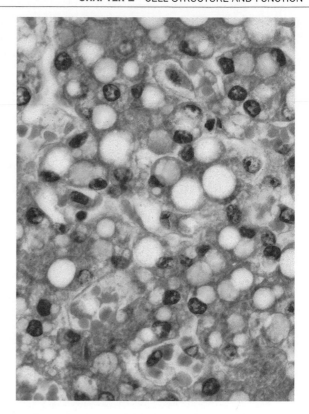

19 Cell injury is often evident by the abnormal appearance of cellular organelles. An example of this is shown in the figure above. There are, however, sufficient normal features in these organelles to identify them as what?

☐ A. Golgi bodies
☐ B. Lysosomes
☐ C. Mitochondria
☐ D. Peroxisomes
☐ E. Polysomes

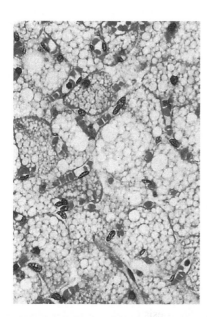

20 The cells in the figure above are highly vacuolated. What accounts for this appearance?

☐ A. Extraction of lipids during routine histologic preparation
☐ B. Highly glycosylated secretory product stored in these cells
☐ C. Poor staining of the hydrophobic lipids
☐ D. Postmortem deterioration of these cells

21 In alcoholic cirrhosis, hepatocytes may have large, unstained spaces in the cytoplasm, as shown in the figure above. Which cytoplasmic component accounts for these unstained spaces?

☐ A. Golgi stacks
☐ B. Lipid
☐ C. Lipofuscin
☐ D. Lysosomes
☐ E. Peroxisomes

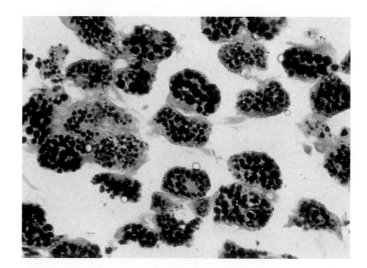

22 The tissue section in the figure above was obtained from tissues treated with osmium tetroxide. The distinctive appearance of cells of this tissue results from the ability of osmium tetroxide to perform what action?

☐ A. Bind to lipids
☐ B. Enhance the penetration of stains into a tissue section
☐ C. Remove water from cells before embedding
☐ D. Soften tissues and enable easier tissue sectioning

23 Certain differentiated cells produce or express cell-type–specific proteins. Staining for these proteins can be used to identify the cell of origin of certain malignant tumors. For example, if a tumor cell is found to express the intermediate filament desmin, from what cells has it most likely developed?
☐ A. Astrocytes
☐ B. Epithelial cells
☐ C. Muscle cells
☐ D. Neurons

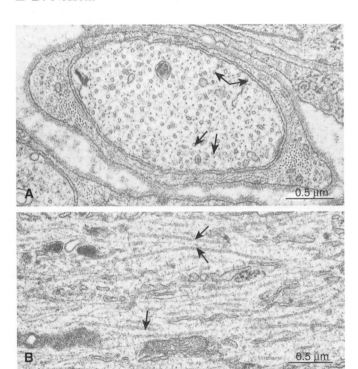

24 The structures indicated by *arrows* in the images above would be expected to label with antibodies to which protein?
☐ A. Actin
☐ B. Clathrin
☐ C. Glial fibrillary acidic protein
☐ D. Myosin
☐ E. Tubulin

ANSWERS

1. A This is the glycocalyx, which consists of integral membrane proteins and other proteins that were glycosylated in the rough endoplasmic reticulum and Golgi apparatus. Both the brush borders of the intestinal villi and the proximal convoluted tubules of the kidney have a particularly prominent periodic acid–Schiff stainable glycocalyx. The center of the lipid bilayer of a membrane is not exposed to the enzymes of the Golgi apparatus and does not become glycosylated by this pathway. Likewise, proteins free in the cytoplasm are not exposed to the enzymes of the Golgi apparatus and do not become glycosylated. **FH pp. 4-5, 31, 278, 315**

2. C Fatty acids and cholesterol are mostly hydrophobic and occupy the middle of the membrane bilayer. The choline, serine, ethanolamine, and sugar groups in glycolipids are polar and are found facing the aqueous environment at the periphery of the membrane. **FH pp. 4-5**

3. B Absence of anchoring protein results in a lack of complement inhibitors on the surface of red blood cells. This causes the red blood cells to be susceptible to complement-mediated cell damage and results in hemolysis of red blood cells. This defect is present in the disease known as *paroxysmal nocturnal hemoglobinuria*. Complement proteins, or their inhibitors, have no direct effect on rate of protein synthesis, DNA transcription, or the function of hemoglobin. Denaturation of hemoglobin occurs when there is insufficient amount of NADPH and glutathione to keep hemoglobin in the reduced state. **FH p. 5**

4. A One inactivated X chromosome is present as a Barr body in normal females. In Turner syndrome, the single functioning X chromosome cannot be inactivated, and there is no Barr body. In Klinefelter syndrome, a genetic disorder affecting males, there are one or more extra X chromosomes. In these cases, there would be one or more Barr bodies. **FH p. 6**

5. D Antibody-secreting plasma cells, like all protein-secreting cells, have abundant rough endoplasmic reticulum. Plasma cells secrete immunoglobulins constitutively, so they have no secretion granules. Lysosomes are common in phagocytic cells, whereas peroxisomes are associated with lipid metabolism. Microtubules are only abundant in long processes, such as cilia and axons, that need structural support. **FH p. 6**

6. C The dark-stained nucleolus includes a complex of the genes for ribosomal RNA plus associated proteins that form ribosomal subunits. This complex enlarges to increase the rate of ribosome production. Exocytosis of transmitter and reuptake of dopamine take place far away from the cell body, at synaptic terminals, and do not require unusually large amounts of protein synthesis. Mitosis takes place only rarely, in neuronal stem cells in restricted areas of the brain, such as the hippocampus. Neurons do not synthesize glycogen; astrocytes synthesize glycogen and then mobilize glycogen to produce lactate for export to neurons. **FH p. 8**

7. E The smooth endoplasmic reticulum contains cytochrome P-450 enzymes, which are involved in the metabolism of various drugs. The Golgi complex has enzymes to add sugar, phosphate, or sulfate groups to proteins; lysosomes contain hydrolytic digestive enzymes; peroxisomes contain oxidative enzymes; and proteasomes contain proteases. **FH pp. 12, 19, 20, 31**

8. A The lipid-rich membranes of the Golgi apparatus stain poorly, and because proteins transit rapidly through the Golgi stacks and do not accumulate in them, they do not stain intensely in this organelle. Lysosomes and mitochondria are widely distributed throughout the cytoplasm, rather than being held near the nucleus. The rough endoplasmic reticulum is very basophilic, rather than light-staining, owing to ribosomal RNA present. Zymogen granules typically are located near the cell membrane at the apical pole of a cell and are eosinophilic because of their high protein content. **FH p. 15**

9. D These proteins come in pairs: one is part of the vesicle, and one is part of the target. Thus, a vesicle from the rough endoplasmic reticulum will only bind to the Golgi apparatus because the rough endoplasmic reticulum–derived vesicle has SNARE proteins, which will only pair with Golgi complex SNAREs. GTPases have many functions in cells but are not involved in targeting vesicles to specific organelles. Lectins are only exposed on the plasma membrane surface, where they often are involved in specific cell-to-cell adhesions. Pore proteins control movement into and out of the nucleus. **FH p. 14**

10. E Secretion granules are homogeneous and often dark-staining owing to their high protein content. Glycogen is present in irregular clusters of particles and does not have the more uniform, rounded appearance of these vesicles. Mitochondria and lipid would be lighter-staining than these. Ribosomes are much smaller than these vesicles. **FH pp. 16, 345**

11. D Phagocytosis, the process by which foreign organisms are destroyed, is mostly carried out by PMNs. A patient with a phagocytic function defect in neutrophils would be expected to have recurrent infections, especially bacterial infections, because bacteria would not be efficiently destroyed. Lack of phagocytic function in PMNs would not directly affect any of the other processes listed. **FH p. 17**

12. A This condition is usually caused by abnormal LDL receptors on the cell surface that have reduced binding to serum LDL or that have reduced internalization capacity. The subsequent steps—delivery to an endosome, conversion to a multivesicular body fusion with a lysosome, and delivery of lysosomal enzymes from the Golgi complex—are not affected. Because LDL in the blood is high, uptake of LDL into cells must have been reduced. **FH p. 17**

13. C The cell shown is a neutrophil (PMN), with an irregular, lobulated nucleus and numerous endocytic vesicles containing ingested bacteria in various stages of digestion after being phagocytosed. Apoptotic cells have highly condensed nuclei, and mitotic cells have highly condensed chromatin. Protein synthesis requires abundant rough endoplasmic reticulum, which is not increased in this cell. Secretory vesicles would be homogeneous and uniform in diameter. **FH p. 18**

14. C Hurler syndrome is a lysosomal storage disease in which undigested material accumulates in lysosomes. The other labeled structures (mitochondria, rough endoplasmic reticulum, glycogen particles, and MVBs) are not affected. Although MVBs are involved in the lysosomal digestion pathway, they function at an early stage, and it is the late-stage lysosomes that accumulate undigested residues. **FH pp. 19-20**

15. C The peroxisome contains catalase, which breaks down the hydrogen peroxide byproducts of its oxidative activity. The cell junction, mitochondria, and glycogen do not contain catalase. Although catalase passes through the Golgi complex as it is synthesized, the levels of catalase in the Golgi complex would not be high. **FH pp. 19-24**

16. B Long-lived cells, including most neurons, accumulate intracellular debris arising from incomplete digestion of material in lysosomes. This debris is termed *lipofuscin*. The other cells are relatively short-lived and are unlikely to accumulate lipofuscin. **FH pp. 20, 139**

17. D The ATP synthase complex is located on the inner mitochondrial membrane (including the cristae). Cells with high energy demands have mitochondria with densely packed cristae. The amount of mitochondrial matrix and the mitochondrial orientation do not correlate with energy demands. The matrix granules are calcium stores and do not relate to energy production. The mitochondria in A are not larger than those in B; note the different scale markers. **FH pp. 21-22**

18. D Mitochondria tucked in among basal infoldings of the plasma membrane are characteristic of cells specialized for ion transport. These folds increase the membrane surface area and allow for increased numbers of ion pumps. The mitochondria are nearby to supply ATP for the energy-requiring pumps. Absorptive cells have a brush border; protein-secreting cells (including antibody secreting cells) have extensive rough endoplasmic reticulum; smooth endoplasmic reticulum is used for glycogen synthesis and detoxification of drugs. **FH p. 23**

19. C Although they have a clear space at one end, these organelles show distinct, characteristic cristae, indicating that they are mitochondria rather than any of the other organelles listed. **FH p. 22, BP p. 5**

20. A The regular, round vacuoles are characteristic of lipid droplets rather than glycosylated secretory products or postmortem degeneration. Routine histologic procedures do not preserve lipids, and they normally are extracted during embedding. **FH p. 25**

21. B In alcoholic cirrhosis, an impaired metabolism of lipids leads to an accumulation of lipid droplets in hepatocytes. Lipid is extracted from cells during tissue processing, leaving behind regular, round, pale vacuoles. Golgi stacks stain poorly, but they generally are confined to the vicinity of the cell nucleus. The proteins present in lysosomes and peroxisomes cause these structures to stain pink with eosin, so they could not account for an unstained region in the cytoplasm. Lipofuscin appears brown, even in unstained tissue. **FH p. 25, BH p. 7**

22. A Osmium tetroxide is used for both light and electron microscopy to stabilize lipids and reduce their elution from tissues by the organic solvents used to prepare tissues for embedding and sectioning. The dark-staining cytoplasmic droplets visible in these cells do not result from any enhancement of stain penetration, dehydration, or softening of tissue components. **FH p. 25**

23. C Desmin is an intermediate filament expressed in muscle tissue. Positive staining for desmin in a tumor would identify it as a neoplasm arising from muscle, leading to an accurate diagnosis. Astrocytes express GFAP intermediate filament protein. Epithelial cells express the intermediate filament cytokeratin. Neurons express neurofilament protein. **FH p. 26**

24. E Microtubules are formed from tubulin. The picture shows hollow, relatively straight tubules. Only microtubules have this appearance. The other proteins form filamentous structures, which are not visibly hollow. **FH pp. 26-28**

FH5 Chapter 2: Cell Cycle and Replication
FH5 Chapter 4: Supporting Connective Tissues
FH5 Chapter 18: Male Reproductive System
BH5 Chapter 7: Displasia and Neoplasia

2

Cell Cycle and Replication

1 As a first step in compacting the chromosomal DNA into shorter, wider structures, the 2-nm wide strands of DNA wind around octomers of what structures?
- ☐ A. Actins
- ☐ B. DNA polymerases
- ☐ C. Histones
- ☐ D. Lamins
- ☐ E. Ubiquitins

2 Some neurons, hepatocytes, and smooth muscle cells are unusually large and possess 4N or even 8N DNA. What process would result in these somatic cells containing these amounts of DNA?
- ☐ A. Apoptosis
- ☐ B. Cytokinesis in the absence of an S phase
- ☐ C. Mitosis in the absence of cytokinesis
- ☐ D. Meiosis

3 During mitosis, cells are under a tight control, which prevents them from entering anaphase unless all kinetochores are bound to microtubules. Without such binding, to what can progression through anaphase lead?
- ☐ A. Broken arms of chromosomes, separated from kinetochores
- ☐ B. Chromatids exchanging DNA
- ☐ C. Daughter cells having unequal numbers of chromosomes
- ☐ D. Daughter cells having unequal sizes
- ☐ E. Excessive shortening of telomeres

4 In the figure below, *arrows* indicate cells that contain dark-staining structures. What are these dark-staining structures?
- ☐ A. Basal bodies
- ☐ B. Crystals of Reinke
- ☐ C. Mitochondria
- ☐ D. Mitotic chromosomes
- ☐ E. Secretory granules

5 On comparing a series of biopsies, shown in the figure below, what does the mitotic figure in C show that is different from mitotic figures in parts A and B?
- ☐ A. Condensed chromosomes
- ☐ B. Metaphase plate
- ☐ C. Stage in which the nuclear envelope is absent
- ☐ D. Stage in which cytokinesis is advanced
- ☐ E. Tripolar spindle

6 Microscopic examination of tissue removed from the breast of a 50-year-old woman reveals numerous cells like the one shown in part C of the figure below. What are these cells most likely to be?
- ☐ A. Fibroblasts
- ☐ B. Inflammatory cells
- ☐ C. Malignant epithelial tumor cells
- ☐ D. Myoepithelial cells
- ☐ E. Normal breast epithelial cells

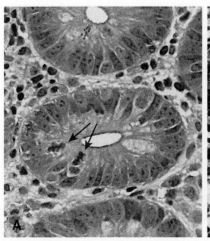
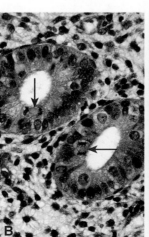
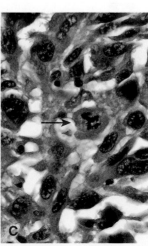

7 The appearance of the cell indicated by the *arrow* in part C of the figure on the previous page suggests that this cell has repressed or inactivated which process?
- ☐ A. Apoptosis
- ☐ B. Energy production
- ☐ C. Motility
- ☐ D. Protein synthesis

8 Some diseases are inherited always through the mother. In these cases, what are the characteristics of the defective genes?
- ☐ A. Dominant when found on the Y chromosome
- ☐ B. Dominant when found on the X chromosome
- ☐ C. Present in mitochondrial DNA
- ☐ D. Recessive when found on the Y chromosome
- ☐ E. Recessive when found on the X chromosome

9 Which feature is specific to the second meiotic division, when compared with mitosis or the first meiotic division?
- ☐ A. Centrioles do not form a spindle
- ☐ B. Chromatids are not connected by centromeres
- ☐ C. Crossing over occurs here
- ☐ D. DNA is not duplicated before division
- ☐ E. Kinetochores do not attach to the spindle

10 A piece of placental tissue was obtained by amniocentesis, and cells from it were grown in culture. Examine the below karyotype, which was obtained from this tissue, and give your diagnosis.
- ☐ A. Abnormal female
- ☐ B. Abnormal male
- ☐ C. Normal female
- ☐ D. Normal male

11 A 3-year-old child was found to have mental retardation and slanted palpebral fissures. A karyotype was performed and is shown in the figure below. What most likely has caused the abnormality?
- ☐ A. Chromosome breakage during mitosis
- ☐ B. Crossing over during meiosis
- ☐ C. Extra chromosome duplication during S phase
- ☐ D. Nondisjunction during meiosis

12 Binding of Fas ligand to the Fas receptor triggers what event?
- ☐ A. Apoptosis
- ☐ B. Necrosis
- ☐ C. Phagocytosis
- ☐ D. Receptor-mediated endocytosis

13 In some tumors of lymph nodes, there is an acquired genetic change resulting in overexpression of bcl-2 protein. What is the most likely consequence of bcl-2 overexpression?
- ☐ A. Excessive proliferation
- ☐ B. Polyploidy
- ☐ C. Prolonged survival
- ☐ D. Trisomies of various chromosomes

14 Which of the following tissues and cells normally would show numerous apoptotic bodies?
- ☐ A. Hepatocytes
- ☐ B. Intestinal tract epithelium
- ☐ C. Myocardium
- ☐ D. Neural tissue
- ☐ E. Plasma cells

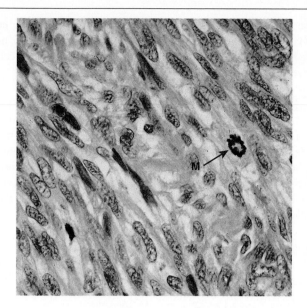

15 The figure above illustrates cells of a malignant tumor. The letter *M* points to what feature commonly found in cancerous tissues?

☐ A. M cell, which presents abnormal antigens to lymphocytes
☐ B. Macrophage carrying out phagocytosis
☐ C. Mast cell after binding IgE
☐ D. Metastatic cell primed for migration away from the tumor
☐ E. Mitotic figure with abnormal ring formation

ANSWERS

1. C DNA wraps around structures made of four pairs of histones. This wrapping forms a strand that is both shorter and wider than the DNA strand alone. DNA polymerase functions in DNA repair. Lamins are intermediate filaments that help maintain nuclear architecture. Actins are involved in cell movement. Ubiquitin functions in intracellular protein degradation. **FH p. 34**

2. C Suppression of cytokinesis through several mitoses results in cells that have several nuclei or a single nucleus with 4N or 8N DNA. Apoptosis is a process of programmed cell death. Cytokinesis in the absence of DNA replication would not increase its DNA content. Meiosis results in the formation of haploid (1N) eggs or sperm. **FH pp. 36, 40-41**

3. C The normal situation is to have paired kinetochores in a centromere, each bound to different microtubules, which pull the chromatids to opposite ends of the spindle. If a kinetochore is unbound, it will not be pulled toward a specific spindle end and may end up in the wrong cell. If a piece of a chromosome breaks from the portion containing the kinetochore, it will move independently; whether that kinetochore is bound to microtubules is irrelevant. Sister chromatid exchange occurs during meiosis. Telomere shortening is not related to

kinetochore binding to microtubules. The relative sizes of the daughter cells are determined by where cytokinesis occurs, not by kinetochore binding to microtubules. **FH p. 36-38**

4. D Mitotic chromosomes are darkly stained because of the highly condensed chromatin. Basal bodies are indeed detectable in epithelial cells, but are smaller and less basophilic than chromosomes. Crystals of Reinke are cytoplasmic inclusions of uncertain origin that are often found in steroid-producing cells. They approximate the size of chromosomes, but because of their high content of protein, they stain intensely pink with eosin rather than blue with hematoxylin. Likewise, secretory granules would also be eosinophilic. Mitochondria are smaller and stain less intensely than chromosomes. **FH pp. 38, 353**

5. E The tripolar spindle shown is indicative of an abnormal mitosis. Parts A and B show normal mitotic cells with condensed chromosomes in metaphase and telophase, respectively. In all three images, the nuclear membrane is absent. Because cytokinesis occurs at the end of telophase, all images show cells too early in mitosis for this process to occur. **FH p. 38**

6. C The finding of tripolar mitosis is abnormal and indicates a neoplastic process; the cells are most probably malignant. Abnormal mitoses are not found in normal breast epithelial cells, inflammatory cells, myoepithelial cells, or fibroblasts **FH p. 38**

7. A In normal cells, the presence of abnormal DNA triggers apoptosis or DNA repair processes. The presence of the tripolar spindle is indicative of a neoplastic cell with mutated DNA, which has inhibited its normal apoptosis pathways. The other processes might be expected to be up-regulated in rapidly growing or migrating tumor cells. **FH p. 38**

8. C All mitochondria are maternally derived because sperm mitochondria do not survive after fertilization. Therefore, all mitochondrial DNA comes from the mother, and genetic defects in mitochondrial DNA are always maternally derived. Mothers do not contribute Y chromosomes to offspring, and both parents contribute X chromosomes to female offspring. **FH pp. 40-41**

9. D DNA is duplicated before meiosis 1, but then two divisions occur without further DNA synthesis, resulting in haploid cells. Crossing over occurs during meiosis 1. The other processes occur in meiosis 1 and in mitosis. **FH p. 40-41**

10. B This is a male because there is one X and one Y chromosome, but there are three chromosomes 21, indicating a trisomy (Down syndrome). **FH p. 42**

11. D Numerical chromosomal abnormalities such as trisomies result from errors in meiosis. Nondisjunction during the first meiotic division or anaphase lag during the second meiotic division results in a trisomy. The karyotype in the figure shows trisomy 21, and there is no evidence of chromosome breakage. These errors in meiosis are usually associated with advanced maternal age. Extra chromosome duplication in S phase is usually seen as an acquired change in human cancers, but would not lead to the above phenotype because such trisomies would be confined to the tumor cells. Crossing over during meiosis is a normal process that results in an increased genetic variability of the gametes. **FH p. 40**

12. A Binding of the Fas ligand to the Fas receptor triggers the caspase cascade and cell death by apoptosis. Necrosis is caused by cell damage. Phagocytosis and receptor-mediated endocytosis are internalization events that are unrelated to the Fas receptor. **FH p. 43**

13. C Apoptosis, a process by which a cell containing abnormal proteins is caused to die, is regulated by proapoptotic and antiapoptotic genes like *bcl-2*. Overexpression of the antiapoptotic protein bcl-2 results in inhibition of apoptosis, which prevents cells from dying, thus prolonging their survival.

The bcl-2 protein does not directly affect proliferation or cell division. It neither triggers endoduplication of the DNA, nor inhibits cytokinesis, processes that result in polyploid cells. Trisomies occur as errors in cell division **FH p. 43**

14. B The epithelium of the intestinal tract has a high rate of turnover, with many cells undergoing death by apoptosis. Dead and dying cells are replaced by proliferation of stem cells, resulting in a continuous renewal of this epithelium. Individual cells in the other choices listed may undergo apoptosis, but they are either terminally differentiated or have a low turnover rate and do not show numerous apoptotic bodies under physiologic conditions. **FH p. 43**

15. E This ring-form mitotic figure is characteristic of the abnormal patterns of cell division seen in tumors. Macrophages and mast cells have pale-staining nuclei and do not divide. M cells are restricted to the epithelium of the intestine. **FH pp. 38, 80, BH p. 76**

PART

2

Basic Tissue Types

Blood

1 A 50-year-old man presents to his physician with complaints of swelling in his legs. On physical examination, there is bilateral swelling of his ankles. A deficiency in which protein most likely caused his edema?
- ☐ A. Albumin
- ☐ B. Antitrypsin
- ☐ C. Ferritin
- ☐ D. Fibrinogen
- ☐ E. Gamma globulin

2 A 25-year-old woman presents with headaches, weakness, and fatigue. Physical examination shows pale conjunctivae. Laboratory studies show anemia. Measurement of which of the following proteins would be useful in evaluating her anemia?
- ☐ A. Albumin
- ☐ B. Antitrypsin
- ☐ C. Ferritin
- ☐ D. Fibrinogen
- ☐ E. Gamma globulin

3 A 30-year-old man presents with poorly controlled bleeding from minor wounds or scrapes. Measurement of which of the following proteins would be useful in evaluating his bleeding?
- ☐ A. Albumin
- ☐ B. Antitrypsin
- ☐ C. Ferritin
- ☐ D. Fibrinogen
- ☐ E. Gamma globulin

4 A 5-year-old boy under examination by a physician has chronic fatigue and skeletal abnormalities. The suspected diagnosis is Fanconi anemia. To confirm this diagnosis, bone marrow is aspirated from the sternum of the child. What is the typical staining procedure used to prepare a bone marrow smear for study?
- ☐ A. Hematoxylin and eosin stain
- ☐ B. Periodic acid–Schiff (PAS) reaction
- ☐ C. Perl reaction
- ☐ D. Toluidine blue stain
- ☐ E. Wright stain

5 A young woman comes to the clinic complaining of a lack of energy and fatigue. You examine a smear of her blood and notice that although the erythrocytes have a normal shape, they are smaller than normal, with an increased central pallor. You immediately suspect she has anemia due to what condition?
- ☐ A. Genetic defect in actin
- ☐ B. Genetic defect in spectrin
- ☐ C. Lack of folic acid
- ☐ D. Lack of iron

6 In a patient born with a spectrin deficiency, which of the following would most likely be present in her red blood cells (RBCs)?
- ☐ A. Decreased ability to carry oxygen
- ☐ B. Fragmented nuclei
- ☐ C. Increased size
- ☐ D. Lack of deformability due to rigid membranes
- ☐ E. Sickled shape

7 A 10-year-old boy was found to have numerous sickled RBCs in a blood smear, indicating he had sickle cell anemia. In such patients, there is an increased removal of RBCs from the circulation. Physical examination of this patient would most likely show an increased size of which organ?
- ☐ A. Heart
- ☐ B. Kidney
- ☐ C. Lymph node
- ☐ D. Pancreas
- ☐ E. Spleen

8 Which bone marrow-derived cells are destroyed by phagocytosis but do not undergo apoptosis?
- ☐ A. Basophils
- ☐ B. Eosinophils
- ☐ C. Erythrocytes
- ☐ D. Lymphocytes
- ☐ E. Mast cells
- ☐ F. Monocytes
- ☐ G. Neutrophils

9 A forensic pathologist was called to investigate a possible murder. Some dried blood was found in a basement of an old abandoned house. After staining the sample with Wright stain, all the pathologist saw were small lymphocytes, polymorphonuclear neutrophils, 3-μm diameter platelets, dark basophils, reddish eosinophils, and erythrocytes that were all nucleated. After reviewing this evidence, he concluded that no person had been murdered there. Why did he conclude that?

☐ A. Human basophils do not stain darkly
☐ B. Human eosinophils do not stain red
☐ C. Human erythrocytes in circulation are not nucleated
☐ D. Platelets are 10 μm in diameter

10 During an automobile accident, a young boy experiences a rupture of the spleen. This resulted in a severe loss of blood. Blood smears obtained a few days after this event will show a large increase in what circulating cells?

☐ A. Megakaryocytes
☐ B. Neutrophils
☐ C. Plasma cells
☐ D. Reticulocytes
☐ E. T lymphocytes

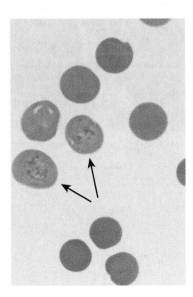

11 A patient was being evaluated to determine the cause of anemia. A supravital stain was performed incubating the patient's peripheral blood with brilliant cresyl blue. The study showed an increased number of the cell types indicated by the *arrows* in the above figure. Which condition would cause this result?

☐ A. Deficiency of vitamin B_{12}
☐ B. Failure of marrow to produce mature RBCs
☐ C. Inadequate intake of iron
☐ D. Lack of erythropoietin production by the kidney
☐ E. Point mutation in hemoglobin gene resulting in sickled RBC

12 A construction worker cuts his arm while working and, because it is not bleeding badly, leaves the cut untreated. A few days later, he notices that his arm is red and swollen. He goes to the clinic, where a blood smear is performed. Which blood cells are likely increased in number?

☐ A. Basophils
☐ B. Eosinophils
☐ C. Lymphocytes
☐ D. Monocytes
☐ E. Neutrophils

13 A father brings his 3-year-old daughter to the pediatrician because the child has had a fever, headache, and sore throat for the past 2 days. After a physical examination, the physician makes a diagnosis of viral pharyngitis and orders a complete blood count, which shows an increased white blood cell (WBC) count. Which of the following blood cell types would most likely be elevated?

☐ A. Basophil
☐ B. Eosinophil
☐ C. Lymphocyte
☐ D. Monocyte
☐ E. Neutrophil

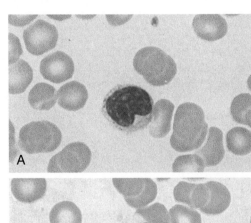

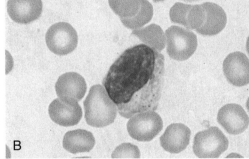

14 The nucleated cells in the figure above may develop into cells that will do what?

☐ A. Removes debris from the free surfaces of the lung alveoli
☐ B. Form platelets
☐ C. Kill larvae of parasitic worms
☐ D. Secrete antibodies
☐ E. Secrete vasoactive substances

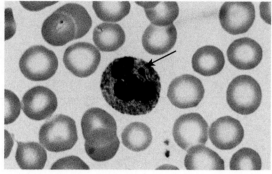

15 In the figure above, what is the small structure labeled with an *arrow*?

- ☐ A. Centriole pair
- ☐ B. Inactivated X chromosome
- ☐ C. Golgi stack
- ☐ D. Lysosome
- ☐ E. Secretion granule

16 A 3-year-old boy presents with recurrent bacterial infections since birth. This is a symptom of chronic granulomatous disease, an X-linked genetic disorder. Laboratory studies show that his neutrophils are unable to generate hydrogen peroxide. Which process is defective in his neutrophils?

- ☐ A. Adhesion to the endothelium
- ☐ B. Degranulation
- ☐ C. Killing of bacteria
- ☐ D. Motility
- ☐ E. Opsonization of antigens

17 A rare congenital disease characterized by recurrent bacterial infections has the further characteristic that the family members who have this disease are unable to produce pus. The basis of the problem has been traced to a leucocyte adhesion deficiency (LAD). An abnormal function of which cells would most severely impede the generation of pus?

- ☐ A. B lymphocytes
- ☐ B. T lymphocytes
- ☐ C. Neutrophils
- ☐ D. Plasma cells
- ☐ E. Platelets

18 Following a competition in which he swam in a polluted river, a patient's blood smear showed that 10% of the leukocytes were eosinophils. Levels of other granulocytes were normal. What condition does this observation suggest?

- ☐ A. Autoimmune reaction
- ☐ B. Bacterial infection
- ☐ C. Parasitic infection
- ☐ D. Viral infection

19 A 21-year-old woman presents to the dermatologist complaining of a skin rash. She notes that the rash occurs every time she eats shellfish. A complete blood count shows an increased WBC count. Which blood cell type would most likely be elevated?

- ☐ A. Basophil
- ☐ B. Eosinophil
- ☐ C. Lymphocyte
- ☐ D. Monocyte
- ☐ E. Neutrophil

20 A patient in your clinic has suffered an immediate hypersensitivity reaction after a bee sting. His hand is red and painfully swollen. This type of reaction is mediated by IgE binding to what cells?

- ☐ A. Basophils
- ☐ B. Eosinophils
- ☐ C. Lymphocytes
- ☐ D. Monocytes
- ☐ E. Neutrophils

21 Which of the bone marrow–derived cells repeatedly migrate out of the blood into connective tissue and then reenter the vasculature?

- ☐ A. Basophils
- ☐ B. Eosinophils
- ☐ C. Erythrocytes
- ☐ D. Lymphocytes
- ☐ E. Monocytes
- ☐ F. Neutrophils
- ☐ G. Mast cells

22 A 15-year-old boy presents with symptoms of easy bruising and poorly controlled bleeding from wounds. Which defect could explain these symptoms?

- ☐ A. Defects in adhesion molecules on platelets
- ☐ B. Defects in adhesion molecules on capillary endothelial cells
- ☐ C. Defects in selectin molecules on lymphocytes
- ☐ D. Excessive reactivity of mast cells to allergens

23 Decreased production of which of the following would be expected as a direct consequence of renal failure?

- ☐ A. Basophils
- ☐ B. Monocytes
- ☐ C. Neutrophils
- ☐ D. Platelets
- ☐ E. RBCs

24 Which of the following cells would be elevated in the blood from a patient taking corticosteroids for the treatment of autoimmune disease?

- ☐ A. Basophil
- ☐ B. Eosinophil
- ☐ C. Lymphocyte
- ☐ D. Monocyte
- ☐ E. Neutrophil

25 Before a bone marrow transplantation to correct an inherited defect in hematopoiesis, the bone marrow of a patient is irradiated to destroy it. Following this procedure, which cells derived from the original marrow can still continue to proliferate in peripheral tissues and organs?

☐ A. Basophils
☐ B. Eosinophils
☐ C. Erythrocytes
☐ D. Lymphocytes
☐ E. Neutrophils

26 Which cells of bone marrow undergo mitosis without cytokinesis?

☐ A. Adipose cells
☐ B. Endothelial cells
☐ C. Fibroblasts
☐ D. Hematopoietic stem cells
☐ E. Megakaryocytes

ANSWERS

1. A Albumin is the most abundant serum protein and plays an important role in maintaining a high plasma osmotic pressure that keeps fluid within the blood vessels. Low levels of albumin result in a net loss of fluid from the intravascular space into the extracellular tissue compartment, resulting in edema. None of the other proteins listed is important in controlling serum osmotic pressure. **FH p. 46**

2. C Ferritin is a plasma protein that forms a complex with iron and regulates iron storage and transport. Ferritin is low in iron deficiency anemia. The other proteins listed are not directly correlated with anemia. **FH p. 46**

3. D Fibrinogen is a plasma protein component of the coagulation cascade that converts to insoluble fibrin, forming a blood clot. This is the only protein listed that participates in the clotting cascade. **FH p. 46**

4. E Wright stain incorporates two dyes to distinguish the typical cells in a blood or bone marrow smear. This provides greater discrimination than either hematoxylin and eosin or toluidine blue, stains that are used in routine staining of light microscopic sections. The Perl reaction identifies iron, whereas the PAS reaction stains sugar groups. **FH p. 46**

5. D A lack of iron causes erythrocytes to be smaller than normal, with an increase in the central pallor. A lack of folate causes them to be larger than normal. Defects in the cytoskeletal proteins spectrin or actin would not affect hemoglobin function. **FH pp. 46-47**

6. D Cytoskeletal proteins such as spectrin play a role in maintaining the integrity of RBC membranes. Lack of spectrin leads to small cells with rigid cell membranes. This lack of membrane deformability results in an inability of the RBCs to penetrate the walls of splenic sinusoids. This is seen in a disorder of RBCs called *hereditary spherocytosis*. An abnormality of cytoskeletal proteins does not directly affect hemoglobin structure or function or nuclear maturation or result in increased cell size. Sickled shape is due to a hemoglobin mutation, not a spectrin defect. Mature RBCs are devoid of nuclei. **FH p. 47**

7. E Abnormal RBCs are removed from the circulation largely by the spleen and to a lesser extent by the liver. Trapping and destruction of the abnormal RBCs would result in splenomegaly. The other organs listed do not play a role in removal of RBCs. **FH pp. 47, 231**

8. C Erythrocytes in their mature form lack most internal organelles and survive by anaerobic glycolysis. They do not undergo apoptosis. The other cells contain mitochondria and enzymes necessary for apoptosis to occur. Splenic macrophages recognize aged RBCs and phagocytose them in the absence of RBC apoptosis. **FH p. 47**

9. C In humans, mature RBCs lack nuclei, unlike the RBCs of animals such as chickens or lizards. The pathologist's findings show that the blood was not of human origin. The characteristics of the other blood cells are consistent with a human origin. **FH p. 47**

10. D When there is acute blood loss, the rate of export of immature erythrocytes (reticulocytes) from the bone marrow to the blood increases. Under such conditions, there is an increase in erythropoietin secretion, which stimulates RBC production specifically. Neutrophils and T lymphocytes would not increase in these conditions. Plasma cells develop in the connective tissues and are not normally present in the blood. Megakaryocytes are found in the bone marrow and also are not normally seen in the blood. **FH p. 48**

11. E This figure shows reticulocytes. The rate of release of reticulocytes from the bone marrow is proportional to the rate of removal of RBCs from the peripheral blood. In sickle cell disease, a point mutation in the hemoglobin gene, causing a single amino acid substitution, results in polymerization of the hemoglobin in a hypoxic environment. This results in sickling and deformity of the RBCs, which are then rapidly removed from the circulation by the spleen. The marrow compensates for this loss by increasing the rate of erythrocyte export. This is reflected in an increased reticulocyte count. Lack of erythropoietin and lack of iron and vitamin B_{12}, which are required for hemoglobin synthesis and DNA maturation, respectively, and failure of the marrow to produce RBCs would all result in a delayed or decreased RBC production and therefore a decreased reticulocyte count. **FH p. 48**

12. E Neutrophils increase in bacterial infections. Neutrophils are the main body defense against bacteria, destroying them by phagocytosis. **FH p. 49**

13. C An elevated lymphocyte count is usually seen in response to viral infections. An elevated neutrophil count indicates an acute inflammatory response and is most commonly seen in association with bacterial infections. **FH p. 49**

14. A The cells are monocytes and will become macrophages in the tissues. One type of macrophage migrates into the alveoli of the lung and cleans off their free surfaces. Platelets are formed from megakaryocytes, eosinophil granules are toxic to the larvae of parasitic worms, plasma cells secrete antibodies, and basophils secrete vasoactive substances. **FH pp. 56**

15. B In this neutrophil, an inactivated, condensed X chromosome can be found as a nuclear appendage called a *drumstick* (Barr body). Centrioles and Golgi stacks generally stain less intensely, rather than more intensely, than other cytoplasmic structures. Lysosomes and secretion granules can be seen in this cell but are smaller than the drumstick. **FH p. 50**

16. C Patients with chronic granulomatous disease have a deficiency of NADPH oxidase, which results in an inability of neutrophils to generate hydrogen peroxide (respiratory burst). This limits the ability of the neutrophil to kill bacteria. None of the other functions would be affected by this deficiency. **FH p. 51**

17. C Neutrophil enzymes are depleted by the phagocytic activity that occurs when they encounter bacteria and the neutrophils then degenerate. Defunct neutrophils are the major component of pus. **FH p. 51**

18. C Increased circulation of eosinophils occurs after infection by helminthic worms because these cells are specialized to attack these organisms. **FH p. 52**

19. B A skin rash is frequently a symptom of an allergic reaction. An elevated eosinophil count is usually seen in response to allergies and parasitic infections. **FH p. 52**

20. A Basophils are WBCs that have receptors for IgE. They contain various proteoglycans, histamine, and other vasoactive substances in their secretory granules. Release of these molecules during degranulation results in an immediate hypersensitivity reaction. **FH p. 54**

21. D Lymphocytes circulate between connective tissue depots, lymph nodes, and spleen by way of the blood. The other choices listed do not, as individual cells, repeatedly cross

the vascular endothelium. A monocyte derivative, the dendritic cell, can also leave the blood supply then reenter it as part of its immune function, but the monocyte itself does not. **FH p. 55**

22. A Platelets play a role in hemostasis by adhering to collagen at a site of vascular injury, forming the platelet plug. Lack of adhesion molecules on platelets would result in bleeding. Bernard Soulier syndrome is an example of an inherited platelet adhesion defect resulting in recurrent bleeding. Defects in adhesion molecules, either on endothelial cells or on WBCs, results in recurrent infections due to inability of WBCs to adhere to endothelium and leave the capillary to go to the site of infection. Excessive reactivity of mast cells to allergens results in hypersensitivity reactions characteristic of such diseases as asthma and anaphylactic shock. **FH p. 57**

23. E Erythropoietin is a growth factor secreted by the kidney that is necessary for erythropoiesis. Erythropoietin production is diminished in renal failure, resulting in decreased production of RBCs (anemia). Because basophils normally make up a small fraction of WBCs in the peripheral blood (1%), a decrease in their number is usually not significant. Neutrophil and monocyte production by the bone marrow requires the growth hormone granulocyte-monocyte colony-stimulating factor (GM-CSF); therefore, a decrease in GM-CSF will result in reduced number of neutrophils (neutropenia) and monocytes (monocytopenia). Megakaryocytes that produce platelets require the growth hormone thrombopoietin, and lack of this growth factor will result in a low platelet count (thrombocytopenia). **FH p. 61**

24. E Corticosteroids increase the rate of release of neutrophils from the marrow and reduce the rate of neutrophil exit from the circulation, resulting in an increase of neutrophils in the peripheral blood. The other WBCs decrease or are not significantly affected by corticosteroids. **FH p. 61**

25. D Lymphocytes are the only blood cells that, under proper stimulation by cytokines, will continue to divide outside the marrow. **FH p. 61**

26. E Megakaryocytes have enlarged, polyploid nuclei owing to a blockade of cell division following numerous rounds of mitosis. The other cells listed undergo mitosis followed by cytokinesis. **FH p. 63**

FH5 Chapter 3: Blood
FH5 Chapter 4: Supporting/Connective Tissues
BH5 Chapter 2: Acute Inflammation
BH5 Chapter 10: Infarction
BH5 Chapter 16: Lymphoid System

4

Supporting/Connective Tissues

1 Two days after a myocardial infarction, the infarcted area shows signs of inflammation and has been invaded by large numbers of leukocytes. Which leukocytes predominate in an acute inflammatory reaction such as this?

- ☐ A. Basophils
- ☐ B. Eosinophils
- ☐ C. Lymphocytes
- ☐ D. Monocytes
- ☐ E. Neutrophils

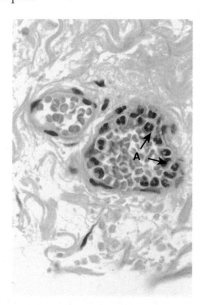

2 In the figure above, numerous cells labeled *A* are adhering to a blood vessel in the early stages of an inflammatory process. What are these cells?

- ☐ A. Fibroblasts
- ☐ B. Lymphocytes
- ☐ C. Mast cells
- ☐ D. Neutrophils
- ☐ E. Plasma cells

3 A 20-year-old man goes to the dermatologist complaining of an itchy reddish lump of a scar that developed when he had a nose ring put in. The dermatologist explained this was a keloid. Which cells formed the keloid?

- ☐ A. Adipocytes
- ☐ B. Chondrocytes
- ☐ C. Fibroblasts
- ☐ D. Mast cells
- ☐ E. Macrophages

4 A newborn was found to have multiple fractures and weak bones due to an inherited disorder of collagen synthesis. Which of the following collagen types would most likely be defective?

- ☐ A. I
- ☐ B. II
- ☐ C. III
- ☐ D. IV
- ☐ E. V

5 To confirm a diagnosis of Marfan syndrome, a patient's genome was assayed for mutations in the fibrillin gene. Results confirmed that the patient was heterozygous for a mutated form of fibrillin. Which process of connective tissue formation would be affected by this mutation?

- ☐ A. Collagen fibril formation
- ☐ B. Elastic fiber formation
- ☐ C. Hyaline cartilage formation
- ☐ D. Integrin binding to the basal lamina
- ☐ E. Reticulin formation

6 A young woman presents with patches of hardened skin, but no other organ involvement is evident, suggesting a mild form of scleroderma. Tests for autoimmune dysfunction confirm that antinuclear antibodies are present, and the hardened areas of skin show increased amounts of typical connective tissue proteins. What protein(s) is (are) responsible for the hardened skin?

- ☐ A. Elastin
- ☐ B. Fibrillin
- ☐ C. Fibrin
- ☐ D. Types I and III collagen
- ☐ E. Type IV collagen and laminin

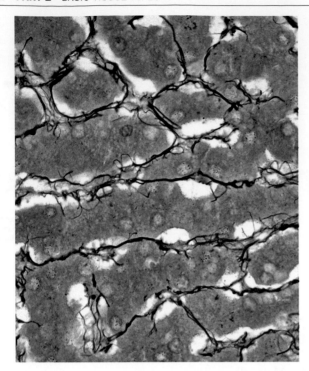

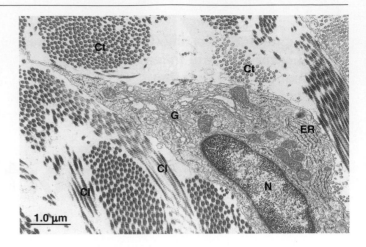

7 The liver biopsy shown above is stained with a silver stain. What is the stained substance that forms the scaffolding of the liver?
- [ ] A. Elastin
- [ ] B. Fibrillin
- [ ] C. Proteoglycan
- [ ] D. Reticulin (type III collagen)
- [ ] E. Type IV collagen

8 A young couple came in for counseling. Recently the wife had suspected Marfan syndrome in her family when her tall, thin sister had an aortic aneurysm due to insufficient elastic tissue. The counselor told them that Marfan syndrome is an autosomal dominant disease and that neither of them exhibited Marfan traits. What is the chance of this couple's child having Marfan syndrome?
- [ ] A. 0%
- [ ] B. 25%
- [ ] C. 50%
- [ ] D. 75%
- [ ] E. 100%

9 The cell shown in the figure above on the right is anchored to the extracellular matrix by the adhesive protein fibronectin. Which plasma membrane protein binds to the fibronectin?
- [ ] A. Connexin
- [ ] B. Desmin
- [ ] C. Integrin
- [ ] D. Laminin
- [ ] E. Myosin

10 What type of cell is shown in the figure above?
- [ ] A. Fibroblast
- [ ] B. Macrophage
- [ ] C. Mast cell
- [ ] D. Plasma cell
- [ ] E. Smooth muscle cell

11 Which component of connective tissue is primarily responsible for binding water in the extracellular matrix?
- [ ] A. Elastic fibers
- [ ] B. Fibrillin
- [ ] C. Sulfated glycosaminoglycans
- [ ] D. Type I collagen
- [ ] E. Type IV collagen

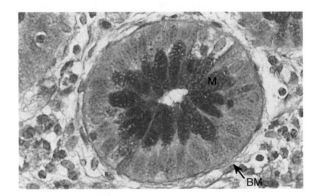

12 The figure above shows a section from a biopsy, which has been stained with the PAS procedure. Which component of the basement membrane is mostly responsible for the pink staining?
- [ ] A. Collagen IV
- [ ] B. Enactin
- [ ] C. Fibronectin
- [ ] D. Laminin
- [ ] E. Proteoglycan

13 To become invasive, a carcinoma must first secrete enzymes to digest what collagen type?

☐ A. I
☐ B. II
☐ C. III
☐ D. IV
☐ E. V

14 As a person ages, the character of the connective tissue of his or her skin changes. Aging of this tissue primarily reflects the changes in the synthetic activity of what cells?
☐ A. Fibroblasts
☐ B. Lymphocytes
☐ C. Macrophages
☐ D. Mast cells
☐ E. Neutrophils

15 The figure on the left illustrates scar tissue from a healed wound. What causes this scar tissue to appear different from the normal, adjacent tissue?
☐ A. Decreased cellularity
☐ B. Increased amount of extracellular ground substance
☐ C. Increased amount of smooth muscle
☐ D. Lack of blood vessels
☐ E. Reduction in the staining intensity and coarseness of collagen fibers

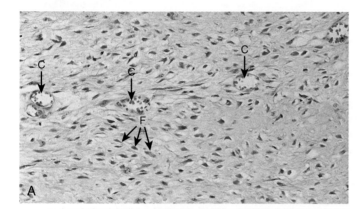

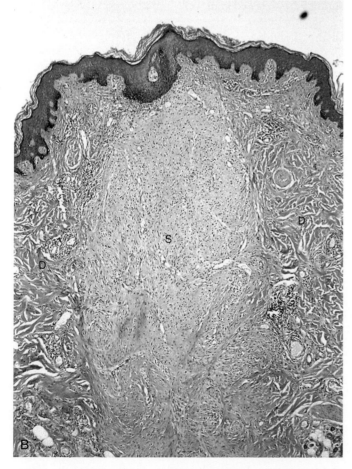

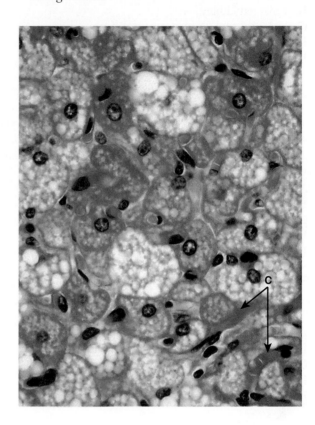

16 The biopsy shown above, taken from near the thoracic aorta, mainly shows cells specialized to do what?
☐ A. Export glycerol and fatty acids for muscle contraction
☐ B. Generate heat by nonshivering thermogenesis
☐ C. Produce peptide hormones
☐ D. Support wound healing
☐ E. Synthesize steroid hormones

17 A 55-year-old obese woman was advised by her physician to lose weight because of an increased risk for disease that results from resistance to which hormone activity?
☐ A. ACTH
☐ B. Adrenalin
☐ C. Growth hormone
☐ D. Insulin
☐ E. Prolactin

18 A 45-year-old man noted a mass on his back. Histologic examination of the mass shows normal adipose tissue. How is this tumor best classified?

☐ A. Angioma
☐ B. Fibroma
☐ C. Leiomyoma
☐ D. Lipoma
☐ E. Myxoma

19 Which of the following would be expected in examining a patient with lysosomal storage disorder?
☐ A. Enlarged heart
☐ B. Enlarged kidney
☐ C. Enlarged muscle
☐ D. Enlarged pancreas
☐ E. Enlarged spleen

20 A 20-year-old man presenting with skin rash and hepatosplenomegaly was being evaluated for the cause of his illness. A biopsy taken from a skin lesion was stained with several dyes. Most informative was the observation that the majority of cells stained metachromatically with toluidine blue, suggesting that the major cell component was what type?
☐ A. Adipocytes
☐ B. Fibroblasts
☐ C. Mast cells
☐ D. Neutrophils
☐ E. Plasma cells

21 One week after a myocardial infarction, debris and dying cells are removed by connective tissue cells. Which cells play the major role in this process?
☐ A. Fibroblasts
☐ B. Macrophages
☐ C. Mast cells
☐ D. Neutrophils
☐ E. Lymphocytes

☐ A. Brown fat cells
☐ B. Fibroblasts
☐ C. Macrophages
☐ D. Mast cells
☐ E. Plasma cells

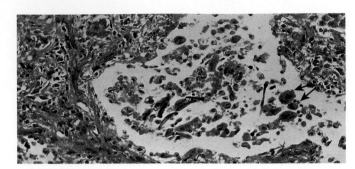

23 The figure above shows an asbestos accumulation in the airways of the lung. The nearby phagocytic cells (*arrows*) differentiate from what cells?
☐ A. Basophils
☐ B. Eosinophils
☐ C. Monocytes
☐ D. Kupffer cells
☐ E. Mast cells

24 Which of the following cells are capable of fusing to form multinucleated giant cells in pathologic situations?
☐ A. Adipocytes
☐ B. Chondrocytes
☐ C. Fibroblasts
☐ D. Macrophages
☐ E. Mast cells

22 In the figure above, normal cells have multiplied excessively to form a tumor. What type of cell predominates here?

ANSWERS

1. E Neutrophils are present in low numbers in normal connective tissues but are the first granulocytes to invade the connective tissue from the blood in large numbers in an acute inflammatory reaction. Although the other cell types participate, they are present in smaller numbers for this type of inflammatory reaction. **FH p. 49, BH pp. 12-14**

2. D The lobulated nuclei of neutrophils are an identifying feature. Lymphocytes, mast cells, and plasma cells all have rounded nuclei. Fibroblasts have flattened nuclei. Fibroblasts and mast cells are never located within a blood vessel. **FH p. 51, BH p. 14**

3. C A keloid is an overproduction of connective tissue that develops during scar formation. Fibroblasts secrete the extracellular matrix of keloids as they do for ordinary connective tissues. Adipocytes are not major contributors to extracellular matrix in such connective tissue. Chondrocytes synthesize cartilage matrix. Mast cells regulate the fluidity of the matrix through regulation of the effective porosity of the local vasculature. Macrophages phagocytize bacteria and particulate matter within ordinary connective tissues. **FH p. 65**

4. A Type I collagen is the type of collagen found in ligaments and bones. There are a number of inherited disorders that have mutations in genes encoding for collagen. The clinical manifestations vary according to the type of collagen fiber affected. Patients born with Osteogenesis Imperfecta have fragile bones resulting in multiple fractures due to a deficiency in the synthesis of type I collagen. Type II collagen is found in hyaline cartilage. Type III collagen is a component of reticulin fibers that make up the delicate connective tissue supporting framework of skin and vascular system and highly cellular tissue such as liver, bone marrow, and lymph nodes. In Ehlers-Danlos syndrome type 4, a defect in type III collagen results in fragile skin and blood vessels, resulting in aneurysms. Type IV collagen is an important constituent of basal laminae and basement membranes. Alport syndrome is a disorder of type IV collagen with thin basement membranes of glomeruli (glomerulonephritis). Deficiency of type V and type I collagen is associated with the classic type of Ehlers-Danlos syndrome. These patients have soft, delicate skin that bruises and scars easily. **FH p. 66**

5. B Fibrillin is a structural glycoprotein, which is required for orderly deposition of elastic fibers. Mutation in this gene results in disrupted elastic fiber deposition as occurs in the genetic disorder Marfan syndrome. **FH pp. 66, 69**

6. D Scleroderma is an autoimmune disorder of the connective tissue characterized by excessive deposition of collagen. Types I and III collagens are found together in the dermis of the skin. A partial list of collagens, as well as other fibrous matrix components and their locations, is presented in **FH p. 66.**

7. D Reticulin forms a delicate supporting framework in the liver and in other solid organs. Certain diseases of the liver result in disruption of this reticulin framework and distort the architecture of the liver. None of the other substances listed stain specifically with silver stains, nor does the pattern of staining fit their distribution in the liver. Elastic fibers (elastin and fibrillin) and basal laminae (type IV collagen and proteoglycans) are largely absent from the liver parenchyma. **FH p. 67**

8. A Although the wife has a family history of Marfan syndrome, she does not carry the mutation. As an autosomal dominant disease, the disorder is expressed even if only a single copy of the allele is present. **FH p. 67**

9. C Integrins are transmembrane proteins that link the cytoskeleton within the cell to adhesive molecules, such as fibronectin, in the extracellular matrix. Connexins form gap junctions, desmins are intermediate filaments in muscle cells, laminins are extracellular adhesive molecules in the basal lamina (lamina densa), and myosins are actin-based motor proteins. **FH pp. 69, 72**

10. A Fibroblasts are elongated, protein-secreting cells, often surrounded by collagen and ground substance. Macrophages would have numerous endosomes and lysosomes. Mast cells are filled with large secretion granules. Plasma cells are round or oval with a round nucleus, and smooth muscle cells contain many actin filaments and dense bodies. **FH p. 72**

11. C The charge distribution on glycosaminoglycans attracts and binds water. Fibers provide mechanical support. Fibrillin is important in formation of elastic fibers. Type IV collagen forms the basement membrane. **FH p. 69**

12. E Proteoglycans contain large amounts of carbohydrates, which stain well with the PAS technique. The other proteins are glycoproteins, but the amount of carbohydrate present in them is small compared with the amount in proteoglycans. **FH p. 70**

13. D A carcinoma arises from epithelial cells. To become invasive, carcinomas must migrate through the basal lamina and basement membrane, which contain collagen type IV. Carcinomas secrete other types of collagenases as well, but must breach the basement membrane first. This allows them to enter underlying connective tissue and subsequently enter nearby blood vessels. The other collagens listed form structural fibers that are not a significant barrier to the movement of cells. **FH pp. 70-71**

14. A All the organic components of connective tissue are synthesized by fibroblasts. The other cells listed protect the connective tissue from microorganisms. **FH p. 72**

15. E The scar tissue(s) in the dermis (D) is noteworthy for increased numbers and activity of fibroblasts (F) and for a lighter staining of extracellular molecules. It is vascularized (C). Smooth muscle does not form a significant part of scar tissue. **FH p. 74, BH p. 23**

16. B Brown fat cells, shown here, metabolize their lipids to generate heat through a nonshivering mechanism. Although somewhat similar in appearance, steroid hormone–secreting cells are found in the adrenal gland and reproductive organs, which are not present in the thorax. White fat cells are distinct from brown fat cells in that they are larger and store lipid in a single central large vacuole. Brown fat cells lack the cytoplasmic basophilia associated with the presence of rough endoplasmic reticulum used in peptide and protein synthesis. **FH pp. 74-77**

17. D Adipocytes, in addition to being storage sites for fat and energy, play a complex role in metabolism. Obesity results in insulin resistance and diabetes. Resistance to the remaining hormones listed is rare but would result in decreased cortisol production (ACTH), growth failure (growth hormone), or lack of production of milk (prolactin). **FH p. 77**

18. D A benign tumor of adipocytes is called a *lipoma*. Benign tumors of blood vessels, fibroblasts, and smooth muscles are classified as angiomas, fibromas, and leiomyomas, respectively. **FH p. 78**

19. E Lysosomal storage disorders result from abnormal deposition of various substance within the lysosomes of macrophages, which leads to their enlargement and proliferation. This results in enlargement of those organs in which macrophages are abundant, including spleen, liver, bone marrow, and lymph nodes. Enlargement of the heart occurs because of increased work load on the heart as a result of excessive pressure or volume. The kidney and pancreas may become enlarged when there is a tumor or cyst occupying their parenchyma. **FH p. 78**

20. C The contents of mast cell granules stain metachromatically with toluidine blue. Other cells in the connective tissue do not stain metachromatically. **FH p. 79**

21. B Macrophages are the major phagocytic cells in the connective tissues and invade an area of damage to remove dying cells and other debris. Although neutrophils are also phagocytic, they are mostly present 1 to 2 days after an infarct. After 1 week, the major removal of material and cells is carried out by macrophages. **FH pp. 80-81, BH p. 106**

22. E Plasma cells are distinguishable owing to their basophilic, agranular cytoplasms and eccentrically positioned nuclei. Macrophages and fibroblasts have irregular or flattened cell nuclei. Brown fat is distinguishable by the multiple small lipid droplets within the cells. Mast cells have a central nucleus and the cytoplasm is filled with large secretion vesicles. **FH p. 80, BH p. 211**

23. C Monocytes are the precursors of the macrophage and dendritic cell lineages. The Kupffer cell is a specialized fixed macrophage of the liver. The other cells listed are not part of the monocyte cell lineage. **FH p. 81**

24. D Macrophages engulf antigens, organisms, and foreign material and play an important role in immunity. When faced with a substance that is difficult to digest, such as mycobacteria, carbon, or asbestos fibers in alveoli, they fuse together to form multinucleate giant cells. These giant cells can wall off the offending cells or materials and protect the body from them. Adipose cells may be very large, but they are single cells. The other cells may enlarge, but do not form multinucleated giant cells. **FH p. 81**

FH5 Chapter 1: Cell Structure and Function
FH5 Chapter 5: Epithelial Tissues
BH5 Chapter 7: Dysplasia and Neoplasia
BH5 Chapter 13: Gastrointestinal System

5

Epithelial Tissues

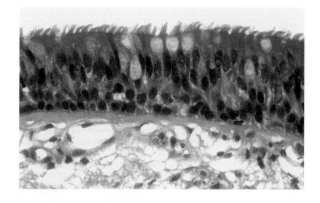

1 Which type of epithelium is seen in the lamina propria shown in the figure above?
☐ A. Pseudostratified columnar epithelium
☐ B. Simple columnar epithelium
☐ C. Simple cuboidal epithelium
☐ D. Simple squamous epithelium
☐ E. Stratified columnar epithelium
☐ F. Stratified cuboidal epithelium
☐ G. Stratified squamous nonkeratinized epithelium
☐ H. Transitional epithelium

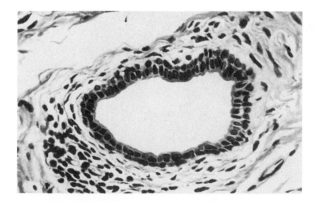

2 The figure at the lower left shows a biopsy specimen taken from a mass near the temporomandibular joint. The type of epithelium lining this hollow structure allows it to be identified as what?
☐ A. Artery
☐ B. Capillary
☐ C. Duct of a salivary gland
☐ D. Thyroid follicle
☐ E. Ureter

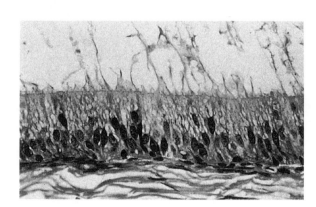

3 Because of an accident in record keeping, the descriptions of several biopsies have been separated from their images. For the one shown above, transmission electron microscopy confirms the absence of microtubules in the apical cell processes. Which of the descriptions match this image?
☐ A. Pseudostratified ciliated columnar epithelium
☐ B. Pseudostratified columnar epithelium with stereocilia
☐ C. Simple columnar epithelium with brush border
☐ D. Stratified columnar epithelium
☐ E. Transitional epithelium

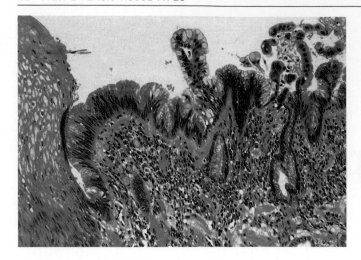

4 In the figure above, the normal stratified squamous epithelium of the esophagus has been replaced by an aberrant type of epithelium, a condition called *Barrett esophagus*. How is the atypical epithelium classified?

- ☐ A. Pseudostratified, ciliated columnar epithelium
- ☐ B. Simple columnar epithelium
- ☐ C. Simple squamous epithelium
- ☐ D. Stratified cuboidal epithelium
- ☐ E. Transitional epithelium

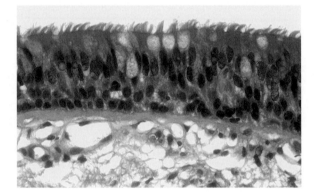

5 The histologic appearance of a biopsy taken from a patient is shown in the above figure. From where was this biopsy most likely taken?

- ☐ A. Bronchus
- ☐ B. Kidney
- ☐ C. Pancreas
- ☐ D. Pleura
- ☐ E. Skin

6 On what would paralysis of ciliary movement have its most immediate effect?

- ☐ A. Epididymal function
- ☐ B. Intestinal absorption
- ☐ C. Mucus removal from lungs
- ☐ D. Salivary secretion
- ☐ E. Sweating

7 Which normally nonkeratinized epithelium may keratinize in response to irritative stresses such as abrasion?

- ☐ A. Endothelium
- ☐ B. Epidermal epithelium
- ☐ C. Intestinal epithelium
- ☐ D. Soft palate epithelium
- ☐ E. Urothelium

8 A histologic section of a biopsy taken from a mass in a 55-year-old woman shows malignant cells arising from transitional epithelial cells. The mass would most likely be found in which of the following sites?

- ☐ A. Colon
- ☐ B. Kidney cortex
- ☐ C. Lung
- ☐ D. Urinary bladder
- ☐ E. Uterus

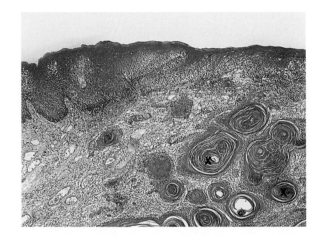

Use the figure above to answer questions 9 and 10.

9 The figure above shows a section of a biopsy of a carcinoma. What type of carcinoma is indicated by the appearance of the regions labeled *X*?

- ☐ A. Adenocarcinoma
- ☐ B. Leiomyosarcoma
- ☐ C. Pheochromocytoma
- ☐ D. Squamous cell carcinoma
- ☐ E. Transitional cell carcinoma

10 The figure above shows a section of a biopsy of a carcinoma. Antibody staining will show the presence of which type of intermediate filaments?

- ☐ A. Desmin
- ☐ B. GFAP
- ☐ C. Keratin
- ☐ D. Neurofilaments
- ☐ E. Vimentin

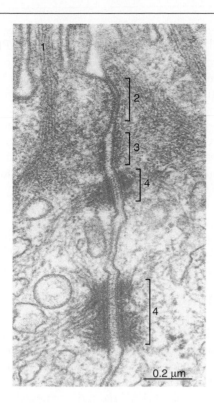

0.2 μm

Use the figure above and the list of proteins below to answer questions 11 to 13.

☐ A. Actin
☐ B. Cadherin
☐ C. Claudin
☐ D. Connexin
☐ E. Desmin
☐ F. Desmoplakin
☐ G. Keratin
☐ H. Laminin
☐ I. Myosin
☐ J. Vimentin

11 Which protein is a major structural component of the structure labeled *2*?

12 Which transmembrane molecule in the structure labeled *3* holds the cells together?

13 Which cytoskeletal element inserts into the membrane at the structures labeled *4*?

14 A mother brings her 3-year-old son to the pediatrician because of recurrent infections. On examination, the child was noted to have dextrocardia and a diagnosis of Kartagener syndrome was made. As the child grows up, which of the following may be seen as a complication of his disease?
☐ A. Decreased visual acuity
☐ B. Disturbance of gait
☐ C. Hair loss
☐ D. Infertility
☐ E. Multiple skin blisters

15 In which structures do the epithelia have a prominent brush border?
☐ A. Esophagus
☐ B. Proximal convoluted tubule
☐ C. Syncytiotrophoblast
☐ D. Trachea
☐ E. Urinary bladder

Questions 16 and 17 refer to the description below.

A microbiologist working with salmonella gets a severe case of diarrhea. Suspecting he has been infected, he goes to the physician for confirmation and treatment. A biopsy of the intestinal epithelium demonstrates that part of the brush border has been damaged, and the supporting cytoskeleton reorganized to permit the salmonella invasion.

16 What primarily makes up the cytoplasmic structure that supports the brush border?
☐ A. Actin
☐ B. Basal bodies
☐ C. Desmin
☐ D. Lamins
☐ E. Microtubules

17 Where does this supporting cytoskeleton normally anchor to the cell periphery?
☐ A. Desmosome
☐ B. Fascia adherens
☐ C. Gap junction
☐ D. Hemidesmosome
☐ E. Zonula adherens

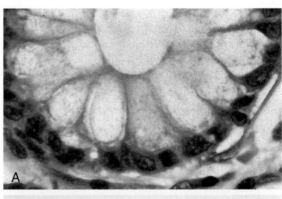

A

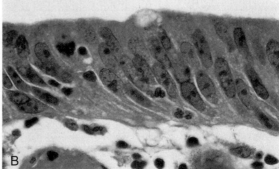

B

18 The micrographs on the previous page illustrate normal (A) and abnormal (B) specimens of the same type of epithelium. What process could account for the development of the epithelial abnormality?

☐ A. Apoptosis
☐ B. Hypertrophy
☐ C. Necrosis
☐ D. Neoplasia
☐ E. Neural stimulation of mucin synthesis

ANSWERS

1. D The larger spaces below the thick basement membrane are blood vessels. Like most blood vessels, they are lined by simple squamous epithelium. **FH p. 83**

2. C Ducts of glands are the only structures in the body lined by stratified cuboidal epithelium. Arteries and capillaries are lined by a simple squamous epithelium, thyroid follicles by a simple cuboidal epithelium, and the ureter by a transitional epithelium. **FH pp. 83-87**

3. B This epithelium has long branched microvilli termed *stereocilia*. That the cells are not ciliated is confirmed by the statement that there are no microtubules in these structures, a necessary component of axonemes. Several irregular layers of nuclei are characteristic of pseudostratified, rather than stratified, columnar epithelium. Transitional epithelium has large rounded cells at the free surface. **FH pp. 84-87, 93**

4. B Here the normal epithelium of the esophagus has been replaced by simple columnar epithelium with its characteristic appearance of a single layer of elongated nuclei. This metaplastic change occurs in response to repeated exposure to stomach acid and increases the risk for the development of adenocarcinoma. **BH p. 144, FH p. 84**

5. A The photomicrograph shows pseudostratified columnar ciliated epithelium. This type of epithelium is almost exclusively seen in the respiratory system and lines the bronchi. The renal tubules and the ducts of the exocrine pancreas are lined by simple cuboidal epithelium. The pleura is lined by flattened squamous cells (mesothelium). The epidermis of the skin is lined by stratified squamous epithelium. **FH p. 85**

6. C Cilia in the pseudostratified columnar epithelium sweep mucus and trapped debris from the airways in the lungs. The processes of intestinal absorption and epididymal function involve microvilli, not cilia. Sweat and saliva are moved along by fluid transport involving ion secretion. **FH pp. 85, 92**

7. D Stresses such as abrasion can change the character of stratified squamous epithelium from nonkeratinized to keratinized. Although such changes can be normal responses to stress, others may be "precancerous." This occurs in parts of the oral cavity, such as the soft palate, in the uterine cervix, and in the esophagus. The epidermis is normally keratinized. **FH p. 86**

8. D Transitional epithelium is found only in the urinary tract. Malignant cells arising from transitional epithelial cells would be found in the urinary bladder. The colon and uterus are lined by glandular columnar epithelium. The mucosa of the respiratory tract, including the bronchioles, is lined by ciliated pseudostratified columnar epithelium, which can undergo squamous metaplasia. The renal tubules in the kidney cortex are lined by cuboidal epithelium. **FH p. 87**

9. D The *X* marks indicate swirls of flattened cells similar to the stratum corneum of normal epidermis. Tumors arising from squamous cells may recapitulate normal differentiation; thus, the presence of swirls of flattened cells in a malignant tumor allows for recognition of the tumor as a squamous cell carcinoma. **FH p. 87**

10. C Carcinomas are of epithelial origin and therefore will have epithelial-type intermediate filaments made of keratin. Tumors of muscle derivation will show positive staining for desmin. Tumors derived from astrocytic cells of the brain would be positive for GFAP and those of neural origin would stain for neurofilaments. Vimentin staining is seen in most tumors derived from connective tissue. **FH p. 87**

11. C This structure is a tight junction, recognizable by its apical location and the close apposition of the two cell membranes. Claudin is a major structural component of tight junctions. **FH pp. 88-91**

12. B This structure is a zonula adherens, recognizable by its location between the tight junction (*above*) and the desmosome (*below*). Cadherins are the molecules that bind to similar molecules in the adjacent cell in both the zonula adherens junction and in desmosomes and mechanically hold the two cells together. **FH pp. 88-91**

13. G This is a desmosome, recognizable by its location as the most basal component of the junctional complex and by the presence of dense cytoplasmic plaques adjacent to the cell membranes at the junction. Keratin intermediate filaments participate in the formation of desmosomes in epithelial cells. **FH pp. 88-91**

14. D In Kartagener syndrome, there is an absence of proteins critical for ciliary motility. About half of the patients with this syndrome have *situs inversus* with dextrocardia because ciliary activity is required for normal right-left asymmetry. The lack of ciliary activity leads to recurrent sinusitis, respiratory infections, and infertility due to malfunction of tails of spermatozoa. The other choices are symptoms unrelated to ciliary movement. Visual acuity is a function of photoreceptors that lack motile cilia. Gait disturbances are related to sensory cells that have microvilli rather than cilia. **FH p. 92**

15. B A brush border is characteristic of the absorptive epithelium forming the proximal convoluted tubules in the kidney. Microvilli are present in many cells, including syncytiotrophoblast and tracheal epithelial cells, but they do not form a prominent brush border in these locations. The esophagus and urinary bladder lack microvilli. **FH pp. 4-5, 93**

16. A The actin cores of the microvilli mesh into the terminal web that supports them. The terminal web also is made primarily of actin. Basal bodies are at the base of cilia. Desmin is found in muscle cells, not epithelial cells. Lamins are found in nuclei. Microtubules form cilia. **FH p. 93**

17. E The actin core of the microvilli meshes into the terminal web. This extends to the edges of the cell at the zonula adherens. Fasciae adherents also include actin filaments, but are found only in cardiac muscle. **FH p. 93**

18. D The cells in part B have multiplied, become stratified, and lost the capacity for mucin synthesis, which is characteristic of neoplasia in the colon. In hypertrophy, cells become larger but not more numerous. Necrosis and apoptosis result in cell death and a decreased, rather than increased, number of cells. **BH p. 78, FH p. 95**

6

Muscle

1 What is the primary contractile cell involved in the closing of a wound that extends into the dermis?
☐ A. Myoepithelial cell
☐ B. Myofibroblast
☐ C. Pericyte
☐ D. Smooth muscle cell
☐ E. Skeletal muscle cell

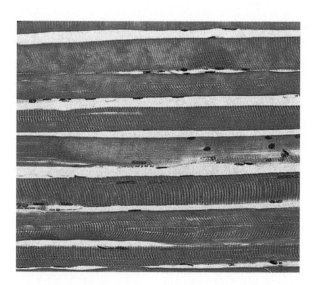

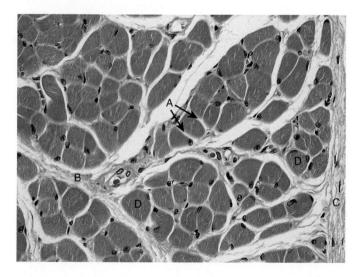

2 Reticular fibers are most prominent in which region of the figure above?

3 The photomicrograph shown above represents tissue from which of the following sites?
☐ A. Aorta
☐ B. Intestinal tract
☐ C. Tongue
☐ D. Urinary bladder
☐ E. Uterus

4 Which of the following tissues would show progressive damage and degeneration in patients with an inherited mutation of the dystrophin gene?

☐ A. Adipose tissue
☐ B. Epidermis
☐ C. Peripheral nerve
☐ D. Skeletal muscle
☐ E. Tendon

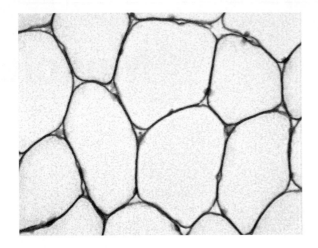

5 The figure above shows a biopsy specimen of skeletal muscle stained with an antibody. Use of an antibody to which protein would give this appearance?

☐ A. Actin
☐ B. Cadherin
☐ C. Dystrophin
☐ D. Tropomyosin
☐ E. Troponin

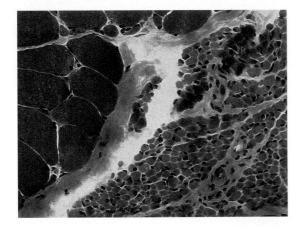

6 The figure above shows a biopsy specimen taken from a thigh muscle. What condition could have resulted in this appearance?

☐ A. Muscular dystrophy
☐ B. Myasthenia gravis
☐ C. Neurogenic muscular atrophy
☐ D. Steroid treatment to improve athletic performance
☐ E. Training for a marathon run

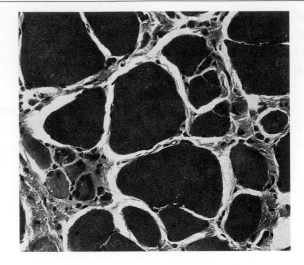

7 The figure above shows a specimen with pathologically increased amounts of connective tissue and aggregations of pink-staining cells that are unusually variable in size. Which disease is illustrated by this figure?

☐ A. Duchenne muscular dystrophy
☐ B. Guillain-Barré syndrome
☐ C. Myasthenia gravis
☐ D. Poliomyelitis
☐ E. Polymyositis

8 In adults, by what mechanism does skeletal muscle repair mainly occur?

☐ A. Endomitosis in a myofiber
☐ B. Fusion of damaged myofibers
☐ C. Fusion of macrophages with damaged myofibers
☐ D. Fusion of satellite cells to make new myofibers

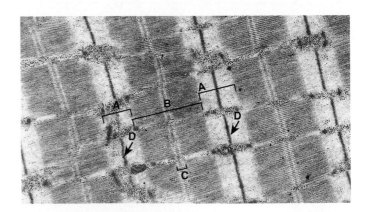

The following two questions refer to the image shown above. Match the letters in the figure with the descriptions given.

9 Myosin, but not actin, is located here.

10 Which structure plays the same role in binding actin as do dense bodies in smooth muscle?

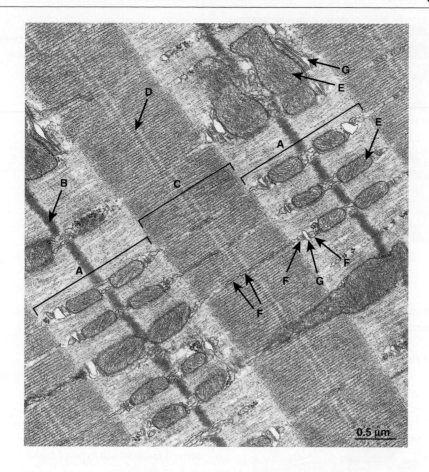

Questions 11 to 13 refer to the figure above. Match the labels on the figure with the descriptions given.

11 Which labeled structure becomes markedly smaller during contraction?

12 Which labeled structure releases calcium when electrically stimulated?

13 Which labeled structure contains extracellular fluid?

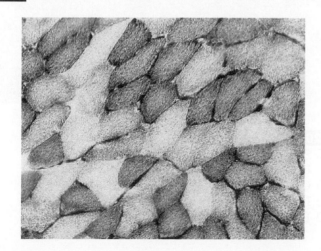

14 The figure at lower left shows a preparation of skeletal muscle stained to differentiate type I/red fibers (stained dark blue) from type II/white fibers (lightly stained). Staining of what component of the cell will give this appearance?
☐ A. Actin
☐ B. Glycogen
☐ C. Mitochondria
☐ D. Sarcoplasmic reticulum

15 Which cell has the highest concentration of mitochondria?
☐ A. Cardiac muscle cell
☐ B. Endothelial cell
☐ C. Fibroblast
☐ D. Plasma cell
☐ E. Smooth muscle cell

16 Which tissue would be most sensitive to an infarction (blockage of blood flow)?
☐ A. Cardiac muscle
☐ B. Hyaline cartilage
☐ C. Loose connective tissue
☐ D. Skeletal muscle, white fibers
☐ E. Smooth muscle

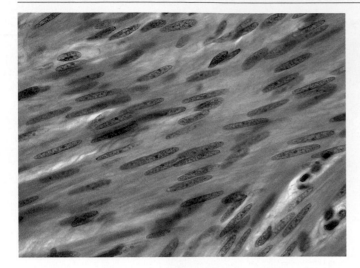

17 The figure above shows a section of a biopsy. From where could this biopsy have been taken?
- [ ] A. Achilles tendon
- [ ] B. Lamina propria of the tongue
- [ ] C. Myometrium
- [ ] D. Sciatic nerve
- [ ] E. Upper esophagus

- [ ] A. Cervical epithelium
- [ ] B. Dense irregular connective tissue
- [ ] C. Dense regular connective tissue
- [ ] D. Peripheral nerve
- [ ] E. Smooth muscle

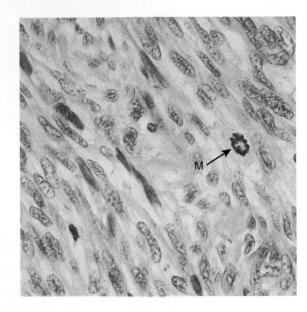

19 The figure above illustrates a malignant tumor (M) derived from which type of tissue?
- [ ] A. Epithelium
- [ ] B. Lymphoid tissue
- [ ] C. Muscle
- [ ] D. Nerve

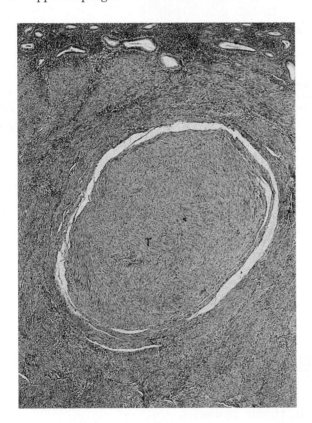

18 The figure above shows a biopsy of a uterine tumor (T). Based on its location and appearance, from what tissue type is the tumor derived?

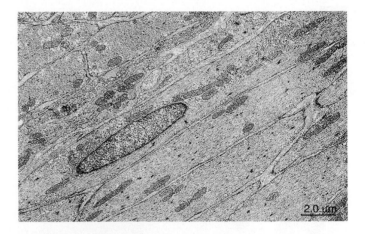

20 In the figure above, what type of cells are shown?
- [ ] A. Epithelial cells
- [ ] B. Fibroblasts
- [ ] C. Satellite cells
- [ ] D. Schwann cells
- [ ] E. Smooth muscle cells

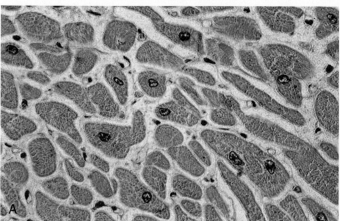

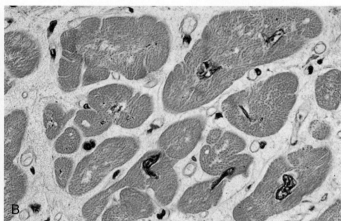

21 The two images above illustrate the normal (A) and pathologic (B) conditions of a tissue. What pathologic process is shown?

- [ ] A. Duchenne-type muscular dystrophy
- [ ] B. Fibrosis of a tendon
- [ ] C. Foreign-body giant cell genesis
- [ ] D. Myocardial hypertrophy
- [ ] E. Smooth muscle hyperplasia in the uterus

following would result in improvement of muscle strength in the affected muscles?

- [ ] A. Administering a drug to increase conduction velocity of axons
- [ ] B. Administering a drug to prevent acetylcholine breakdown
- [ ] C. Exercise that will increase muscle workload
- [ ] D. Nerve stimulation by acupuncture
- [ ] E. Stimulation of sympathetic ganglia

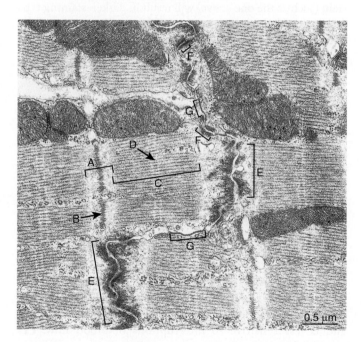

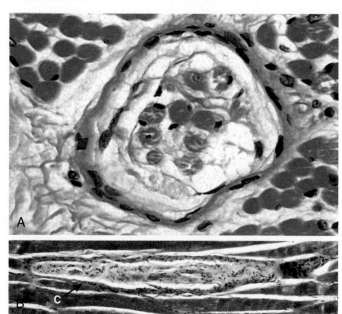

Questions 22 and 23 refer to the figure above. Match the labels on the figure with the descriptions given.

22 Which labeled structure is enriched in both actin and cadherin?

23 Which labeled structure is required for passing the excitatory impulse from cell to cell?

24 A patient presents with fatigue and muscle weakness. She was diagnosed with myasthenia gravis. Which of the

25 The figure above shows a cross section (A) and a longitudinal section (B) of a large, encapsulated structure. (The letter *C* in part B indicates the location of the cross section shown in part A.) What is this structure?

- [ ] A. Encysted larva of *Trichinella spiralis*
- [ ] B. Infected hair follicle
- [ ] C. Muscle spindle
- [ ] D. Pacinian corpuscle
- [ ] E. Pulmonary tubercle enclosing mycobacteria

ANSWERS

1. B Wound closure is facilitated by the contractile action of myofibroblasts. None of the other cell types play a significant role in wound closure. **FH p. 101**

2. A This is the endomysium, a connective tissue layer that immediately surrounds the muscle cells (D). It primarily consists of reticular fibers. The thicker, stronger type I collagen fibers form a larger proportion of the perimysium (B) and epimysium (C). **FH pp. 102-103**

3. C The photomicrograph demonstrates unbranched muscle fibers showing cross striations and flattened nuclei at the periphery. This morphology indicates that these are skeletal muscle fibers. Of the choices above, only the tongue contains skeletal muscle. **FH p. 103**

4. D Dystrophin is a protein that is critical for proper skeletal muscle function. A mutation in the dystrophin gene leads to muscle weakness and wasting. An example of this is seen in Duchenne muscular dystrophy. The other tissues are not significantly affected by mutations in the dystrophin gene. **FH p. 104**

5. C Dystrophin contributes to the complex of molecules that anchor the contractile elements to the plasma membrane. It is found at the periphery of the cell. Actin, tropomyosin, and troponin are associated with the thin filaments, which are distributed throughout the cytoplasm. Antibodies to them would stain the whole cell. Skeletal muscle does not form intercellular junctions, so it would not be expected to stain with antibodies to cadherin. **FH pp. 101-109**

6. C The fibers on the left are normal, whereas the ones on the right have atrophied. The atrophy of a group of muscle fibers suggests a dysfunction of motor units supplying those fibers. This type of pathology is seen in neurogenic muscular atrophy as occurs with the loss of spinal motor neurons. In muscular dystrophy, the atrophy is haphazard, rather than confined to a group of muscle fibers. In myasthenia gravis, because the disease is intermittent, muscle biopsies usually reveal no significant pathology. Anabolic steroid use and marathon training would cause hypertrophy, not atrophy. **FH pp. 103-104, 135, BH p. 312**

7. A Muscle fibers of highly variable diameter are present in muscular dystrophy. In both polio and Guillain-Barré syndrome, there is neurogenic muscle atrophy, affecting a group of muscle fibers rather than random fibers affected in muscular dystrophy. Lymphocytic infiltration characteristic of polymyositis is not present here. **FH pp. 103-104, BH p. 313**

8. D In response to damage to myofibers, adults stem cells, termed *satellite cells*, fuse together to form new myofibers. Myofibers are postmitotic and do not fuse with each other or with macrophages. **FH p. 104**

9. C This is the H band. It is the region of the A band where myosin filaments are present but where actin filaments are absent. **FH pp. 106-107**

10. D This is the Z line. It contains alpha-actinin and anchors the plus ends of the actin filaments. Its function is similar to the function of the dense bodies in smooth muscle. **FH pp. 107, 114-115**

11. A The I band narrows during contraction owing to the increased overlap of the thin filament by the thick filaments. **FH pp. 107, 109**

12. F This is the sarcoplasmic reticulum. It stores calcium, which is released upon stimulation of the cell. The calcium binds to troponin, allowing contraction to occur. Mitochondria (E) store calcium, but do not release it during normal muscle stimulation. **FH pp. 108, 109**

13. G T-tubules are invaginations of the plasma membrane and therefore contain extracellular fluid. **FH pp. 108, 109**

14. C Type I fibers have significantly more mitochondria than type II fibers. Preparations stained with a mitochondrial stain (such as the one above) will result in darker-staining type I fibers and lighter-staining type II fibers. The other cellular structures would not be expected to differ much between the two cell types or would be more concentrated in the type II fibers. **FH p. 111**

15. A The cardiac muscle cell contains numerous mitochondria with closely packed cristae for continuous production of ATP. None of the other cells have as many mitochondria with as many cristae. **FH pp. 116-119**

16. A Because cardiac muscle must continue to contract throughout life, it cannot survive for even a short time if isolated from oxygen and nutrients. White skeletal muscle fibers do not need extensive vascularization because they make use of anaerobic pathways. Cartilage is not vascularized. Chondrocytes obtain nutrients by diffusion from capillaries outside the cartilage and are specifically adapted to a low oxygen environment. Smooth muscle is less heavily vascularized than either of the other types of muscle and is less sensitive to interruptions of blood flow. **FH pp. 116-119**

17. C The homogenous appearance of the tissue plus the elongated, but not flattened, nuclei identify this tissue as smooth muscle. The myometrium is composed of large amounts of smooth muscle. The other choices contain little or no smooth muscle. **FH pp. 112-113**

18. E The tumor is in the myometrium, which is composed mainly of smooth muscle. The cells in the tumor have the homogenous appearance of elongated smooth muscle cells, consistent with their origin from the myometrium. Such benign tumors, called *leiomyomas* (fibroids), are commonly found in the uterus. **FH pp. 112-113, BH p. 225**

19. C The proliferation of spindle cells with abundant, eosinophilic cytoplasm and pale-staining, cigar-shaped nuclei, seen here, is characteristic of leiomyosarcomas, which are derived from smooth muscle. Tumors derived from nerve can also show spindle cell proliferation, but lack the eosinophilic cytoplasm and cigar-shaped nuclei. Tumors of epithelial cells and lymphocytes do not show spindle cells and have round or oval nuclei. **FH p. 113, BH p. 76**

20. E The pale-staining, actin-rich cytoplasm and pale appearance of these elongated nuclei are characteristic of smooth muscle cells. Stratified squamous epithelial cells have a similar general shape, but show an abundance of desmosomes and a smaller extracellular space. Fibroblasts would be surrounded by collagen fibers, satellite cells of ganglia would be adjacent to neurons, and Schwann cells would be adjacent to myelinated axons, all absent here. **FH p. 114**

21. D The centrally positioned nuclei and relatively large fiber diameter with eosinophilic cytoplasm indicate that these cells are hypertrophied cardiac muscle cells. Myofibrils are evident within the cells, eliminating smooth muscle as a possibility. In Duchenne-type muscular dystrophy, the affected fibers may enlarge, but they are skeletal muscle fibers with flattened, peripherally located nuclei. **FH p. 117, BH p. 61**

22. E Like the zonula adherens, the fascia adherens is the site where actin filaments insert onto the cell membrane and the two membranes are held together by cadherin molecules.

The I band (A) is enriched in actin, but not cadherin. Desmosomes (F) are enriched in cadherin and desmin intermediate filaments. **FH p. 120 (see also p. 90)**

23. G This is a gap junction, recognizable by the close apposition of the plasma membranes of the two adjacent cells. Gap junctions are sites of low electrical resistance, allowing the action potential to pass from one cell to the next. **FH p. 120 (see also p. 91)**

24. B Myasthenia gravis is an autoimmune disease caused by binding of autoantibodies to acetylcholine receptors. This results in depletion of receptors and inability of the neurotransmitter acetylcholine to transmit excitatory signals across the motor end plate. Administration of a cholinesterase inhibitor will allow the neurotransmitter to bind competitively to the receptors and prolong its effect. Because the problem is lack of conduction across the motor end plate, increasing the conduction velocity of axons, nerve stimulation by acupuncture, or muscle exercise would not improve muscle strength in myasthenia gravis. The sympathetic ganglia are part of the autonomic nervous system and do not innervate skeletal muscle. **FH p. 135**

25. C The small intrafusal fibers and a capsule are characteristic features of muscle spindles. The fact that the structure is surrounded by skeletal muscle fibers eliminates hair follicles and pacinian corpuscles, which are normally surrounded by connective tissue. A pulmonary tubercle, likewise, would not be surrounded by muscle. The intrafusal fibers cut in cross section do not resemble a single encysted nematode of *Trichinella spiralis*. **FH p. 150**

Nervous Tissues

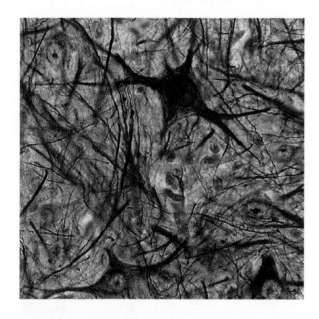

1 In the figure above, cells have been stained using immunocytochemistry and a brown chromogen to demonstrate a specific type of filament. What filaments are they likely to be?
☐ A. Actin filaments
☐ B. Desmin filaments
☐ C. Keratin filaments
☐ D. Myosin filaments
☐ E. Neurofilaments

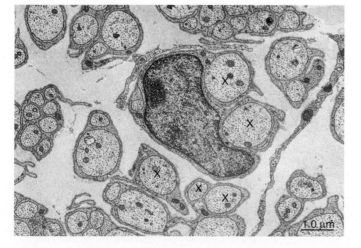

2 What is the large nucleated cell in the figure at bottom left?
☐ A. Astrocyte
☐ B. Fibroblast
☐ C. Neuron
☐ D. Oligodendrocyte
☐ E. Schwann cell

3 The structures labeled X in the figure at bottom left are enriched in which protein?
☐ A. Alpha-actinin
☐ B. Desmin
☐ C. Keratin
☐ D. Tubulin
☐ E. Vinculin

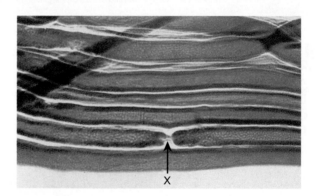

4 The figure above shows a whole mount preparation of a myelinated nerve. What is the structure labeled X?
☐ A. Early indication of a demyelinating disease
☐ B. Node of Ranvier
☐ C. Schmidt-Lanterman cleft
☐ D. Site of localized nerve damage
☐ E. Site where nerve branching will occur

5 A 20-year-old woman complains of weakness of her left leg and visual disturbances. She notes that she had similar episodes 8 months ago but did not seek medical attention at that time because her symptoms seemed to subside on their own. She admits that they appear to be more severe this time. A thorough neurologic examination shows that she has multiple sensory and motor deficits. An MRI shows scattered lesions in many parts of the central nervous system. What else would a microscopic examination of the lesions show?

☐ A. Cystic spaces
☐ B. Demyelination
☐ C. Lewy bodies
☐ D. Motor neuron loss
☐ E. Neurofibrillary tangles

6 Which of the following would best explain the cause of the weakness in the above patient?

☐ A. Congenital absence of nodes of Ranvier
☐ B. Depletion of receptors on motor end membranes
☐ C. Lack of neurotransmitter
☐ D. Lack of sympathetic ganglia
☐ E. Reduced conduction velocity of axons

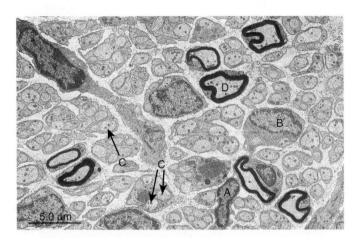

7 In what way do the structures labeled *C* in the figure above differ from the structure labeled *D*?

☐ A. Are not associated with Schwann cells
☐ B. Have a more rapid anterograde transport
☐ C. Have a slower conduction velocity
☐ D. Lack microtubules
☐ E. Possess ribosomes

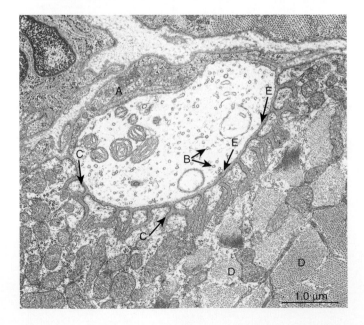

Use the figure at bottom left to answer the next two questions.

8 A 40-year-old man complains of muscle weakness and fatigue. He has a prior history of virus infections, and his family has a history of autoimmune disorders. Blood tests demonstrate the presence of autoantibodies for acetylcholine receptors. Using the letters in the figure, identify where these antibodies will bind.

9 A 35-year-old man complains of muscle weakness shortly after eating home-canned vegetables. The physician suspects botulism. Use the letters in the figure to identify where this botulism toxin exerts its effects.

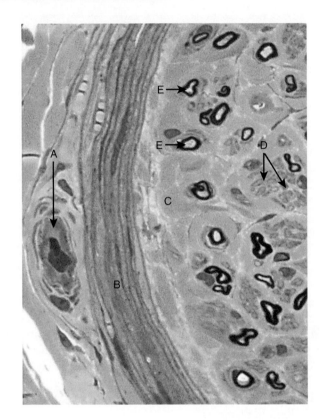

10 Guillain-Barré syndrome is caused by an autoimmune attack on peripheral nerves. Which structure, in the figure above, was breached to permit access of these antibodies to their targets?

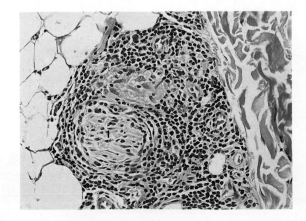

11 A 15-year-old boy was found to have multiple depigmented patches of skin and a loss of sensation in the affected areas. The figure at bottom right of the previous page shows a skin biopsy taken from a lesion and indicates substantial lymphocyte infiltration around the structure labeled *1*. What is this structure?

☐ A. Dense irregular connective tissue
☐ B. Hair follicle
☐ C. Meissner corpuscle
☐ D. Pacinian corpuscle
☐ E. Peripheral nerve

12 A biopsy section taken from the brain of a patient with tissue damage due to a stroke would show proliferation of which of the following cells?

☐ A. Astrocytes
☐ B. Endothelial cells
☐ C. Ependymal cells
☐ D. Neurons
☐ E. Oligodendrocytes

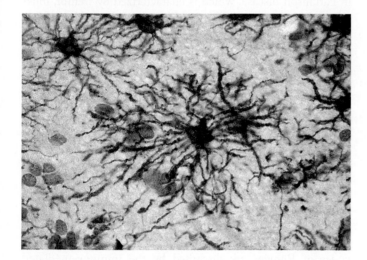

13 The figure above illustrates a tissue section stained using immunocytochemistry to illustrate a component of the cytoskeleton. This component consists of intermediate filaments composed of a protein called GFAP. Which cells contain this type of intermediate filament?

☐ A. Astrocytes
☐ B. Epithelial cells
☐ C. Microglia
☐ D. Neurons
☐ E. Oligodendroglia

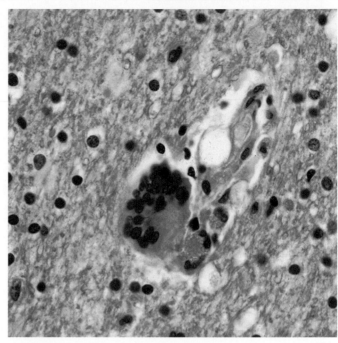

14 The figure above is an autopsy specimen taken from the central nervous system. There are many small, round nuclei visible throughout the figure. To what do these nuclei belong?

☐ A. Fibroblasts
☐ B. Glia
☐ C. Lymphocytes
☐ D. Monocytes
☐ E. Neurons

15 A 65-year-old woman complains of headache and confusion 1 month after a fall. Her physician determines that her symptoms were caused by bleeding due to torn cerebral veins. Where would the bleeding accumulate?

☐ A. Epidural space
☐ B. Pia mater
☐ C. Scalp
☐ D. Subarachnoid space
☐ E. Subdural space

16 If a patient is found to have a tumor derived from Merkel cells, in which of the following sites is the tumor most likely to be located?

☐ A. Cerebral cortex
☐ B. Ependymal layer
☐ C. Meninges
☐ D. Neuromuscular junctions
☐ E. Skin

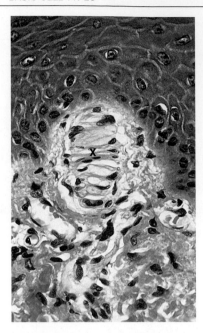

17 The structure labeled *X* in the figure above functions in which sensation?

☐ A. Cold
☐ B. Heat
☐ C. Pain
☐ D. Pressure
☐ E. Touch

ANSWERS

1. E The large, pale, round nuclei with prominent nucleoli identify the stained cells as neurons. Desmin and keratin filaments are found only in muscle and epithelial cells, respectively. Actin is usually detectable in isolated stress fibers or as bundles beneath the cell membrane and would not have a distribution that fills the cytoplasm in this pattern. Myosin is much sparser in neurons than the abundant neurofilaments shown here. **FH p. 126**

2. E This figure shows a section through numerous axons in a peripheral nerve. Axons are distinguished by their round profiles and light-appearing cytoplasm. The nucleated cell enveloping several axons is a Schwann cell. Nuclei of neurons are large, pale, and rounded and have prominent nucleoli. The abundant extracellular space in this figure is characteristic of the peripheral nervous system and not the central nervous system, so the cell nucleus shown in the figure cannot be that of a central nervous system astrocyte or oligodendrocyte. Fibroblasts would not envelop axons as is seen here. **FH p. 128**

3. D Tubulin is concentrated in the axons (*X*), giving structural support to the long cellular processes and providing a transportation system between the axon terminal and the cell body of the neuron. Alpha-actinin and desmin are proteins

found only in muscle. Keratin and vinculin are restricted to epithelial cells and connective tissue cells, respectively. **FH p. 128**

4. B Nodes of Ranvier are normal, nonpathologic sites where two Schwann cells are joined and the myelin is interrupted. The nodes are important functionally because they allow for rapid passage of the electrical impulse along a myelinated nerve. Clefts of Schmidt-Lanterman arise from irregularities within the myelin sheath, rather than at the ends of a myelin sheath, shown in the figure. The axons appear healthy, with no signs of damage or disease. **FH p. 128**

5. B The patient has the characteristic clinical presentation of multiple sclerosis with remitting clinical course and multifocal central nervous system involvement. The hallmark of multiple sclerosis is demyelination. Cystic spaces in the brain are characteristic of an old infarct. They usually occur in older individuals, and the clinical presentation, depending on the size and location of the infarct, is usually localized rather than multifocal. Lewy bodies are inclusions in neurons seen in Parkinson disease, which is characterized by tremor, muscle rigidity, stooping, and a shuffling gait. Motor neuron loss occurs in diseases like amyotrophic lateral sclerosis, resulting in progressive muscle weakness and paralysis. Neurofibrillary tangles are aggregates of abnormal protein found in neurons of patients with Alzheimer disease. The tangles result in loss of neurons in the frontal cortex and cingulate gyrus; thus, these patients present with cognitive dysfunction and memory loss. **BH p. 306**

6. E In nervous tissue, the myelin sheath insulates and protects the underlying axons and greatly enhances their conduction velocity. In multiple sclerosis, there is an immune-mediated destruction of myelin sheaths, resulting in slowing of conduction velocity in the affected nerves. Impulses often do not reach their targets, resulting in muscle weakness. The nodes of Ranvier are disrupted by the immune-mediated destruction; however, the congenital absence of the nodes is quite rare. Receptors on motor end plates and neurotransmitters are unaffected in multiple sclerosis. A lack of conduction would result in paralysis, not weakness. A lack of sympathetic ganglia would impair the function of glands but not the function of postural muscles. **FH p. 130**

7. C The unmyelinated fibers at *C* have a slower conduction velocity owing to a diminished insulation and lack of nodes of Ranvier that facilitate saltatory conduction. Both myelinated and unmyelinated fibers are associated with Schwann cells, and all nerve fibers possess microtubules that mediate anterograde transport. Ribosomes are excluded from the axoplasm of all fibers. **FH p. 130**

8. C The acetylcholine receptors are located on the muscle cell membrane at motor end plates. **FH p. 134**

9. E The botulism toxin inhibits the binding of the synaptic vesicles to the presynaptic membrane. **FH p. 134-135**

10. B The cells of the perineurium form a blood-nerve barrier. These cells, joined by a network of tight junctions, separate the epineurium and surrounding connective tissue away from the endoneurium and the nerve fibers. Blood vessels of the endoneurium also participate in a blood-nerve barrier by having robust tight junctions, which would deny access of antibodies to neural tissue. Blood vessels (A) outside of the perineurium do not display barrier properties. **FH p. 136-137**

11. E This structure is a peripheral nerve. This patient has leprosy (Hansen disease). As shown in the figure above, nerves become surrounded by lymphocytes, leading to their destruction and to loss of sensation in the skin. Meissner corpuscles are located next to the stratified squamous epithelium of the skin (not visible here), and pacinian corpuscles are much larger than a single peripheral nerve, as are hair follicles. **FH p. 138, BH p. 42**

12. A Astrocytes are a type of neuroglia that play an important role in repair of central nervous system tissue after injury or damage. Neurons in most brain regions are postmitotic and do not proliferate. Oligodendrocytes are not thought to be very responsive to tissue damage. Endothelial cell proliferation and granulation tissue formation are important components of healing in chronic inflammation of many tissue types. However, in the brain, the blood-brain barrier prevents many cells from entering and damaging brain tissue. Healing after injury occurs mainly by proliferation of astrocytes. Ependymal cells line the ventricles but do not respond to injury. **FH p. 140**

13. A Glial fibrillary acidic protein (GFAP), a form of intermediate filament, is specific to astrocytes. The abundant, branched processes of these cells identify them as protoplasmic astrocytes. **FH p. 141**

14. B These are glial cells, recognizable by their small, round nuclei. Neuronal nuclei are much larger than the cell nuclei shown and are euchromatic with prominent nucleoli. Fibroblasts, lymphocytes, and monocytes are not abundant in the central nervous system. **FH p. 140, BH p. 305**

15. E Veins and venous sinuses are found in the subdural space that lies between the dura mater and arachnoid space. Venous bleeding would accumulate in the subdural space. Some parts of the skull are thinner than others and as a result of head trauma, arteries that lie close to the skull rupture, and blood accumulates in the epidural space (the space between the dura mater and the skull). Therefore, most epidural hemorrhages are arterial in nature and tend to accumulate rapidly. The pia mater is a thin membrane that covers the brain parenchyma. The vessels of the pia mater are usually of very small caliber and may not account for significant bleeding. The subarachnoid space lies between the arachnoid membrane and the pia matter and contains cerebrospinal fluid. Arteries cross the subarachnoid space to reach the brain parenchyma and can rupture because of trauma or aneurysms and result in subarachnoid hemorrhages, but these also are arterial in nature. Bleeding from veins in the scalp would result in superficial hematomas. **FH p. 146**

16. E In the skin, free nerve endings are found along the dermal-epidermal junction associated with non-neuronal cells, called *Merkel cells*. A tumor arising from Merkel cells would be found in the skin. Although Merkel cells are derived from the neural crest, they are found only in the skin and not in the other structures listed. **FH p. 148**

17. E The beehive-like appearance of an encapsulated nerve ending just under the epidermis is characteristic of Meissner corpuscles. These corpuscles are sensitive to touch. Sensations of cold, heat, and pain are communicated to the central nervous system from unencapsulated nerve endings. Pressure and vibratory sensations are detected by large pacinian corpuscles. **FH p. 149**

Organ Systems

FH5 Chapter 8: Circulatory System
BH5 Chapter 8: Atherosclerosis
BH5 Chapter 9: Thrombus and Embolism
BH5 Chapter 10: Infarction
BH5 Chapter 11: Cardiovascular System

8

Circulatory System

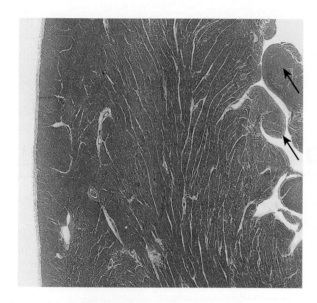

1 In the figure above, which of the following describes the function of the structures shown by the *arrows*?
- ☐ A. Anchor the chordae tendineae
- ☐ B. Divide the ventricular cavity
- ☐ C. Initiate impulse conduction
- ☐ D. Secrete pericardial fluid
- ☐ E. Supply blood to myocardium

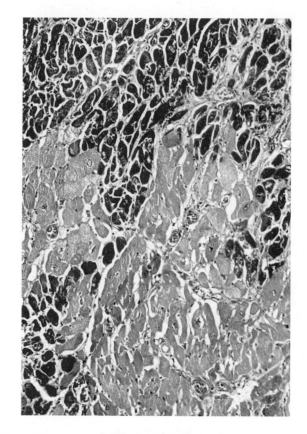

2 A microscopic section of the heart of a 61-year-old man with chest pain is shown. What caused the cellular damage represented by the pale-staining areas?
- ☐ A. Blockage of the atrioventricular node
- ☐ B. Calcification of the aortic valve
- ☐ C. Inflammation of the pericardium
- ☐ D. Thrombosis of the coronary artery
- ☐ E. Vegetation of the tricuspid valve

3 A 55-year-old man presenting to the emergency room with severe chest pain was admitted with a diagnosis of myocardial infarction. Laboratory tests and electrocardiogram confirmed the diagnosis. One week later, the patient died suddenly. Examination of the heart at autopsy reveals areas of left ventricular myocardium showing loose edematous tissue with macrophages, few capillaries, and fibroblasts. Based on these findings, which of the following would account for the sudden death of the patient?

☐ A. Aneurysm formation
☐ B. Aortic dissection
☐ C. Myocardial rupture
☐ D. Pulmonary infarction
☐ E. Severe hypertension

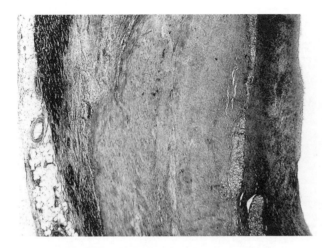

4 A histologic section obtained from the left ventricular myocardium of a 65-year-old woman who was hospitalized for a severe myocardial infarction 9 months earlier is shown in the figure above. Which of the following may be seen as a complication of the pathology shown in the image?

☐ A. Aneurysm formation
☐ B. Aortic dissection
☐ C. Hypertension
☐ D. Mitral stenosis
☐ E. Myocardial rupture

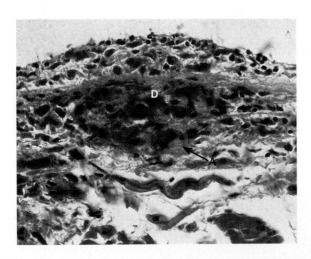

5 The figure at the bottom left shows a portion of the endocardium recovered from a patient who had suffered from an acute episode of rheumatic fever. What structure is labeled by the letter *D*?

☐ A. Aschoff body, composed of macrophages and lymphocytes
☐ B. Atherosclerotic coronary artery
☐ C. Hypertrophied cardiac muscle cells
☐ D. Myocardial infarct
☐ E. Thrombotic vegetation

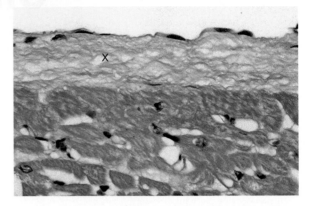

6 In the figure above, what would an acute inflammation in the region labeled X be called?

☐ A. Aortitis
☐ B. Endocarditis
☐ C. Myocarditis
☐ D. Pericarditis
☐ E. Vasculitis

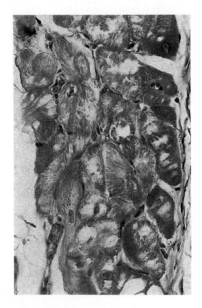

7 A histologic section of myocardium shows fibers with pale-staining central areas as shown in the figure above. Which of the following best describes these fibers?

☐ A. They are usually found in the epicardium
☐ B. They connect with each other by gap junctions
☐ C. They contain few mitochondria
☐ D. They have abundant T-tubules
☐ E. They secrete pericardial fluid

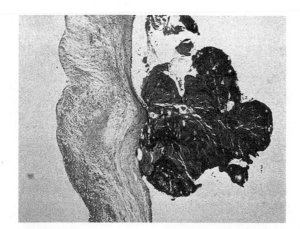

8 A 65-year-old woman, hospitalized for metastatic breast carcinoma, was found to have shortness of breath. A murmur was heard on cardiac examination. A microscopic section of the mitral valve is shown in the figure above. Which of the following complications might be seen in this patient?
☐ A. Cerebral infarct
☐ B. Myocardial rupture
☐ C. Pericarditis
☐ D. Pulmonary embolism
☐ E. Sepsis

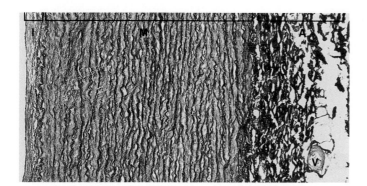

9 The figure above shows a section of an aorta. What makes up the brown-stained structures in the region labeled *M*?
☐ A. Collagen type I
☐ B. Collagen type III
☐ C. Collagen type IV
☐ D. Elastin
☐ E. Proteoglycan

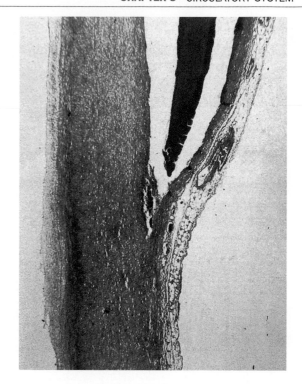

10 A 54-year-old man expires soon after complaining of sudden onset of chest pain that radiated to his back. A microscopic section taken from his aorta is shown in the figure above. What is the cause of the pathogenesis?
☐ A. Atherosclerosis
☐ B. Cystic medial necrosis
☐ C. Inflammation
☐ D. Muscular hypertrophy
☐ E. Thrombus formation

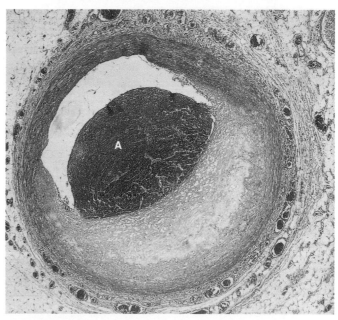

11 What does the letter *A* in the above figure label?
☐ A. Hamartoma
☐ B. Hemangioma of the skin

Continued on next page

☐ C. Hemorrhage into an atherosclerotic plaque
☐ D. Inflamed valve
☐ E. Venous thrombosis

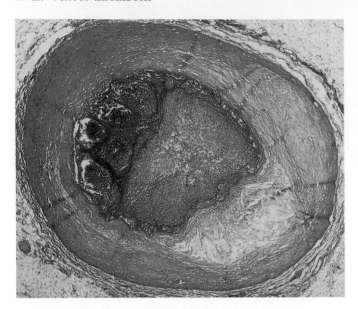

12 A cross section of the coronary artery from a 70-year-old man is shown in the figure above. Which of the following would be a risk factor for the pathology shown?
☐ A. Autoimmune disease
☐ B. Hypertension
☐ C. Marfan syndrome
☐ D. Severe malnutrition
☐ E. Strenuous exercise

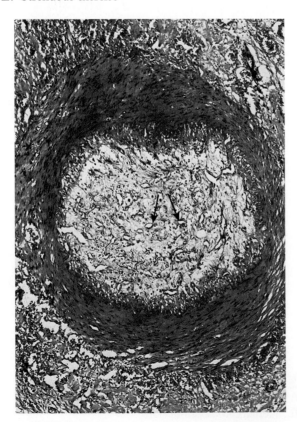

13 Which of the following best describes the changes shown by the *arrows* in the cross section of this artery occluded by a thrombus (bottom left)?
☐ A. Dissolution
☐ B. Embolization
☐ C. Organization
☐ D. Propagation
☐ E. Recanalization

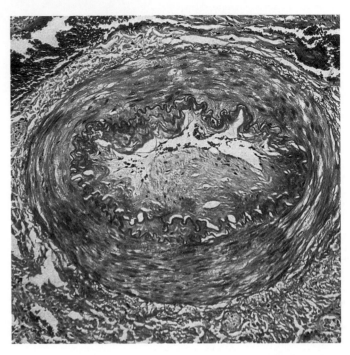

14 The figure above shows a kidney biopsy specimen from a patient with essential (primary) hypertension. Which feature listed below is a result of this condition?
☐ A. An abnormally thickened tunica adventitia
☐ B. An abnormally thin tunica media
☐ C. An abnormally thin tunica intima
☐ D. Duplication of the internal elastic lamina
☐ E. Loss of the external elastic lamina

15 A 59-year-old woman complains of severe headache and blurring of vision in her left eye. Physical examination reveals pain and tenderness over the left temporal artery. A biopsy of the temporal artery is shown at the top of the next page. What is the most likely diagnosis?
☐ A. Giant cell arteritis
☐ B. Henoch-Schönlein purpura
☐ C. Kaposi sarcoma
☐ D. Microscopic polyarteritis
☐ E. Polyarteritis nodosa

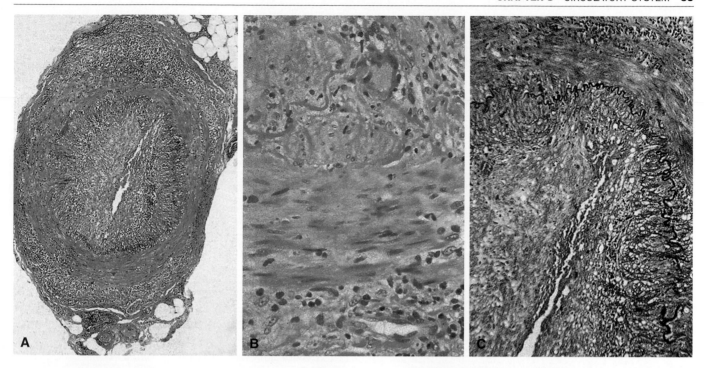

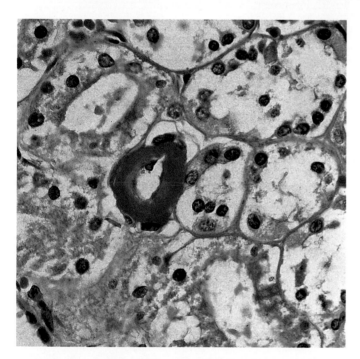

16 A 57-year-old man with a history of hypertension develops progressive renal failure. A kidney biopsy was performed, and a microscopic section is shown in the figure above. What is the cause of the change shown in the arteriole?

☐ A. Atherosclerotic plaque formation
☐ B. Deposition of basement membrane–like material
☐ C. Intimal proliferation
☐ D. Muscular hypertrophy
☐ E. Thrombus formation

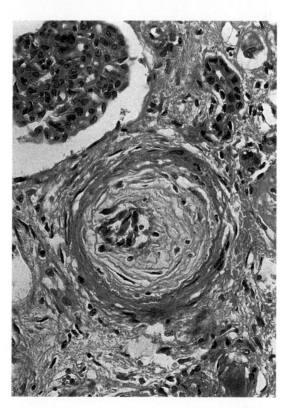

17 A 25-year-old man presents to the emergency room with severe headache and renal failure. His blood pressure is 150/100 mm Hg. A renal biopsy is performed, and a microscopic section is shown in the figure above. What is the cause of the change in the artery?

☐ A. Atherosclerotic plaque formation
☐ B. Deposition of basement membrane–like material
☐ C. Intimal proliferation
☐ D. Muscular hypertrophy
☐ E. Thrombus formation

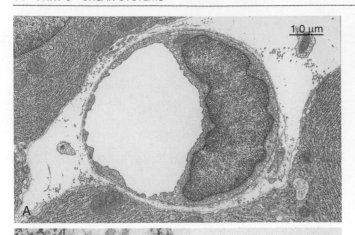

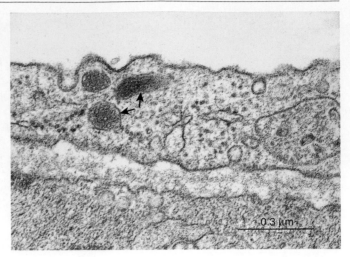

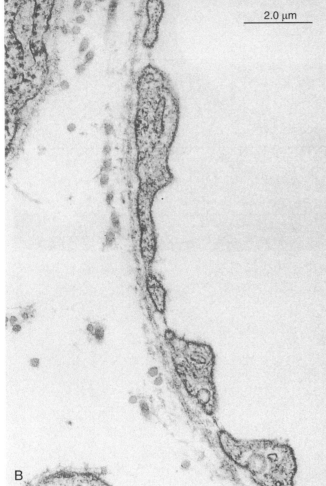

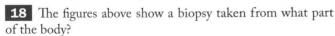

18 The figures above show a biopsy taken from what part of the body?

- ☐ A. Adrenal gland
- ☐ B. Biceps brachii
- ☐ C. Lamina propria of the stomach
- ☐ D. Liver
- ☐ E. Renal cortex

19 Which of the following best describes the function of the substance stored in Weibel-Palade bodies shown by the *arrows* in the above electron micrograph image of an endothelial cell?

- ☐ A. Mediate vasoconstriction
- ☐ B. Promote thrombus formation
- ☐ C. Regulate blood pressure
- ☐ D. Stimulate collagen production
- ☐ E. Suppress acute inflammation

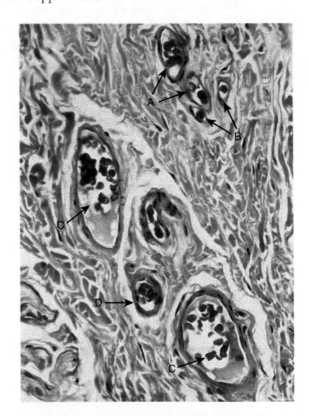

Use the figure above to answer questions 20 and 21.

20 Which labeled structure in the figure above is the main site of emigration of white blood cells from the circulation?

21 Which labeled structure in the figure on the previous page has a major role in controlling blood flow through the microcirculation?

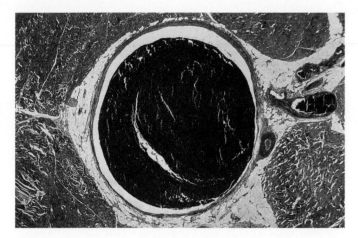

Use the figure above to answer questions 22 and 23.

22 A cross section of the popliteal vein from a 75-year-old woman is shown above. Which of the following would most likely be a predisposing factor for the development of this condition?
- [ ] A. Atherosclerosis
- [ ] B. Diabetes
- [ ] C. Extensive immobility
- [ ] D. Hypertension
- [ ] E. Rheumatic fever

23 Which of the following may be seen in the patient described above as a complication of the pathology shown in the figure?
- [ ] A. Systemic hypertension
- [ ] B. Lymphatic obstruction
- [ ] C. Myocardial infarction
- [ ] D. Pulmonary embolism
- [ ] E. Renal failure

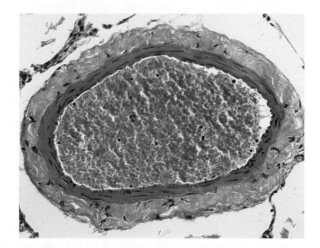

24 The figure above illustrates what type of vessel?
- [ ] A. Arteriole
- [ ] B. Capillary

- [ ] C. Elastic artery
- [ ] D. Lymphatic vessel
- [ ] E. Medium-sized vein

25 A 38-year-old man consults a dermatologist because of multiple, violet-colored skin lesions that developed on his arms and back. The dermatologist takes a biopsy of one of the back lesions. A microscopic section shows proliferation of sheets of stromal cells with interspersed, slitlike vascular spaces and extravasation of red blood cells. Based on the microscopic findings, which of the following conditions is most likely be present in this patient?
- [ ] A. AIDS
- [ ] B. Diabetes
- [ ] C. Hypertension
- [ ] D. Renal failure
- [ ] E. Vasculitis

ANSWERS

1. A The *arrows* show papillary muscles that protrude into the left ventricular cavity, but do not divide it. These provide attachment points for the chordae tendineae. The interventricular septum divides the ventricular cavity into the right and left ventricles and is composed of a solid wall of cardiac muscle. In the right atrium, the sinoatrial node, which is composed of modified myocytes, initiates the electrical impulse in the heart. The pericardium secretes pericardial fluid, and the coronary arteries supply blood to the myocardium. **FH p. 152**

2. D The image shows an area of myocardial infarction. Thrombosis of the coronary artery leads to infarction of the myocardium that is supplied by the blocked vessel. There is no indication of inflammation or abnormal vegetative growth. Blockage of the atrioventricular node may be caused by certain medications or by electrolyte imbalance. This causes slowing of electrical conductivity in the heart with resultant arrhythmia, not myocardial infarction. Inflammation of the pericardium (i.e. pericarditis) may be caused by infectious agents, autoimmune diseases, or renal failure. It is characterized by an inflammatory infiltrate of the pericardium and may be accompanied by a pericardial effusion. The latter, in large amounts, may cause heart failure owing to compression, not myocardial infarction. Although pericarditis may occur secondary to a myocardial infarct, it does not cause infarction of the myocardium. Vegetations of the tricuspid valve may embolize into the pulmonary circulation, blocking vessels and causing pulmonary infarction. Emboli from the mitral valve (not the tricuspid) can enter the coronary arteries and cause a myocardial infarct. Calcification of the aortic valve causes left ventricular hypertrophy, not myocardial infarction. **BH p. 106-107, FH p. 153**

3. C Five to 10 days after an infarction, the damaged myocardium is composed of a loose, edematous mesh with few capillaries and fibroblasts before its replacement by granulation tissue. Because of the soft consistency of the tissue, the myocardium is most vulnerable to rupture at this time, which results in sudden death. Aneurysms can form over an area of a myocardial infarct and can rupture, resulting in sudden death. However, aneurysms will not likely cause sudden death within a week after a myocardial infarct because they take many months to form. Dissection of the thoracic aorta, usually caused by hypertension, can cause sudden death, but it rarely occurs simultaneously with a myocardial infarct. Pulmonary infarctions may cause sudden death if they occur over large areas of the lung bilaterally; however, they are not directly associated with a myocardial infarction. Hypertension can precipitate a myocardial infarction, and blood pressure may remain elevated following the infarct. In these cases, sudden death is due to arrhythmias or left ventricular failure rather than myocardial rupture. **BH pp. 106-107, FH p. 153**

4. A The figure shows an old infarct, with a large part of the myocardium replaced by a pale-staining, dense collagenous scar. Continuous contraction of the surrounding myocardium over several months causes stretching and distention of the scar, resulting in formation of an aneurysm. When a healed myocardial infarct ruptures months after the insult, it is usually due to such an aneurysm. Dissection of the thoracic aorta, usually caused by hypertension, is not a complication of a healed myocardial infarct. The area of a healed infarct in the myocardium weakens the heart and may result in congestive heart failure, not hypertension. Mitral stenosis occurs as a result of congenital deformity or as a complication of inflammation of the valve and is not a complication of a myocardial infarction. Myocardial rupture is a complication of a myocardial infarct; however, rupture usually occurs 1 week after an infarction when the dead tissue is soft and has not yet been replaced by fibrous tissue. **BH p. 108, FH p. 153**

5. A Aschoff bodies are characteristic inflammatory lesions seen in the interstitium of the myocardium or endocardium of patients with rheumatic fever. Atherosclerotic plaques would be present in the intima of a coronary artery and not in the myocardial interstitium. Surrounding cardiac muscle cells are normal in size and show no damage to cytoplasm or nuclei, as would be seen in an infarct. Aggregates of fibrin and red blood cells, as might be seen in a thrombus, are not seen here. **BH p. 122, FH p. 153**

6. B A very thin layer of connective tissue located next to pink-staining cardiac muscle tissue and covered by a simple squamous epithelium is the endocardium of the heart, not the pericardium; inflammation here thus would be endocarditis. Myocarditis is an inflammation of the myocardium. The muscle cells are much too large to be smooth muscle, as would be expected in vasculitis or aortitis. **FH pp. 154-155, BH pp. 122-124**

7. B The image shows Purkinje fibers, which are modified cardiac muscle fibers. They contain abundant mitochondria and glycogen; the latter accounts for the pale cytoplasm.

They are adapted for rapid conduction of electrical signals and are joined by extensive gap junctions. They have no T-tubule system. Purkinje fibers are found in the endocardium, not in the epicardium. The serous lining cells of the pericardium secrete pericardial fluid. **FH p. 155**

8. A The image shows nonbacterial fibrin thrombi on the mitral valve, an entity referred to as *marantic endocarditis*. These thrombi can embolize and cause infarcts in the systemic circulation (e.g., a cerebral infarct). Sepsis is an unlikely complication because the thrombi are nonbacterial. Cardiac valve thrombi do not cause myocardial rupture or pericarditis. Thrombi on the tricuspid valve may cause pulmonary embolism. Mitral valve thrombi will not cause a pulmonary infarct unless the person has an atrial septal defect, a congenital defect with abnormal communication between the right and left atria. In the latter case, the person would have been symptomatic earlier in life. **FH p. 156, BH p. 123**

9. D The tunica media in the aorta is composed of alternating layers of smooth muscle and elastic fibers. The preparation has been stained with a stain specific for elastic fibers. Elastic fibers are stained dark-brown to black. Although collagens I, III, and IV and proteoglycans are present in the wall of the aorta, they do not form regular, distinctive layers in the tunica media. **FH p. 157**

10. B The clinical presentation and the image shown are characteristic of aortic dissection. Dissecting aneurysms of the thoracic aorta frequently show noninflammatory degeneration of the smooth muscle and elastic tissue of the media known as *cystic medial necrosis*. This weakens the wall of the aorta, leading to rupture and dissection. Atherosclerosis may result in aneurismal dilation, more commonly of the abdominal aorta, but the dilation is due to damage to the intima. Inflammation of the aorta may cause the aorta to weaken and rupture; however, it would be characterized by infiltration of white blood cells in the wall of the vessel rather than cystic medial necrosis. Muscular hypertrophy of the media, most commonly seen in small arteries and arterioles, occurs in conditions with high blood pressure. A thrombus, composed of blood, fibrin, and platelets, would be present in the lumen adherent to the intima and would cause occlusion, not dissection. **BH p. 114, FH p. 157**

11. C The image shows a vessel with an atherosclerotic plaque in the tunica intima. The vessel is clearly a muscular artery, as illustrated by its thick tunica media, so a venous thrombosis or valve cannot be possible choices. A hemangioma would show multiple dilated vessels. A hamartoma is an excessive proliferation of normal tissue. **BH p. 92, FH p. 158**

12. B The artery shows occlusion of the lumen by a thrombus superimposed on an atherosclerotic plaque. Hypertension is a major risk factor for the development of atherosclerosis. Other risk factors include smoking, diabetes, and hypercholesterolemia. Autoimmune diseases and severe malnutrition are not direct risk factors for atherosclerosis. Patients with

Marfan syndrome have an increased risk for developing aortic dissection, but not atherosclerosis. Strenuous exercise may cause muscle damage, but exercise, in general, reduces risk for atherosclerosis. **BH p. 93, FH p. 158**

13. E The proliferation of blood vessels (*arrows*) within the lumen of a thrombosed vessel is indicative of *recanalization*, a process that attempts to restore the patency of the vascular lumen. In *organization*, the thrombus is replaced by fibrous tissue, which occludes the lumen. In *dissolution*, there is a complete removal of the thrombus due to digestion by macrophages. *Propagation* of a thrombus is characterized by deposition of additional red blood cells, fibrin, and platelets on the thrombus, causing it to grow and extend along the wall of the vessel. Embolization is the process by which thrombi dislodge and travel in the bloodstream to tissues far away from where they originated. **BH p. 101, FH p. 158**

14. D In benign hypertension, the internal elastic lamina duplicates to make two distinct layers. In addition, the tunica intima and tunica media both thicken, as shown in the figure. The tunica adventitia is normal. **FH p. 158, BH p. 112**

15. A Giant cell arteritis is a systemic disease of blood vessels involving medium-sized arteries of the head (A). Infiltration of the vessel wall by lymphocytes, plasma cells, and giant cells (B) and degeneration of the internal elastic lamina (C), as well as the clinical presentation given above, are characteristic findings. Henoch-Schönlein purpura is a vasculitis of small to medium-sized arteries due to immune complex (IgA) deposition and infiltration by neutrophils and lymphocytes. It is a disease primarily occurring in children and is clinically characterized by purpura and joint and abdominal pain. Kaposi sarcoma is a vascular neoplasm (not a vasculitis) composed of a proliferation of spindle cells and small blood vessels. It presents as a skin lesion or tumor mass, not as a pain in the temporal region. In polyarteritis nodosa and microscopic polyarteritis, there is a prominent vasculitis involving medium-sized arteries and arterioles, respectively. The walls of the affected vessels are infiltrated by neutrophils and lymphocytes. Giant cells are uncommon, and these diseases do not commonly affect the temporal arteries. Clinically, they present with purpura, but not as pain in the temporal region. **BH p. 116, FH p. 158**

16. B Hypertension results in thickening of arterioles due to deposition of basement membrane–like material in the wall, especially in the arterioles of the kidneys. These are recognized by their pink-staining homogeneous appearance. This results in luminal narrowing, which may further aggravate the hypertension due to increased vascular resistance. An atherosclerotic plaque would be found deposited within the intima. The plaque would be pale-staining and composed of cholesterol crystals and foamy macrophages. Intimal proliferation also occurs in conditions with very high blood pressure and would be cellular rather than homogeneous and pink. Muscular hypertrophy of the media occurs as a response to hypertension in muscular arteries, not arterioles. A thrombus would

be present in the lumen, adherent to the intima. It appears red because it is composed of blood, fibrin, and platelets. **BH p. 112, FH p. 159**

17. C The artery in the image shows arterial changes caused by malignant hypertension. The arterial wall thickening is due to concentric proliferation of intimal cells. These can be recognized by their location on the luminal side of the internal elastic membrane. In contrast to essential or secondary hypertension, the media in malignant hypertension remains largely unchanged. **BH p. 113, FH p. 159**

18. C Fenestrated capillaries such as the one shown in the figure are found in the lamina propria of the digestive tract, in the kidney, and associated with glands. Here, the surrounding cells have highly developed rough endoplasmic reticulum, typical of exocrine (not endocrine) gland cells, such as the chief cells in the gastric mucosa. The liver has sinusoids instead of capillaries, and muscle has continuous-type capillaries. **FH p. 161**

19. B Weibel-Palade bodies are membrane-bound organelles that store von Willebrand factor, which promotes formation of a thrombus by causing platelets to adhere to damaged endothelium. Weibel-Palade bodies also contain adhesion molecules, which play a role in initiating (not suppressing) inflammation. A variety of other substances, not associated with Weibel-Palade bodies, are found in and secreted by endothelial cells that play a role in regulating blood flow (nitric oxide) and collagen formation (endothelial derived growth factor). **FH p. 162**

20. A These are postcapillary venules, recognizable by their thin walls and larger diameter than capillaries. In addition to thin walls, these vessels have very slow blood movement, making them the ideal site for emigration of white blood cells out of the vascular space. **FH p. 163**

21. D This is an arteriole, recognizable by its relatively small size and the presence of one or two layers of smooth muscle in its wall. Selective contraction of arterioles determines the distribution of the blood flow into the microcirculatory bed. **FH pp. 159, 163**

22. C The image shows a thrombus in a vein. Venous thrombosis is caused by stasis of blood flow and may be seen as a complication in patients who are bedridden or relatively immobile. Both diabetes and hypertension can cause arterial (not venous) occlusion owing to accelerated atherosclerotic plaque deposition in arteries. Rheumatic fever is an inflammatory disorder that follows streptococcal infections. It is not associated with venous thrombosis. **BH p. 97, FH p. 164**

23. D Thrombosis in the deep veins of the lower extremities may give rise to emboli that occlude the branches of the pulmonary artery. Such an embolus causes infarction in the lung or sudden death if it is large enough to occlude the major branch of the pulmonary artery. Lymphatic obstruction is caused by inflammatory disorders of the lymphatics, not by venous thrombosis. Emboli from deep veins of the leg cause pulmonary not myocardial infarction because they are halted in the pulmonary circulation before they get to the heart. Emboli originating from the left side of the heart can enter the systemic circulation, causing renal infarcts and possible renal failure. Systemic hypertension is caused by arterial, not venous, disorders. **BH p. 97-98, FH p. 164**

24. E This large vessel shows the proportionately thicker tunica adventitia and thinner tunica media that distinguish veins from their companion arteries. This vessel contains blood, so it cannot be a lymphatic vessel, and it is much too large to be a capillary or arteriole. **FH p. 164**

25. A The microscopic finding described is consistent with Kaposi sarcoma, a vascular tumor commonly seen in AIDS patients. None of the other listed conditions have an association with an increased risk for developing Kaposi sarcoma. Patients with diabetes are predisposed to develop skin ulcers, especially on the foot, owing to poor blood supply caused by atherosclerotic peripheral vascular disease. In renal failure, retention of waste products in the blood may cause itching and irritation of the skin. Reddish papules may be seen in patients with vasculitis, but they tend to be smaller and more numerous than those seen in Kaposi sarcoma. Microscopically, vasculitis is characterized by an inflammatory infiltrate in the wall of the arteries. **BH p. 119**

FH5 Chapter 9: Skin
FH5 Appendix 2: Notes on Staining Techniques
BH5 Chapter 16: Lymphoid and Haematopoietic Systems
BH5 Chapter 21: Skin

9

Skin

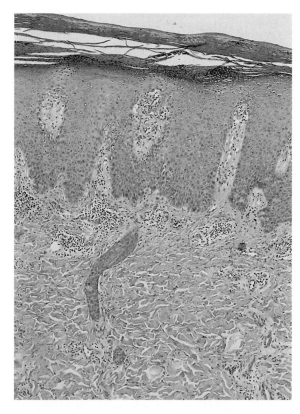

Use the figure above to answer the next two questions.

1 A 20-year old man presents with skin lesions on his legs. A section of the biopsy, shown above, reveals which abnormality?

☐ A. Absence of the stratum lucidum
☐ B. Diffuse separation between the papillary dermis and stratum basale
☐ C. Elongated rete pegs
☐ D. Extensive type I collagen in the dermis
☐ E. Peeling of the stratum corneum

2 Based on the microscopic findings from the patient, which of the following would best describe the clinical appearance of his skin lesion?

☐ A. Erythematous, scaly patches
☐ B. Fine papules
☐ C. Nodules with central crater
☐ D. Numerous blisters
☐ E. Pigmented nodules

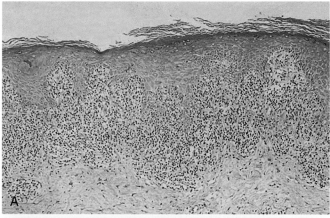

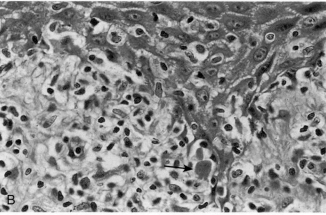

3 A 46-year-old man presents to his dermatologist with purple, pruritic papules on his wrists and ankles. The dermatologist takes a biopsy of one of the lesions. A low-power image of the microscopic finding is shown in A on the previous page. High-power magnification (B) shows dead basal cells (*arrow*). Which of the following is the most likely diagnosis?

- ☐ A. Keratoacanthoma
- ☐ B. Lichen planus
- ☐ C. Psoriasis
- ☐ D. Pyogenic granuloma
- ☐ E. Wart

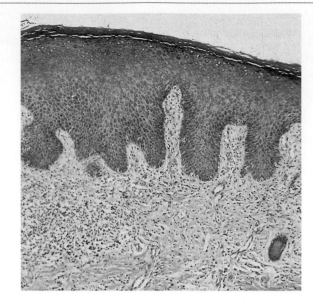

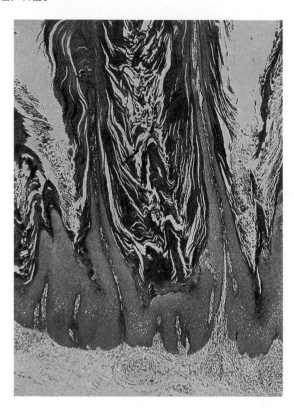

4 A microscopic section of a skin biopsy taken from a papillary, exophytic lesion on the hand of a 22-year-old man is shown in the figure above. What is the cause of this lesion?

- ☐ A. Hypersensitivity reaction
- ☐ B. Melanocytic proliferation
- ☐ C. Penetrating injury
- ☐ D. Sun damage
- ☐ E. Viral infection

5 A 52-year-old woman presents with chronic dermatitis on her thigh. A section from a biopsy is shown in the figure on the right. Which layer is most abnormally thickened?

- ☐ A. Stratum corneum
- ☐ B. Stratum granulosum
- ☐ C. Stratum spinosum (prickle cell layer)
- ☐ D. Stratum basale
- ☐ E. Basement membrane

6 As keratinocytes mature and migrate through the epidermis, their cytoplasmic content changes. Based on their appearance in sections stained with hematoxylin and eosin, the cytoplasmic components of the cells of the stratum granulosum make what change when they become cells of the stratum corneum?

- ☐ A. From being highly glycosylated to being nonglycosylated
- ☐ B. From being mostly protein to being mostly lipid
- ☐ C. From being nonphosphorylated to being phosphorylated
- ☐ D. From being primarily acidic to being primarily basic
- ☐ E. From containing much rough endoplasmic reticulum to containing little rough endoplasmic reticulum

7 The "prickles" in the prickle cell layer of the epidermis can be stained with an antibody to which protein?

- ☐ A. Actin
- ☐ B. Desmin
- ☐ C. Keratin
- ☐ D. Myosin
- ☐ E. Tubulin

8 A 65-year-old woman presents with multiple lesions on her arms, chest, and oral mucosa. Immunofluorescence studies performed on a biopsy of one of the skin lesions demonstrate an antibody directed against a hemidesmosomal antigen. Which of the following would best describe the clinical appearance of her skin lesions?

- ☐ A. Erythematous, scaly patches
- ☐ B. Fine papules
- ☐ C. Nodules with central craters
- ☐ D. Numerous blisters
- ☐ E. Pigmented nodules

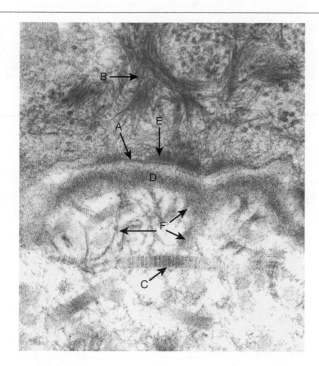

Use the figure above to answer the next two questions.

9 The above figure shows the basal surface of a keratinocyte in the stratum basale. Which component shown is formed from type VII collagen?

10 The above figure shows the basal surface of a keratinocyte in the stratum basale. Which label indicates keratin filaments?

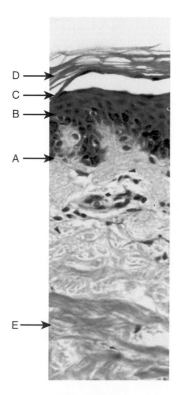

11 A microscopic image taken from a biopsy of a 20-year-old man is shown above. If this section of live tissue were incubated with tyrosine, where would most of the black-stained cells be located?

12 A biopsy of a pigmented skin lesion in a 55-year-old man shows proliferation of melanocytes. Which of the following findings would indicate a poor prognosis and a greater chance of metastatic spread?
☐ A. Clusters of dysplastic melanocytes throughout the epidermis
☐ B. Continuous line of dysplastic melanocytes in the stratum basale
☐ C. Nests of uniform, small melanocytes in the stratum basale and papillary dermis
☐ D. Nodular proliferation of dysplastic melanocytes deep into the reticular dermis

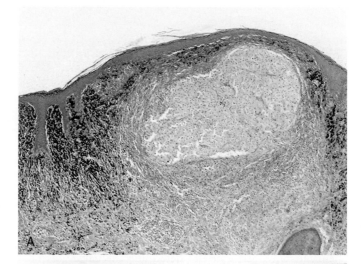

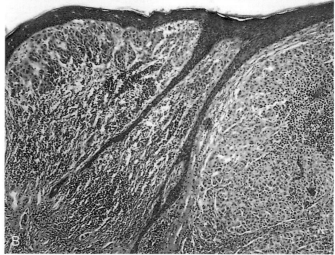

13 A 55-year-old man presented with a darkly pigmented nodular skin lesion on his left leg. Biopsy was performed on the lesion, and the microscopic images are shown in the figure above. Which of the following is the most likely predisposing factor?
☐ A. Chronic sun exposure
☐ B. Environmental toxin
☐ C. Repeated trauma
☐ D. Skin popping
☐ E. Tattoo application

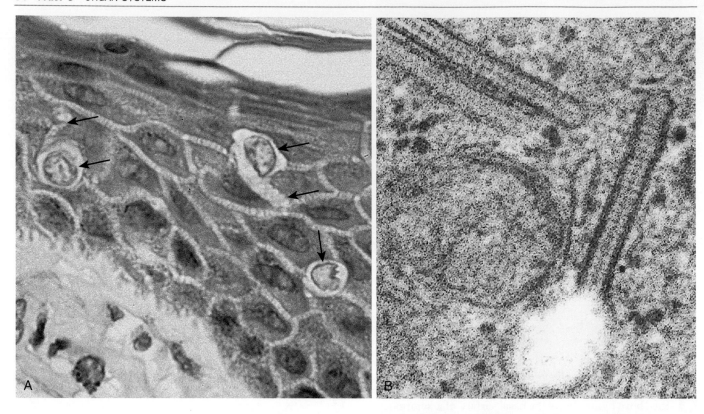

The next question refers to part B of the figure above.

14 A 1-year-old girl presents with bone pain, skin lesions, and hepatosplenomegaly. A skin biopsy shows extensive proliferation of cells in the dermis and epidermis. Immunohistochemical stains performed to determine the nature of these cells showed positive staining for antibody to CD1a. An electron micrograph of a cell taken from the lesion is shown in part B of the figure above. The lesion arose from which cell type?

☐ A. Langerhans cell
☐ B. Macrophage
☐ C. Melanocyte
☐ D. Merkel cell
☐ E. Squamous cell

The next question refers to parts A and B of the figure.

15 The cells indicated by the *arrows* in part A of the figure above have been demonstrated to contain the structures shown in the electron micrograph in part B. What is the primary function of these cells?

☐ A. Antigen presentation
☐ B. Detection of light touch
☐ C. Detection of pain
☐ D. Synthesis of keratin
☐ E. Synthesis of melanin

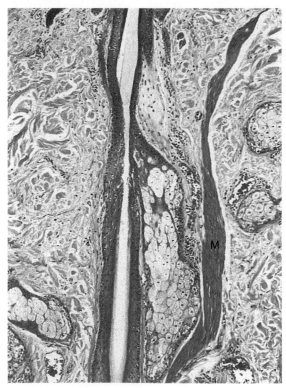

16 The muscle labeled *M* in the figure above is stimulated to contract by what means?

☐ A. Cold
☐ B. Dryness
☐ C. Heat
☐ D. Pain
☐ E. Pressure

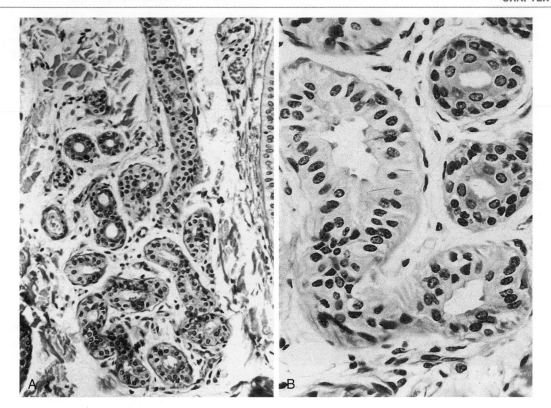

17 The structures shown in the figure above play a major role in what function?

☐ A. Keeping the skin moist
☐ B. Keeping the skin oily
☐ C. Protection from ultraviolet irradiation
☐ D. Secreting pheromones
☐ E. Thermoregulation

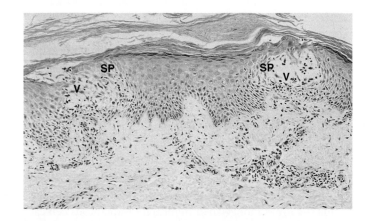

18 In the figure above, the epidermis has abnormalities labeled by the letters *SP* and *V*. What causes these abnormalities?

☐ A. Deposition of abnormal keratins
☐ B. Development of epidermal edema
☐ C. Hyperplasia of keratinocytes
☐ D. Invasion of lymphocytes into the epidermis
☐ E. Thinning of the stratum spinosum

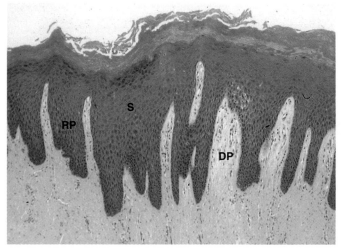

19 What is the term for the abnormal skin condition illustrated in the figure above? Rete pegs (RP), the stratum spinosum (S) and dermal papillae (DP) are labeled.

☐ A. Acanthosis
☐ B. Basal cell carcinoma
☐ C. Parakeratosis
☐ D. Spongiosis
☐ E. Viral wart

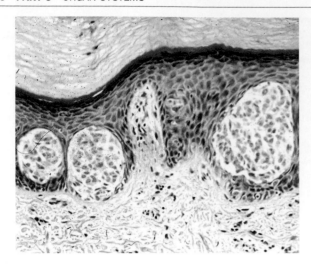

20 In the figure above, what is the source of the accumulations of pale-staining cells within the epidermis?
- ☐ A. Hair follicles
- ☐ B. Keratinocytes
- ☐ C. Langerhans cells
- ☐ D. Melanocytes
- ☐ E. Sebaceous glands

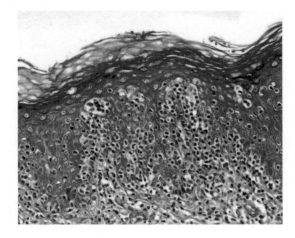

21 In the figure above, the epidermis has developed anatomic abnormalities. What is the cause of these abnormalities?
- ☐ A. Deposition of abnormal keratins
- ☐ B. Development of epidermal edema
- ☐ C. Hyperplasia of keratinocytes
- ☐ D. Invasion of lymphocytes into the epidermis
- ☐ E. Thinning of the stratum spinosum

For questions 22, 23, and 24, match the characteristic microscopic description of skin tumors with the diagnosis listed below.

- ☐ A. Basal cell carcinoma
- ☐ B. Cutaneous T-cell lymphoma
- ☐ C. Dermatofibroma
- ☐ D. Lipoma
- ☐ E. Melanoma
- ☐ F. Neurofibroma
- ☐ G. Squamous cell carcinoma in situ

22 Nests of cells with scant cytoplasm extending from the epidermis to the dermis, deep blue-staining nuclei with cells at the periphery of the tumor arranged in a palisade pattern.

23 Loss of organization and stratification of the epidermis with dysplasia involving full thickness of the epidermis.

24 Ill-defined, irregular proliferation of spindle cells in the dermis with scattered foamy histiocytes and thickening of the overlying epidermis.

ANSWERS

1. C Rete pegs are the regions of epidermis that extend downward into the connective tissue of the dermis. In this biopsy, the rete pegs are abnormally long. A stratum lucidum is often not visible, and its absence in not abnormal. There is no obvious separation between the papillary dermis and the stratum basale. Extensive type I collagen in the dermis and peeling of the stratum corneum are found in normal skin. **FH p. 168, BH p. 269**

2. A The figure shows acanthosis, parakeratosis, microabscesses, and dilated capillaries in dermal papillae, which are characteristic microscopic findings of psoriasis. The thickened epidermis and the dilated vessels appear as erythematous scaly patches. Fine papules may be seen in association with a variety of diseases but are not characteristic of psoriasis. Nodules with central crater may be seen in molluscum contagiosum, a viral infection of the skin or in keratoacanthoma, a low-grade squamous cell carcinoma. Numerous blisters are seen in allergic contact dermatitis or blistering disorders, such as pemphigus vulgaris or bullous pemphigoid. Many diseases of the skin, ranging from benign to malignant present as pigmented nodules, but the latter are not typical presentation of psoriasis. **BH p. 269, FH p. 168**

3. B Lichen planus is a type of inflammatory dermatitis with a characteristic clinical presentation, including purple, pruritic papules and distinct microscopic findings with hyperkeratosis, hydropic degeneration of the basal layer with dead basal cells called *Civatte bodies*, and a dense, bandlike inflammatory infiltrate in the dermis. Keratoacanthoma is a low-grade, well-differentiated squamous cell carcinoma of the skin. Clinically, it presents as a dome-shaped nodule with a central crater, and microscopically, the crater is filled with keratin surrounded by proliferating squamous cells. The other features seen in lichen planus are lacking. Unlike lichen planus, psoriasis presents as erythematous, scaly patches, and microscopically, there is acanthosis, parakeratosis, microabscesses, and dilated capillaries in dermal papillae. Pyogenic granuloma is a glistening, red papule that grows rapidly, and microscopically, it is characterized by a proliferation of small blood vessels. Wart, also known as *verruca*, is a dome-shaped papule with a rough surface. **BH p. 269, FH p. 168**

4. E Warts are usually small, rough, exophytic lesions that are caused by the human papillomavirus (HPV). Microscopically, they are characterized by finger-like projections of the epidermis, with hyperkeratosis and prominence of the granular layer. Hypersensitivity reactions are characterized by red, itchy rashes with swelling, edema, and inflammation of the epidermis and dermis. Melanocytic proliferations occur as nests of cells in the epidermis or dermis and usually result in darkly pigmented lesions. A penetrating injury would cause bleeding and a defect in the skin. Sun damage to the skin, called *actinic keratosis*, causes a red, scaly, crusty lesion with parakeratosis, dysplastic epithelium, and solar elastosis. **FH p. 168, BH p. 270**

5. C Although all layers are somewhat thickened, the stratum spinosum shows the most thickening, forming deep rete pegs. **FH p. 168, BH pp. 266, 269**

6. D The keratohyaline granules of keratinocytes contain acidic, phosphorylated protein that stains dark purple with hematoxylin and eosin (H&E) staining. As the cells move into the stratum corneum, phosphate groups are removed and the protein becomes basic. The cells of the stratum corneum stain intensely pink in H&E-stained slides. Staining of the stratum granulosum is due to the negative charges on the proteins and not the presence of rough endoplasmic reticulum. **FH pp. 169, 428**

7. C The cells of the stratum spinosum (prickle cell layer) contain many keratin intermediate filament bundles (tonofibrils) that insert into desmosomes found within the "prickles" joining adjacent cells. Actin, myosin, and tubulin are present in small amount in these cells and do not form distinct bundles. Desmin is not present in epithelial cells. **FH pp. 169-171**

8. D Bullous pemphigoid is an autoimmune skin disorder characterized by autoantibodies to hemidesmosomal antigens. The resulting dysfunctional hemidesmosomes do not properly anchor the epidermis to the underlying basement membrane and dermis, resulting in the formation of blisters. Abnormal hemidesmosomes would not cause the other conditions listed. **FH p. 172, BH p. 268**

9. F These are anchoring fibrils, which are made of type VII collagen. They help anchor the basal lamina (D) to the underlying dermis by forming looping networks of thin, non-banded fibrils. Weakened or absent anchoring fibrils can result in blistering, that is, separation at the epithelial-dermal junction. **FH p. 172**

10. B Thick bundles of filaments within cells of the epidermis are formed from keratin. The keratin anchors the hemidesmosomes (E) into the cytoskeleton. In diseases in which these filaments are defective, the cytoplasm tears away from the hemidesmosomes. **FH p. 172**

11. A This procedure only will stain melanocytes because they are the only cells in the epidermis that contain the enzyme tyrosinase, needed in the formation of melanin. Addition of tyrosine to these cells will result in increased production of melanin and a dark appearance. Melanocytes are located in the stratum basale of the epidermis. Most of the cells in the epidermis are keratinocytes, which are unable to synthesize melanin. **FH p.173**

12. D Melanoma is a malignant tumor characterized by proliferation of atypical or dysplastic melanocytes. The Breslow thickness, which measures the depth of the proliferating tumor cells from the granular layer of the epidermis to the deepest extension in the dermis, directly correlates with the likelihood of metastasis and a poor prognosis. Choices A and B describe abnormal melanocytes confined to the epidermis. After the malignant cells grow down into the dermis, the chance of metastasis increases in proportion to the depth of invasion. Nests of uniform, small melanocytes in the basal layer and upper dermis are most likely benign nevi because melanocytes in melanoma show cellular variation and dysplastic features. **BH pp. 273-277, FH p. 173**

13. A The biopsy specimen shows a large dermal growth due to infiltration by malignant cells that show evidence of melanin production (brown pigment), characteristic of a malignant melanoma. Excessive exposure to the sun is thought to be the major risk factor for the development of malignant melanoma. None of the other choices is associated with the development of this disease. Environmental toxins may cause skin rashes. Repeated trauma, as well as skin popping by intravenous drug abusers, results in ulceration and scarring of the skin. Tattoo application adds pigmentation to the skin, but does not stimulate tumor formation. **BH p. 275-277, FH 173**

14. A Langerhans cells show positive staining with antibody to CD1a. They also contain characteristic tennis racquet–like cytoplasmic organelles with cross striations called *Birbeck granules*. The other cells listed do not contain Birbeck granules and do not stain with CD1a. Moreover, the clinical presentation is characteristic of Langerhans cell histiocytosis, which is due to malignant proliferation of Langerhans cells. **FH p. 174**

15. A The cells indicated are Langerhans cells, identified by the presence of Birbeck granules in the cytoplasm. Langerhans cells are antigen-presenting cells that can endocytose antigens, process them, and present them to T cells, activating an immune response. They do not carry out any of the other functions listed. **FH p. 174**

16. A This is the arrector pili muscle, recognized as a bundle of smooth muscle cells in the dermis, which is associated with hair follicles and sebaceous glands. These arrector pili muscles contract when the skin is cold, raising the hairs, forming insulating spaces of trapped air, and hence conserving heat. **FH p. 178**

17. E The image shows eccrine sweat glands, which primarily function in thermoregulation. These are recognized by their small-diameter lumens and stratified cuboidal epithelium in their duct portions. The apocrine sweat glands (pheromone production) have a larger diameter in their secretory portions, and sebaceous glands (oily secretion) are composed of clusters of pale-staining cells that lack a lumen. Melanin in the skin protects against ultraviolet ray damage. The stratum corneum is the major barrier to the loss of water from the skin. **FH p. 179**

18. B In acute dermatitis, fluid accumulates within the stratum spinosum and forces keratinocytes apart. These areas appear as light, low-density areas or empty spaces in the epidermis. The epidermis is otherwise normal in appearance, with no evidence of lymphocyte infiltration. **FH p. 181, BH p. 268**

19. A This skin specimen shows morphologically normal cells forming abnormally thick layers of the epidermis. This condition is termed *acanthosis*. In parakeratosis, cell nuclei would be visible in the stratum corneum; in spongiosis, the stratum spinosum would be edematous; and in basal cell carcinoma, the epidermis would have abnormally numerous basal cells. **BH p. 267, FH p. 181**

20. D This figure shows junctional nevi, a benign proliferation of melanocytes. These proliferating cells are typically located in the stratum basale. Histologically, the hallmark of junctional nevi is the well-defined nests composed of cells with homogeneous cytoplasm containing melanin pigment (not shown in the figure). Keratinocytes would have dense eosinophilic cytoplasm and would be located throughout the epidermis. Langerhans cells typically show grooved nuclei and are located mainly in the stratum spinosum; moreover, they do not form well-defined nests, nor do they contain melanin.

Hair follicles and sebaceous glands would be found in the dermis, not the epidermis. **FH p. 181, BH p. 274**

21. D The distinctive small, round, dark-staining nuclei of lymphocytes present in this section are indicative of abnormal infiltration of the epidermis by lymphocytes, as may be seen in T-cell lymphomas of the skin. Hyperplasia of the keratinocytes would result in a markedly thickened epidermis, whereas thinning of the stratum spinosum would result in a thin, flattened layer of epidermis, which may be seen in atrophic conditions. Edema results in a lighter-staining area of epidermis. **FH p. 181, BH p. 207**

22. A Basal cell carcinoma arises from the basal cells of the epidermis and shows the characteristic microscopic findings as described above. Peripheral palisading of tumor cells is not a characteristic feature of any of the other choices listed. **BH p. 272**

23. G Squamous cell carcinoma *in situ*, also called Bowen disease, is characterized by full-thickness dysplasia in the epidermis with an intact basement membrane. Of the choices listed, basal cell carcinoma is the only other tumor of the epidermis that can show epithelial disorganization and dysplasia. However, in basal cell carcinoma, the proliferating cells in the epidermis are confined to the basal layer and show the characteristic peripheral palisading as they grow downward into the dermis. **BH p. 272**

24. C Dermatofibroma is a common benign tumor found in the dermis and is characterized by the proliferation of spindle cells in the dermal collagen. Spindle cell proliferation and foamy histiocytes would not be seen in the other choices listed. In cutaneous T-cell lymphoma, there is a malignant proliferation of lymphocytes in the epidermis and dermis. Lipoma, a benign tumor of adipocytes, is composed of a proliferation of mature adipocytes. Melanoma is composed of a proliferation of dysplastic melanocytes, and neurofibroma is a benign proliferation of nerve. **BH p. 278-279**

FH5 Chapter 5: Epithelial Tissues
FH5 Chapter 10: Skeletal Tissues
FH5 Chapter 16: Urinary System
BH5 Chapter 22: Skeletal System

10

Skeletal Tissues

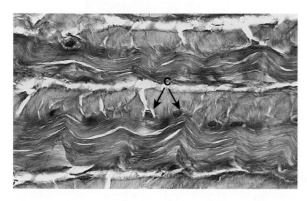

1 What condition causes damage to the tissue shown in the figure above?
- ☐ A. Fracture of a long bone
- ☐ B. Guillain-Barre syndrome
- ☐ C. Prolapsed disk
- ☐ D. Rheumatoid arthritis
- ☐ E. Tendonitis

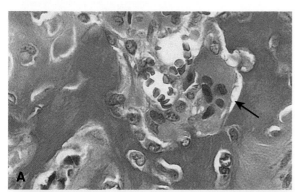

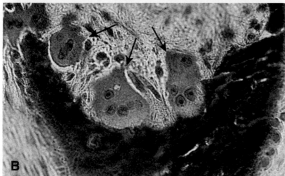

Use the figure at bottom left to answer the next two questions.

2 What is the source of the cells labeled by the *arrows*?
- ☐ A. Lymphocytes
- ☐ B. Mesenchymal stem cells
- ☐ C. Monocytes
- ☐ D. Muscle satellite cells
- ☐ E. Osteoprogenitor cells

3 A markedly decreased activity of the cells indicated by the *arrows* in the images at bottom left would most likely result in which of the following?
- ☐ A. Cartilage destruction
- ☐ B. Hypercalcemia
- ☐ C. Osteosclerosis
- ☐ D. Reduced bone mass
- ☐ E. Unmineralized bone

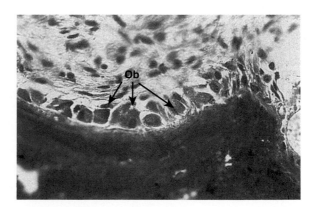

4 In the figure above, a layer of pink-staining material can be seen beneath osteoblasts (Ob). What type of material is this?
- ☐ A. Highly mineralized
- ☐ B. Highly vascular
- ☐ C. Keratinized
- ☐ D. Osteoid
- ☐ E. Rich in type II collagen

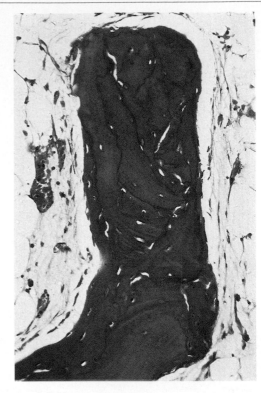

5 In the figure above, polarizing microscopy has been used to show the layered arrangement of collagen in lamellar bone (L) and the disordered collagen fibers in woven bone (W). In what condition is woven bone particularly prominent?

☐ A. Acromegaly
☐ B. Dwarfism
☐ C. Paget disease
☐ D. Slowly growing bone of the ribs
☐ E. Vitamin D deficiencies

6 A 55-year-old man with end-stage renal disease has difficulty walking and complains of generalized bone pain that is more pronounced in the left hip. Radiologic studies show lytic bone lesions. A bone biopsy was performed, and a microscopic section shows thin bony trabeculae with a marked increase in the number and activity of osteoclasts. Which of the following conditions is most likely to be present in the patient?

☐ A. Acute osteomyelitis
☐ B. Diabetes mellitus
☐ C. Hyperparathyroidism
☐ D. Osteosarcoma
☐ E. Paget disease

7 A 60-year-old man is found to have a severe skeletal deformity with bowing of his legs. A microscopic section of his bone is shown in the figure above. What is the cause of this pathology?

☐ A. Chronic inflammation
☐ B. Excess osteoblastic and osteoclastic activity
☐ C. Increased parathyroid hormone
☐ D. Lack of vitamin D
☐ E. Neoplastic proliferation

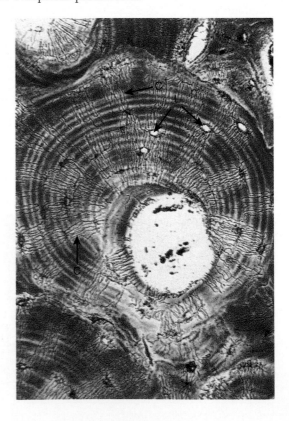

8 In living bone, which protein is found within the structures labeled *C* on the bottom of the opposite page? Lacunae (L) are labeled.
- ☐ A. Cadherin
- ☐ B. Collagen
- ☐ C. Connexin
- ☐ D. Desmin
- ☐ E. Myosin

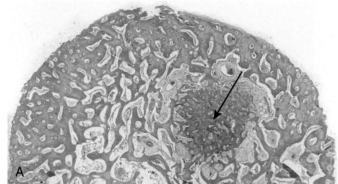

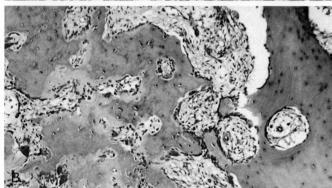

9 In the figure above, a dark mass (*arrow*) can be seen within the marrow cavity of a bone. What disease does this mass indicate?
- ☐ A. Chondrosarcoma
- ☐ B. Multiple myeloma
- ☐ C. Osteoid osteoma
- ☐ D. Osteoporosis
- ☐ E. Paget disease

10 Mineral deposits in most tissues are abnormal and are an indication of some type of pathology. In bone, mineral deposits are normal. What fosters mineral precipitation in bone?
- ☐ A. Active transport of calcium by osteoblasts
- ☐ B. Alkaline phosphatase on matrix vesicles
- ☐ C. Osteonectin in the membranes of osteoblasts
- ☐ D. Secretion of a special form of collagen
- ☐ E. The acidic extracellular matrix in bone-forming areas

11 A 10-year-old boy presents with complaints of diffuse bone pain, markedly bowed legs, and a history of frequent bone fractures. What disease does this most likely indicate?
- ☐ A. Osteoarthritis
- ☐ B. Osteomalacia
- ☐ C. Osteomyelitis
- ☐ D. Osteoporosis
- ☐ E. Rheumatoid arthritis

12 What would treatment of the above patient most likely involve?
- ☐ A. Decreasing his activity
- ☐ B. Increasing his activity
- ☐ C. Increasing protein in his diet
- ☐ D. Increasing vitamin C in his diet
- ☐ E. Increasing vitamin D in his diet

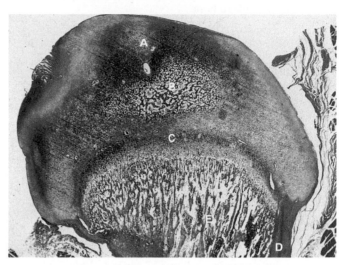

13 Childhood trauma in which labeled region, shown above, is of particular concern to the orthopedic surgeon?

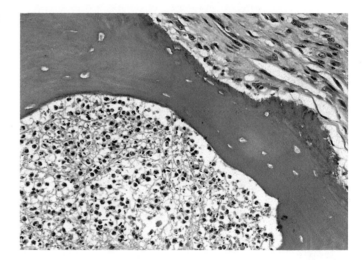

14 During a car accident, a 20-year-old man suffered a compound fracture of the tibia, which later became infected. A sectioned biopsy of the tibia is shown above. Which feature on this figure indicates the bone is necrotic?
- ☐ A. There is extensive osteoclast activity
- ☐ B. Osteocytes are absent
- ☐ C. Osteoblasts are inactive
- ☐ D. The adjacent marrow is filled with adipocytes

15 A 72-year-old woman has difficulty walking and has a stooped posture. What would microscopic examination of her vertebral bone most likely show?

- ☐ A. Bone with prominent cement lines
- ☐ B. Excess osteoid formation
- ☐ C. Osteoblastic proliferation
- ☐ D. Reduced number and size of bone trabeculae
- ☐ E. Unmineralized bone

For questions 16 and 17, match the clinical presentations described below with the most likely bone tumors.

- ☐ A. Chondrosarcoma
- ☐ B. Chordoma
- ☐ C. Ewing tumor
- ☐ D. Multiple myeloma
- ☐ E. Osteoid osteoma
- ☐ F. Osteosarcoma

16 A 15-year-old boy presents with a lytic lesion of the distal femur. The lesion is composed of pleomorphic cells producing osteoid, and there is evidence of metastasis to the lungs.

17 A 20-year-old man presents with a small, painful lesion on the left leg. The pain is relieved by aspirin. The lesion is composed of irregular masses of osteoid rimmed by osteoblasts.

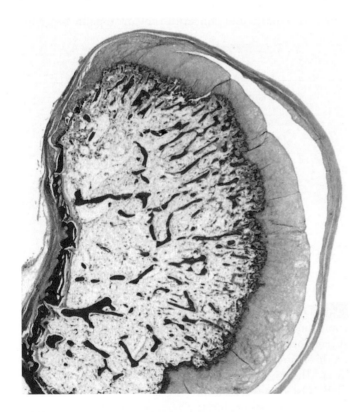

18 In the figure above, what condition does the overall appearance of this bone indicate?

- ☐ A. Degenerative changes of osteoarthritis
- ☐ B. Granulation tissue of rheumatoid arthritis
- ☐ C. Hypertrophy of growth plate cartilage
- ☐ D. Osteochondroma
- ☐ E. Osteoporosis

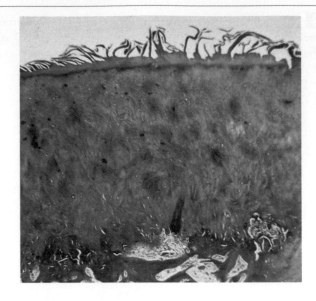

19 A 59-year-old man complains of severe pain in the right knee with difficulty walking. He had been in good health until a few months before his presentation, when he noticed an increasing amount of pain, confined to the right knee. Physical examination showed mild swelling of the knee joint with limitation of movement. The rest of the physical examination was unremarkable. A biopsy of the right knee is shown above. What is the most likely cause of the pathology shown?

- ☐ A. Autoimmune-mediated injury
- ☐ B. Bacterial infection
- ☐ C. Crystal deposition
- ☐ D. Degeneration of cartilage
- ☐ E. Synovial membrane proliferation

20 What is the most likely diagnosis for the disease in the above patient?

- ☐ A. Gout
- ☐ B. Osteoarthritis
- ☐ C. Osteoid osteoma
- ☐ D. Rheumatoid arthritis

21 A 50-year-old man presents with pain of several months' duration in the left great toe. Physical examination reveals a small nodule on the toe, at the interphalangeal joint, that was reddish in color and painful to touch. Laboratory studies show an elevated uric acid level in the serum. What would a biopsy of the nodule most likely show?

- ☐ A. Acute inflammation with bacterial colonies
- ☐ B. Chronic inflammation with multinucleated giant cells
- ☐ C. Degenerated cartilage
- ☐ D. Excessive proliferation of cartilage
- ☐ E. Lymphocytic infiltration of synovium

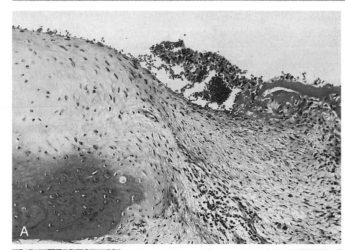

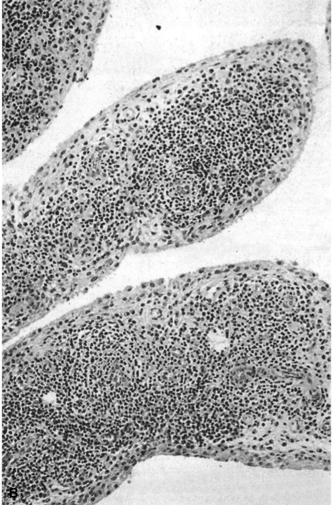

Use the clinical vignette that follows to answer the next two questions.

A 30-year-old woman presents with joint pain and stiffness involving her fingers and wrists. She states that the pain and stiffness improve as she goes about her work during the day. She also noted a small nodule near her left elbow. The nodule is nontender. A biopsy of her interphalangeal joint is shown in the figure above.

22 What is the most likely diagnosis of disease in this patient?
☐ A. Gout
☐ B. Osteoarthritis
☐ C. Paget disease
☐ D. Rheumatoid arthritis
☐ E. Septic arthritis

23 What is the most likely cause of the pathogenesis of her symptoms?
☐ A. Autoimmune reaction
☐ B. Bacterial infection
☐ C. Congenital disorder
☐ D. Crystal deposition
☐ E. Wear and tear

ANSWERS

1. C The tissue shown is fibrocartilage, which is recognized by the round chondrocyte nuclei (C) between layers of collagen fibers. It is present in the anulus fibrosus of the intervertebral disk. Rupture of the anulus fibrosus causes the condition *prolapsed disk*. Age-related changes in the fibrocartilage, combined with mechanical trauma, can predispose to this rupture. The other disorders do not affect the anulus fibrosus. **FH pp. 189, 205**

2. C The cells are osteoclasts, which can be recognized by their multiple nuclei, large size, and location adjacent to bone extracellular matrix. They belong to the macrophage family and develop from monocytes. **FH pp. 189-190**

3. C These are osteoclasts, which are phagocytic bone cells. They play an important role in bone resorption during bone growth and repair. Decreased activity of osteoclasts would result in unopposed osteoblastic activity and thickening of bone, which is called *osteosclerosis*. Cartilage destruction results from physical damage, not osteoclastic activity. It is a result of wear and tear associated with age or excess physical activity with repeated injuries. Hypercalcemia and reduced bone mass results from increased, not decreased, osteoclastic activity. Unmineralized bone is caused by a deficiency of vitamin D. **FH p. 190**

4. D At the surface of a developing bone, between the bone and the layer of osteoblasts, is a layer of unmineralized bone matrix, termed *osteoid*. The unmineralized matrix, which is secreted by the osteoblasts, does not mineralize for several hours after it is secreted and is therefore visible at the surface of a developing bone. Osteoid is rich in type I collagen but does not contain type II collagen, keratin, or blood vessels. **FH p. 190**

5. C Rapidly formed bone has disordered collagen, unlike the mature lamellar bone of the normal skeleton. Woven bone is rapidly deposited in conditions of increased bone turnover, as in Paget disease. In dwarfism or in vitamin D deficiencies, bone formation is slowed but has normal lamellae.

In acromegaly, excess bone formation takes place slowly rather than rapidly. **FH pp. 191, 201**

6. C Secondary hyperparathyroidism occurs in renal failure, which leads to marked osteoclastic activity, diffuse destruction of bone with lytic lesions, and a predisposition to fractures. Acute osteomyelitis can also cause localized (not generalized) lytic lesions, and the pathology is due to inflammation-induced infarction of bone rather than increased osteoblastic activity. A microscopic section would show dead bone and neutrophils infiltrating the bony trabeculae. Patients with diabetes mellitus are predisposed to developing skin ulcers. Deep, untreated ulcers may extend to the bone and result in acute osteomyelitis. In osteosarcoma, a localized lytic lesion may be present; however, the destruction is caused by malignant tumor cells and not by osteoclasts. In the early osteolytic phase of Paget disease, there may be lytic lesions due to bone resorption by osteoclasts; however, the increased osteoclastic activity is an inherent defect in osteoclasts and is not associated with renal failure. **FH p. 191, BH p. 281**

7. B The figure shows osteosclerosis with prominent cement lines in a mosaic pattern, characteristic of Paget disease. This disease results from uncontrolled osteoclastic bone resorption and excess osteoblastic activity, leading to haphazard bone remodeling. Although an infectious agent has been implicated in the pathogenesis of Paget disease, the mechanism is not due to chronic inflammation. Increased parathyroid hormone activity would cause bone thinning (not sclerosis) due to increased osteoclastic activity. Lack of vitamin D would result in bone of normal thickness but soft in consistency owing to lack of mineralization. Benign tumors of bone may have excess deposition of bone; however, the prominent cement lines and the mosaic pattern characteristic of Paget disease are lacking. In malignant bone tumors, there is a proliferation of malignant osteoblasts accompanied by deposition of small islands of delicate osteoid. **FH p. 191, BH p. 284**

8. C These structures are canaliculi within the bone matrix, and they contain the fine processes of the osteocytes. The processes of two adjacent osteocytes meet within the canaliculi and are joined by gap junctions, which are formed from the protein connexin. None of the other proteins are found in significant amounts in bone. **FH pp. 91, 193**

9. C The abnormal tissue is an osteoid osteoma, with dense, sclerotic bone surrounded by a rim of actively proliferating osteoblasts. It shows the flattened lacunae characteristic of bone, but not of cartilage (as would be seen in a chondrosarcoma). Cancerous plasma cells typical of multiple myeloma are not present. In osteoporosis, the bone would be markedly thinner. The characteristic cement lines and haphazard pattern of bone deposition seen in Paget disease are not present here. **FH p. 195, BH p. 286**

10. B Matrix vesicles pinch off from osteoblasts and have alkaline phosphatase in their membranes. This enzyme increases the free phosphate for mineral deposits and decreases the amount of inhibitory pyrophosphate present. Both actions foster mineral precipitation. Active transport of calcium would not play a significant role in mineral deposition because there is little within the cells. Osteonectin may foster mineral precipitation, but it is a secreted protein and is not present in the membranes of osteoblasts. Osteoblasts secrete collagen type I, the same type that is found in unmineralized connective tissues. An acidic environment would tend to dissolve hydroxyapatite crystals, not promote their formation. **FH p. 196**

11. B The symptoms are those of osteomalacia, or "soft bones," due to inadequate mineralization. Osteoarthritis occurs in older patients, and patients present with joint pain and reduction of mobility of the weight-bearing joints. Osteomyelitis would be characterized by pain limited to the affected bone and may be accompanied by swelling of the overlying soft tissue. Patients may also have fever and other signs of inflammation. Osteoporosis also presents with skeletal deformity and increased incidence of fracture; however, it typically occurs in elderly women and preferentially affects the vertebrae and the proximal femur. This pathogenesis is due to an imbalance in bone formation and loss rather than lack of mineralization. **FH p. 197, BH pp. 281, 283**

12. E Childhood osteomalacia (rickets) is often due to inadequate calcium absorption, which in turn is caused by inadequate vitamin D in the diet. Decreasing physical activity would further aggravate bone abnormality by increasing bone loss. Although increasing physical activity would promote bone formation, without vitamin D, the new bone would be weak and prone to deformity and fracture. Protein and vitamin C are important in providing an overall balanced diet; however, they do not play a direct role in mineralization of bone. **FH pp. 196-197, 302, BH pp. 281, 283**

13. C This is the epiphyseal plate, which is the site where linear growth of a long bone occurs. Trauma to this region may lead to abnormal growth. Trauma to the other regions is less likely to lead to inadequate bone growth. **FH p. 199**

14. B The lacunae in the bone fragment are empty, indicating the osteocytes are dead. The necrotic bone is surrounded by inflammatory cells. There is no sign of intense osteoclastic activity, and inactive osteoblasts are often seen in normal mature bone. Adipocytes are not seen in this figure. **BH p. 282, FH p. 201**

15. D The clinical presentation is characteristic of osteoporosis. Osteoporosis is commonly seen in postmenopausal women and is characterized by reduced bone mass leading to deformity and susceptibility to fracture. Bone with prominent cement lines is seen in patients with Paget disease. It is more common in males, and patients complain of bone pain due to nerve compression by the enlarging bone. Excess osteoid formation occurs in benign bone tumors such as osteoid osteoma and osteoblastoma. The tumors occur in young patients, and the clinical presentation is due to localized pain. Osteoblastic proliferation is seen in these benign bone tumors, and it can also occur around new bone formation during healing of a fracture. Unmineralized bone is caused by vitamin D deficiency and results in skeletal deformity in children and adults. Although osteoporosis and osteomalacia in adults have overlapping clinical presentations, in osteomalacia, patients complain of generalized pain and muscle weakness, which are not typical of osteoporosis. **BH p. 283**

16. F Most cases of osteosarcoma occur in children and adolescents. The knee is the most common location, and the tumors frequently metastasize early in the course of the disease. Histologically, the tumors are characterized by pleomorphic cells with delicate islands of pink osteoid. Chondrosarcomas are malignant tumors of cartilage and are most commonly seen in older adults. Microscopically, they are characterized by formation of malignant cartilage, not osteoid. Chordomas are malignant tumors derived from notochord, most commonly affecting the sacrum. Microscopically, they are characterized by a proliferation of large cells with abundant, vacuolated cytoplasm. Ewing tumor is also a bone (or soft tissue) tumor that occurs in young adults. In contrast to osteosarcoma, Ewing tumor is characterized by a uniform proliferation of small round blue (basophilic) cells. Multiple myeloma is a malignant hematopoietic tumor seen in older adults and is characterized by a neoplastic proliferation of plasma cells in the bone marrow. The plasma cells produce osteoclastic activating factors, which in turn erode bone, resulting in lytic lesions. **BH pp. 285-286**

17. E Osteoid osteoma is a benign tumor that has a characteristic clinical presentation of a small painful lesion, most commonly occurring in the lower leg, and which is relieved by aspirin. Histologically, it is composed of partially mineralized, irregular masses of osteoid, rimmed by osteoblasts. All the other tumors listed are malignant tumors with characteristic clinical presentations and histologic findings. **BH pp. 285-286**

18. D The greatly thickened layer of cartilage overlying the abnormally protruding bone is typical of an osteochondroma. The cartilage in osteoarthritis would show degenerative changes. A growth plate or granulation tissue is not seen in this figure, and the normal bone density rules out osteoporosis. **BH p. 287-288**

19. D The figure shows fibrillation and flaking of the articular cartilage, which are early signs of degeneration of the articular cartilage, resulting from excessive wear and tear. Autoimmune-mediated injury of joints with synovial proliferation occurs in rheumatoid arthritis. Bacterial infection characterized by white blood cell infiltration of bone is the cause of the pathology in osteomyelitis, whereas crystal deposition in joints accounts for the signs and symptoms of gout. There is no indication of inflammation (autoimmune disease or bacterial infection), nor are crystal deposits visible. The synovial membrane is not visible in the image. **BH p. 288, FH p. 203**

20. B The patient has osteoarthritis. Osteoarthritis is characterized by the degeneration and loss of articular cartilage without significant inflammation at the early stages. Patients with gout present with intense pain and redness of the affected joint. Osteoid osteoma presents with a small painful lesion that is relieved by aspirin. Histologically, it is composed of partially mineralized, irregular masses of osteoid, rimmed by osteoblasts. Rheumatoid arthritis affects the small joints of the hands and wrist and is characterized by lymphocytic infiltrate of the synovium. **BH p. 288, FH p. 203**

21. B The patient has gout, which is characterized by deposition of uric acid crystals in joints, causing acute inflammation. Chronic inflammation develops over time, with a multinucleated giant cell reaction to the crystals. The other conditions listed are not associated with elevated uric acid levels. Acute inflammation with bacterial colonies occurs in osteomyelitis, which may affect any joint. Degeneration of cartilage is seen in osteoarthritis, which affects the large weight-bearing joints of the hips and knees. Excessive proliferation of cartilage occurs in benign and malignant tumors of cartilage. The toe is not a common site of these tumors. Lymphocytic infiltrate of the synovium occurs in rheumatoid arthritis, which affects the small joints of the hands and wrist. **BH p. 289**

22. D The clinical presentation and the presence of a dense lymphocytic infiltrate in the synovium are characteristic of rheumatoid arthritis. Gout is characterized by inflammation of the joints due to deposition of uric acid crystals and most commonly affects the toe. Osteoarthritis affects the large weight-bearing joints of the hips and knees and shows destruction of articular cartilage. Paget disease presents with bone pain affecting various bones of the body and is characterized by markedly thickened and brittle bone. Septic arthritis, caused by bacterial infection, usually affects a single joint and is characterized by fever, pain, and swelling of the affected joint. **FH p. 203, BH p. 290**

23. A Rheumatoid arthritis is an autoimmune disorder. The destruction of cartilage is secondary to inflammation, not wear and tear. The disease has no association with bacterial infection or crystal deposition, nor is it a congenital disorder. **BH p. 290, FH p. 203**

FH5 Chapter 3: Blood
FH5 Chapter 11: Immune System
BH5 Chapter 4: Infections of Histological Importance
BH5 Chapter 7: Dysplasia and Neoplasia
BH5 Chapter 16: Lymphoid and Haematopoietic Systems

11

Immune System

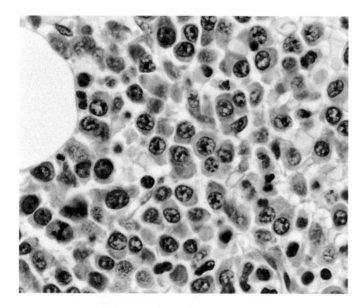

Use the figure above to answer the next two questions. (Note that both questions 1 and 2 refer to this figure, but the questions are independent.)

1 The figure above shows a biopsy of bone marrow obtained from a patient with multiple myeloma. Molecules produced by these cancerous cells reach abnormally high levels in the bloodstream. What type of molecule would you expect to be overproduced here, based on the appearance of these cells?
- ☐ A. Hyaluronic acid
- ☐ B. Immunoglobulins
- ☐ C. Interleukin-2
- ☐ D. Leptin
- ☐ E. Tumor necrosis factor

2 A 65-year-old man presents with fatigue and bone pain. The skeletal radiograph shows multiple lytic bone lesions. Bone marrow biopsy was performed and shows sheets of cells, as seen in the figure opposite. Based on the bone marrow findings, which of the following may be present in the urine of this patient?
- ☐ A. Bacterial colonies
- ☐ B. Bence Jones protein
- ☐ C. Granular casts
- ☐ D. Sodium urate crystals
- ☐ E. White blood cells

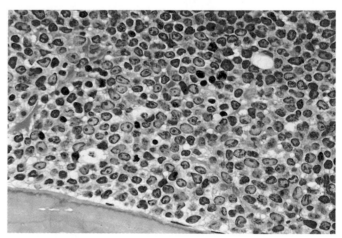

3 The micrograph above illustrates a biopsy of bone marrow from a patient presenting with anemia and episodes of bleeding. What pathologic condition is shown here?
- ☐ A. Acute myeloid leukemia
- ☐ B. Chronic lymphocytic leukemia
- ☐ C. Myelofibrosis
- ☐ D. Multiple myeloma
- ☐ E. Sickle cell anemia

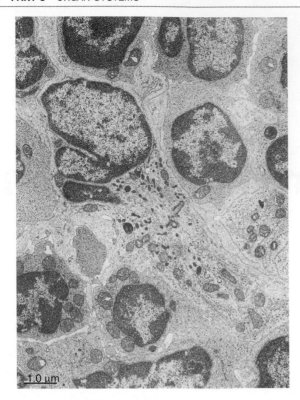

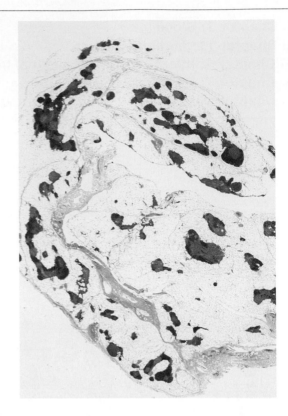

4 Based on its morphology and the identity of the surrounding cells, what most likely is the large cell in the center of the figure above?

☐ A. Antigen-presenting cell in a lymph node
☐ B. Kupffer cell in the liver
☐ C. Langerhans cell in the epidermis
☐ D. M cell in the intestinal mucosa
☐ E. Phagocytic cell in the red pulp of the spleen

5 The proteasome is responsible for processing of peptide fragments that perform what function?

☐ A. Act as a second adhesive site for binding T-killer cells
☐ B. Are stored in the lumen of vesicles immediately beneath the dendritic cell plasmalemma until they are ready for exposure on the cell surface
☐ C. Are used by T cells to identify healthy target cells
☐ D. Bind to MHC I proteins
☐ E. Stimulate B-cell activation

6 A 40-year-old woman is in for a routine radiograph. The radiologist reports that there is a large mediastinal mass. A thymoma is suspected, and a biopsy of the mass is performed. Staining of a section of the biopsy with an antibody to which protein will be most useful in confirming the diagnosis?

☐ A. Actin
☐ B. Desmin
☐ C. Keratin
☐ D. Tubulin
☐ E. Vimentin

7 The figure above shows a biopsy of the thymus from a 70-year-old asymptomatic woman. What is the most likely diagnosis?

☐ A. B-cell lymphoma
☐ B. Congenital thymic aplasia
☐ C. Degeneration due to AIDS
☐ D. Normal thymic involution
☐ E. Thymic lipoma

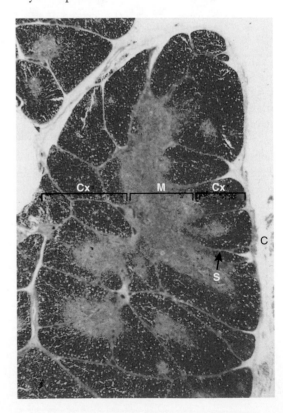

8 What is a unique feature of the figure shown at the bottom of the previous page? The cortex (Cx), medulla (M), septa (S), and capsule (C) are labeled.
- ☐ A. Afferent lymphatic vessels
- ☐ B. Central arteries
- ☐ C. Hassall corpuscles
- ☐ D. High endothelial venules
- ☐ E. Lymphatic nodules

9 A patient presents with recurrent infections and cardiac and facial abnormalities suggesting DiGeorge syndrome. After verifying the disease by identifying a chromosome 22 deletion, the thymus is imaged. It appears to be unusually small. Which function of the immune system is directly impacted?
- ☐ A. Cell-mediated immunity
- ☐ B. Mast cell degranulation
- ☐ C. Plasma cell formation
- ☐ D. Phagocytosis of bacteria
- ☐ E. Viral protein accumulation in dendritic cells

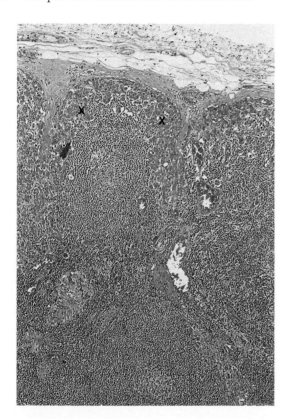

10 Metastatic malignant cells (X) have invaded the organ shown above. Which organ is it?
- ☐ A. Appendix
- ☐ B. Lymph node
- ☐ C. Peyer patch
- ☐ D. Spleen
- ☐ E. Thymus

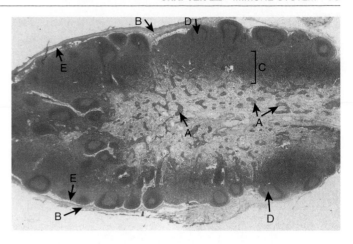

Use the figure above to answer the next two questions.

11 What is a unique feature of the organ shown above?
- ☐ A. Afferent lymphatic vessels
- ☐ B. Central arteries
- ☐ C. Hassall corpuscles
- ☐ D. High endothelial venules
- ☐ E. Nodules

12 Which letter on the figure above indicates the site of B-cell activation, maturation, and clonal expansion?

For questions 13 and 14, match the descriptions below with the immune cells listed.

- ☐ A. B lymphocyte
- ☐ B. Eosinophil
- ☐ C. Langerhans cell
- ☐ D. Macrophage
- ☐ E. Mast cell
- ☐ F. Neutrophil
- ☐ G. Plasma cell
- ☐ H. T lymphocyte

13 Cytotoxic cell that requires presensitization

14 Cell that recognizes antigen through its transmembrane immunoglobulin

15 A 32-year-old woman with fatigue, weight loss, and generalized lymphadenopathy underwent a lymph node biopsy, which showed effacement of the lymph node architecture. A diagnosis of lymphoma was made, and flow cytometry studies were performed and showed the neoplastic cells to be positive for CD3 and CD4. What most likely was the origin of the lymphoma?
- ☐ A. B lymphocytes
- ☐ B. Dendritic cells
- ☐ C. Mast cells
- ☐ D. Plasma cells
- ☐ E. T lymphocytes

16 A 23-year-old man presents with cervical lymphade-nopathy. A lymph node biopsy was performed and shows a granulomatous inflammation. Which of the following is the most likely etiologic agent?

- ☐ A. *Borrelia burgdorferi*
- ☐ B. Cytomegalovirus
- ☐ C. Epstein-Barr virus
- ☐ D. *Helicobacter pylori*
- ☐ E. *Mycobacterium tuberculosis*

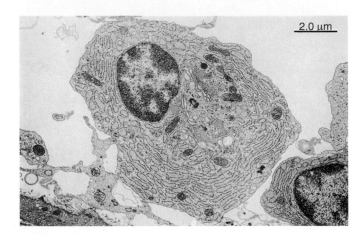

17 The function of the cell shown in the figure above is the synthesis and secretion of what?

- ☐ A. Complement
- ☐ B. Histamine
- ☐ C. Immunoglobulin
- ☐ D. Lactoferrin
- ☐ E. Lysozyme

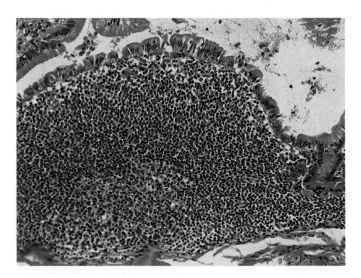

18 What is the location of the lymphoid tissue seen in the figure above?

- ☐ A. Intestine
- ☐ B. Lymph node
- ☐ C. Palatine tonsil
- ☐ D. Spleen
- ☐ E. Thymus

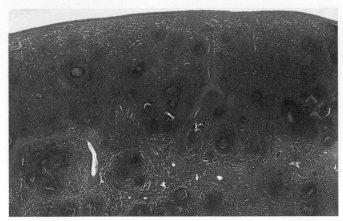

19 A 55-year-old woman is injured in an automobile accident, requiring removal of the organ shown in the figure above. What is a unique feature of this organ?

- ☐ A. Afferent lymphatic vessels
- ☐ B. Central arteries
- ☐ C. Hassall corpuscles
- ☐ D. High endothelial venules
- ☐ E. Nodules

20 What changes would be expected in the above patient as a result of this operation?

- ☐ A. An increased susceptibility to blood-borne, encapsulated pathogens
- ☐ B. An increased risk for Addison disease
- ☐ C. An increased risk for autoimmune disease
- ☐ D. A need for frequent dialysis
- ☐ E. A substantial drop in blood platelets

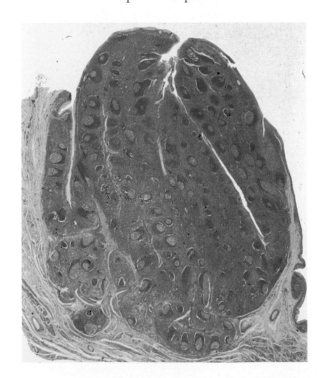

21 What specialized feature distinguishes the organ shown at the bottom of the previous page?
☐ A. Afferent lymphatic vessels
☐ B. Central arteries
☐ C. Hassall corpuscles
☐ D. Hemicapsule
☐ E. High endothelial venules

22 A 32-year-old man presents with anemia and spleno-megaly. Which of the following is the most likely cause of his anemia?
☐ A. Aplastic anemia
☐ B. Chronic hemolytic anemia
☐ C. Iron deficiency anemia
☐ D. Renal failure
☐ E. Sideroblastic anemia

23 A 50-year-old woman presents to her physician with complaints of abdominal pain, nausea, and vomiting. Endo-scopic examination of the stomach shows a small nodular lesion in the gastric antrum. A biopsy was performed, and based on the microscopic findings, a diagnosis of lymphoma was made. This patient most likely had an infection by which of the following organisms?
☐ A. *Borrelia burgdorferi*
☐ B. Cytomegalovirus
☐ C. Epstein-Barr virus
☐ D. *Helicobacter pylori*
☐ E. *Mycobacterium tuberculosis*

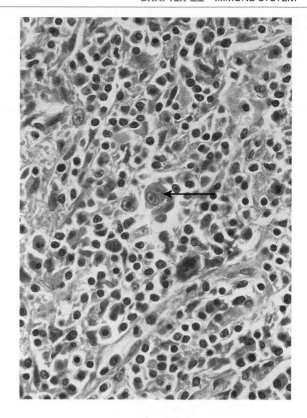

25 A 25-year-old man presents with fatigue, shortness of breath, and weight loss. The chest radiograph shows a medi-astinal mass. A biopsy of the mass was performed, and the microscopic finding is shown in the figure above. Which of the following is the most likely diagnosis?
☐ A. Diffuse large B-cell lymphoma
☐ B. Follicular lymphoma
☐ C. Hodgkin lymphoma
☐ D. Lymphoblastic lymphoma
☐ E. Small lymphocytic lymphoma

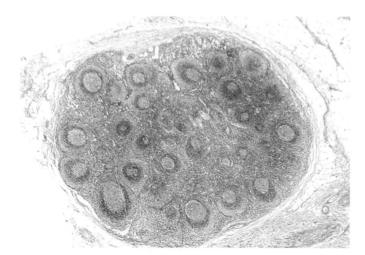

24 A 32-year-old man with a history of intravenous drug use complains of fatigue, weight loss, and diarrhea. Physical examination reveals generalized lymphadenopathy. A biopsy of a cervical lymph node was performed, and a microscopic section is shown in the figure above. His CD4 count was very low, and serologic studies for HIV-1 virus were positive. What disease is the patient at increased risk for developing?
☐ A. Acute myeloid leukemia
☐ B. Chronic lymphocytic leukemia
☐ C. Multiple myeloma
☐ D. Myelofibrosis
☐ E. Non-Hodgkin lymphoma

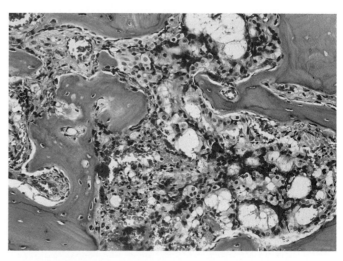

Use the figure above to answer the next two questions.

26 A 75-year-old man presents with weight loss and bone pain in his right hip. The radiograph of the pelvis shows a sclerotic lesion, which was later biopsied. A microscopic section of the sclerotic lesion is shown in the figure on the previous page. The cells in the marrow were positive for pan-cytokeratin by immunohistochemical staining. What is the most likely diagnosis?

- ☐ A. Acute leukemia
- ☐ B. Non-Hodgkin lymphoma
- ☐ C. Metastatic carcinoma
- ☐ D. Multiple myeloma
- ☐ E. Paget disease of bone

27 Which of the following is most likely to be present in the above patient?

- ☐ A. Elevated serum sodium
- ☐ B. Enlarged, hard prostate gland
- ☐ C. Generalized lymphadenopathy
- ☐ D. Monoclonal immunoglobulin in the serum
- ☐ E. Myeloblasts in the peripheral blood

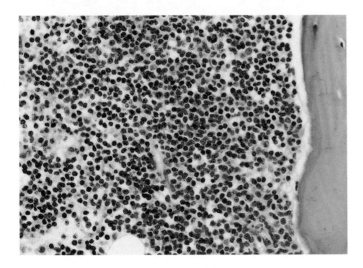

28 A 65-year-old woman presented with fatigue and abdominal pain. On physical examination, she was noted to have bilateral cervical lymphadenopathy and splenomegaly. Laboratory studies show anemia and thrombocytopenia. A bone marrow biopsy was performed, and the microscopic image is shown above. What is the most likely diagnosis?

- ☐ A. Chronic lymphocytic leukemia
- ☐ B. Chronic myeloid leukemia
- ☐ C. Hodgkin lymphoma
- ☐ D. Multiple myeloma
- ☐ E. Metastatic carcinoma

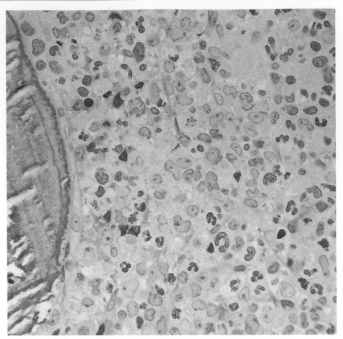

Use the figure above to answer the next two questions.

29 A 50-year-old man presents to his primary care physician with complaints of abdominal fullness and early satiety. Physical examination reveals splenomegaly but no lymphadenopathy. A complete blood count shows an elevated white blood cell count. A bone marrow biopsy was performed and is shown in the figure above. Which of the following is the most likely diagnosis in the above patient?

- ☐ A. Chronic lymphocytic leukemia
- ☐ B. Chronic myeloid leukemia
- ☐ C. Hodgkin lymphoma
- ☐ D. Multiple myeloma
- ☐ E. Metastatic carcinoma

30 Examination of the peripheral smear from the above patient would most likely show an increased number of what?

- ☐ A. Basophils and their precursors
- ☐ B. Eosinophils and their precursors
- ☐ C. Lymphocytes and their precursors
- ☐ D. Monocytes and their precursors
- ☐ E. Neutrophils and their precursors

31 A 35-year-old woman presents with fatigue, weight loss, and abdominal pain. Examination of the peripheral blood shows anemia with low white blood cell and platelet counts. Review of her records reveals that she had a bone marrow biopsy performed 2 years ago that was notable for mild fibrosis. Bone marrow biopsy was repeated, and the microscopic finding shows replacement of the marrow by marked fibrosis, as shown in the figure on the following page. Which of the following would most likely be present in this patient?

- ☐ A. Enlarged spleen and liver
- ☐ B. Loss of reflexes in the lower extremity
- ☐ C. Lower leg skin ulcers
- ☐ D. Multiple lytic bone lesions
- ☐ E. Sickle cells in the peripheral blood

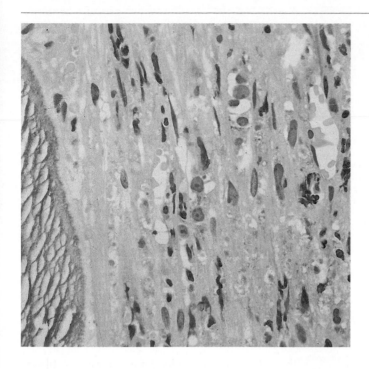

ANSWERS

1. B These cells are plasma cells, with a basophilic cytoplasm and an eccentrically positioned, round nucleus. The excessive proliferation of plasma cells in the bone marrow results in overproduction of immunoglobulins. Hyaluronic acid is mainly synthesized by fibroblasts, interleukin-2 by lymphocytes, leptin by fat cells, and tumor necrosis factor by macrophages. **FH p. 59, BH p. 211**

2. B The patient has multiple myeloma, a disease characterized by lytic bone lesions and marrow infiltration by neoplastic plasma cells. The plasma cells produce a monoclonal immunoglobulin, and the light chain component of the immunoglobulin may be detected in the urine as Bence Jones protein. Bacterial colonies and white blood cells are seen in the urine of patients with urinary tract infections. Granular casts are seen in pyelonephritis or glomerulonephritis. Sodium urate crystals are present in the urine of patients with gout. **BH p. 211**

3. A In acute myeloid leukemia, primitive blast cells with irregularly shaped nuclei, a high nuclear-to-cytoplasmic ratio, and dispersed, fine chromatin are found in marrow, as seen in the figure. This marrow is not enriched in lymphocytes, fibroblasts, or plasma cells, as would be seen in lymphocytic leukemia, myelofibrosis, or multiple myeloma, respectively. In sickle cell anemia, the marrow shows maturing erythroid hyperplasia, not primitive blasts. **FH p. 59, BH p. 211-212**

4. A The central cell is well endowed with digestive organelles typical of phagocytic cells. The surrounding cells, which have large nuclei and little cytoplasm, are characteristic small lymphocytes. The only choice that matches this combination is that of an antigen-presenting cell in a lymph node. Kupffer cells are phagocytic but surrounded by hepatocytes. Langerhans cells are surrounded by keratinocytes and contain Birbeck granules. M cells are adjacent to intestinal absorptive cells. Macrophages in the red pulp of the spleen would be surrounded by erythrocytes. **FH pp. 212-213**

5. D Proteasomes digest proteins in the nucleus and cytosol. Digested polypeptides from viral proteins and abnormal cell proteins are bound to MHC I proteins and expressed on the cell's plasma membrane. MHC I proteins containing these fragments are recognized by T cells, which kill infected cells. In dendritic cells, the peptide fragments are bound to MHC II in vesicles beneath the plasmalemma until presented on the cell surface, but these are membrane bound, not in the lumen. **FH p. 212**

6. C A thymoma is a tumor of the epithelial cells that make up the framework of the thymus. Often these tumors are asymptomatic. Keratin is an epithelia-specific intermediate filament protein that can be used to determine whether the mass is a thymoma. Because the proliferating cells in thymoma are epithelial cells, the other markers are either negative or would be present in small amounts compared to keratin. Desmin and vimentin are intermediate filament proteins from muscle and mesenchymal cells respectively. Actin and tubulin would be seen in all types of cells and are not specific for epithelia. **FH p. 215, 216**

7. D The figure shows a normal thymus from an older patient. After middle age, the thymus is well into the process of involution, with most of the lymphoid tissue replaced by adipose tissue. In B-cell lymphoma involving the thymus, there is a proliferation of numerous lymphocytes that completely replace the normal thymic tissue. The normal lobular architecture and Hassall corpuscles are lost. Although the thymus may show degenerative changes (involution) in HIV, the patient would be expected to show signs and symptoms of HIV. The thymus would be absent in congenital thymic aplasia and in thymic lipoma, the thymus would be uniformly replaced by fatty tissue rather than the intermingling with residual lymphoid tissue islands as seen here. **FH p. 216**

8. C This organ is the thymus, recognizable by its lobular architecture, with each lobule having a cortex and medulla. Hassall corpuscles, solid bodies formed of concentric layers of epithelial cells, are a unique feature of the thymus. Central arteries are only present in the spleen. High endothelial venules are present in numerous areas of lymphoid tissue, where they provide for selectivity in lymphocyte circulation and are not unique to any organ. Nodules are B-lymphocyte rich areas that form in various tissues during an active immune response. They are rare in the normal thymus and usually form under pathologic conditions. **FH p. 216**

9. A T-cell maturation occurs in the thymus. Abnormal thymus formation can result in T-cell deficiency and hence in a deficiency in cell-mediated immunity. The other processes are not dependent on the thymus. **FH pp. 216-217**

10. B This shows the characteristic subcapsular sinus of the lymph node. In this figure, the subcapsular sinus is filled with malignant cells. Structural features of the other structures listed—appendix (crypts), Peyer patches (crypts and villi), spleen (central arteries), and thymus (Hassall corpuscles)—are not present. **BH p. 81, FH p. 220**

11. A Only the lymph node, recognizable by its nodular cortex and medullary sinuses and cords, is connected to afferent lymphatic vessels. These can enter through the capsule anywhere to drain into the subcapsular sinuses. **FH p. 221**

12. D B cells undergo stimulation, maturation, and clonal expansion in the nodules (follicles). These are recognizable as rounded structures with pale centers. **FH p. 220**

13. H A subset of T cells are cytotoxic and are able to kill virus-infected cells and some cancer cells. They require interaction with antigen-presenting cells and helper T cells (presensitization) to become activated. B lymphocytes and plasma cells also require presensitization to become active. However, they are not directly cytotoxic. Instead, they activate the complement system or effector phagocytic cells that can in turn destroy organisms. Macrophages, neutrophils, and eosinophils are also capable of cytotoxicity; however, they are part of the innate immune system and do not need presensitization. Langerhans cells present antigens to B and T cells to activate them. Mast cells are part of the innate immunity system and play a role in acute inflammation. **FH p. 209**

14. A A transmembrane immunoglobulin is the antigen receptor for B lymphocytes. Only B cells have transmembrane immunoglobulins. Binding of antigen to the surface immunoglobulin leads to activation of the B cell. **FH p. 209**

15. E Transmembrane proteins and molecules found on white blood cells are assigned a CD (cluster of differentiation) designation and are used to identify the various cells of the immune system because a particular expression pattern is associated with each cell type. CD3 and CD4 are found on T lymphocytes. CD19 and CD20 are expressed on B cells. Dendritic cells express CD21 (follicular dendritic cells) and S100 (interdigitating dendritic cells). Mast cells express CD117, whereas CD38 is found on plasma cells. **FH p. 214**

16. E Infections by *Mycobacterium tuberculosis* typically show granulomatous inflammation. Granulomatous inflammation is not seen in any of the other infectious agents listed. **FH p. 218**

17. C The cell shown in the figure is a plasma cell. It is oval in shape, has a lot of rough endoplasmic reticulum, and a

clock-face distribution of chromatin in the nucleus. It secretes immunoglobulins but has no secretion granules because it secretes constitutively. Histamine, lactoferrin, and lysozyme-secreting cells have obvious secretion granules. Complement is secreted by hepatocytes, which, as epithelial cells, are closely associated with their neighbors. **FH p. 226**

18. A The simple columnar epithelium associated with these lymphocytes is found only in the intestines. No columnar epithelial lining is associated with the thymus, lymph nodes or spleen, and palatine tonsils have a stratified squamous epithelium. **FH p. 228**

19. B The spleen shown on p. 80 is characterized by the presence of central arteries, red and white pulp, and sinusoids. Choices A, B, and C are unique to lymph nodes, spleen, and thymus, respectively. High endothelial venules are present in numerous areas of lymphoid tissue, where they provide for selectivity in lymphocyte circulation. Nodules are B-lymphocyte rich areas seen in a variety of immune tissues. **FH p. 229**

20. A The spleen acts as a blood filter, removing blood-borne pathogens, particularly encapsulated ones. The spleen normally stores about 30% of the body's platelets. Some splenectomy patients show a substantial increase in circulating platelets. Addison disease results from loss of the adrenal glands, not the spleen. The spleen plays a role in innate immunity, but its absence has not been associated with an increased risk for autoimmune diseases. Patients with renal failure have a need for frequent dialysis, and the absence of the spleen has no direct bearing on renal function. **FH p. 229**

21. D The palatine tonsil shown in the figure is characterized by the presence of a hemicapsule. Lymph node, spleen, and thymus are uniquely identified by the choices A, B, and C, respectively. High endothelial venules are present in numerous areas of lymphoid tissue where they provide for selectivity in lymphocyte circulation. **FH p. 228**

22. B The spleen plays an important role in removal of aged or defective red blood cells. In chronic hemolytic anemias, excessive destruction of red blood cells leads to splenomegaly. The other choices listed cause a hypoproliferative anemia, with decreased production (not hemolysis) of red blood cells and are not associated with splenomegaly. In aplastic anemia, the decreased red cell production is due to failure of stem cells and replacement of marrow by fat. In iron deficiency and renal failure, red blood cell production is decreased owing to lack of iron and erythropoietin respectively. Sideroblastic anemia is due to failure of heme synthesis. **FH p. 229**

23. D *Helicobacter pylori* infection of the stomach is associated with the development of mucosa-associated lymphoid tissue (MALT) lymphomas, peptic ulcers, and gastric adenocarcinomas. Epstein-Barr virus (EBV) is also associated with the development of lymphomas. However, EBV-associated lymphomas are more commonly seen in the lymph nodes rather then the stomach. *Borrelia burgdorferi* has been linked to the development of MALT lymphoma in the skin (not the stomach) in association with Lyme disease. Infections with cytomegalovirus and mycobacteria are not directly linked to the development of lymphomas. **FH p. 231**

24. E Patients with AIDS have a markedly increased propensity to develop certain tumors, most commonly non-Hodgkin lymphoma and Kaposi sarcoma. These neoplasms are thought to be driven by the presence of Epstein-Barr virus and human herpes virus type 8 that are increased in HIV patients. HIV infection has not been associated with a significantly increased risk for developing the other disorders listed. **BH pp. 44, 198-200**

25. C The figure shows classic Reed-Sternberg cells (arrow) admixed with lymphocytes, eosinophils, and neutrophils. Reed-Sternberg cells are the neoplastic cells in Hodgkin lymphoma and are only seen in this entity. Both diffuse large B-cell and lymphoblastic lymphoma can involve the mediastinum. However, Reed-Sternberg cells, the hallmark cells of Hodgkin lymphoma, are not seen. As the name implies, diffuse large B-cell lymphoma is composed of a diffuse proliferation of numerous large B cells. In lymphoblastic lymphomas, the normal thymus is replaced by proliferation of immature lymphoid precursors (lymphoblasts). Follicular, lymphoplasmacytic, and small lymphocytic lymphomas rarely occur in the mediastinum. Follicular lymphoma is characterized by a nodular proliferation of follicles. In lymphoplasmacytic lymphoma, there is a diffuse proliferation of lymphocytes and plasma cells. Small lymphocytic lymphoma is characterized by a diffuse proliferation of small lymphocytes. **BH pp. 208-209**

26. C The figure shows replacement of the marrow by epithelial cells as evidenced by the positive cytokeratin stain. Epithelial cells are not normally found in the marrow, and their presence is indicative of metastatic carcinoma. All the other choices listed are associated with pathology in the bone marrow; however, cytokeratin staining is not observed in any of them. In acute leukemia, the marrow is replaced by a proliferation of immature hematopoietic cells (i.e., blasts). Non-Hodgkin lymphoma and multiple myeloma are characterized by a proliferation of mature lymphocytes and plasma cells, respectively. Dense sclerotic bone that expands and occupies the marrow cavity is seen in Paget disease; however, epithelial cells are not present. **BH p. 210**

27. B Most metastatic tumors to bone show destructive, lytic lesions. In this case, the bone shows osteosclerosis, which is most often seen in metastasis from carcinoma of the prostate. Physical examination of the prostate in patients with prostate cancer usually reveals an enlarged, hard prostate. Serum calcium, not sodium, may be elevated in patients with metastatic prostate cancer. Generalized lymphadenopathy is most commonly seen in patients with

lymphoma. Prostate carcinoma can metastasize to regional lymph nodes, in which case the lymphadenopathy is evident in the regional (pelvic) lymph nodes, but generalized lymphadenopathy due to tumor spread is uncommon. Monoclonal immunoglobulin in the serum is seen in patients with neoplastic proliferation of plasma cells. Proliferation of myeloblasts in the bone marrow and peripheral blood is seen in patients with acute myeloid leukemia. **BH p. 210**

28. A The marrow shows infiltration by small mature lymphocytes, which is seen in chronic lymphocytic leukemia. This disease is commonly seen in elderly people and is characterized by lymphadenopathy, splenomegaly, and an increased number of small mature lymphocytes in the peripheral blood and bone marrow. Replacement of the marrow by these lymphocytes results in anemia and thrombocytopenia. Chronic myeloid leukemia is characterized by a neoplastic proliferation of the myeloid series in the bone marrow and peripheral blood. Hence, examination of the marrow and peripheral blood would show an increase of neutrophils and their precursors, not small lymphocytes. Marrow involvement by Hodgkin lymphoma may be seen in patients with advanced disease. In this case, the diagnostic Reed-Sternberg cells may be seen in the bone marrow. Multiple myeloma is characterized by a proliferation of plasma cells, whereas metastatic carcinoma would show evidence of epithelial cells infiltrating the marrow cavity. **BH p. 212**

29. B The peripheral blood and bone marrow findings are characteristic of chronic myeloid leukemia. All the other diseases listed can involve the bone marrow; however, none of them would show a proliferation of myeloid cells as seen in the figure. **BH p. 213**

30. E The marrow shows marked myeloid hyperplasia with proliferation of neutrophils and their precursors, characteristic of chronic myeloid leukemia. Myelocytes and metamyelocytes, at various stages of maturation, appear in the peripheral blood in increased numbers. Basophils can be seen in increased numbers in the peripheral blood of patients with chronic myeloid leukemia; however, only mature basophils (not their precursors) are increased. Eosinophils are increased in allergic conditions and the hypereosinophilic syndrome. In the latter case, the marrow would show a marked increase of eosinophils, which is not seen in this biopsy. An increase in lymphocytes and their precursors would occur in lymphomas, with the marrow showing an increase in lymphoid, not myeloid cells. Monocytes and their precursors are increased in monocytic leukemias, which would be reflected in the marrow by an increase in cells of the monocytic, rather than neutrophils, series. **BH p. 213**

31. A Progressive fibrosis of the marrow is seen in chronic idiopathic myelofibrosis. This is partly compensated by extramedullary hematopoiesis in the spleen, liver, and lymph nodes, resulting in hepatosplenomegaly and lymphadenopathy. The other signs and symptoms listed are not characteristic of myelofibrosis. Loss of reflexes in the extremities may be seen in patients with vitamin B_{12} deficiency. In this case, the marrow would show megaloblastic erythroid hyperplasia, not progressive myelofibrosis. Sickle cells in the peripheral blood and leg ulcers are characteristically seen in patients with sickle cell anemias, and the marrow shows normoblastic erythroid hyperplasia without fibrosis. Multiple lytic lesions of bone are most often seen in multiple myeloma, characterized by a proliferation of plasma cells in the marrow, which may be accompanied by mild but not progressive fibrosis. **BH p. 214**

FH5 Chapter 12: Respiratory System
BH5 Chapter 3: Chronic Inflammation
BH5 Chapter 4: Infections of Histological Importance
BH5 Chapter 12: Respiratory System
BH5 Chapter 15: Urinary System

12

Respiratory System

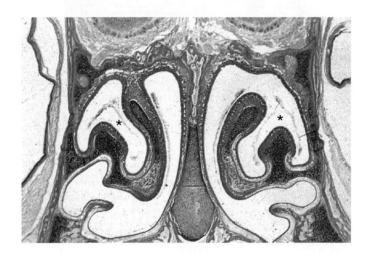

1 The mucosa lining the irregular spaces (*) seen in the figure above has what particular characteristic?

☐ A. A parakeratinized epithelium
☐ B. A supporting layer of skeletal muscle
☐ C. A very rich blood supply
☐ D. Large numbers of elastic fibers
☐ E. Very long microvilli on the surface epithelium

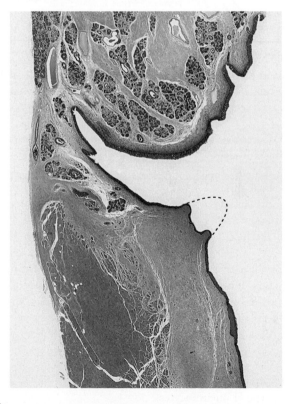

2 The figure above shows a coronal section through the larynx. The *dotted line* indicates a region that has been surgically removed. In the normal larynx, what would occupy the missing region?

☐ A. Bundle of smooth muscle
☐ B. Elastic ligament
☐ C. Hyaline cartilage
☐ D. Large accumulation of lymphocytes
☐ E. Mucosal fold containing mixed mucosal glands

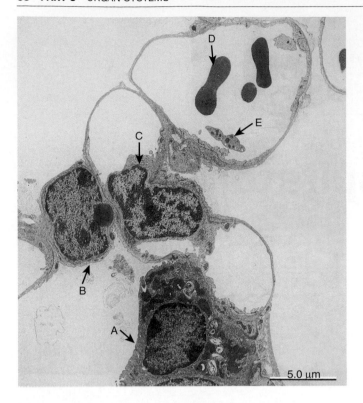

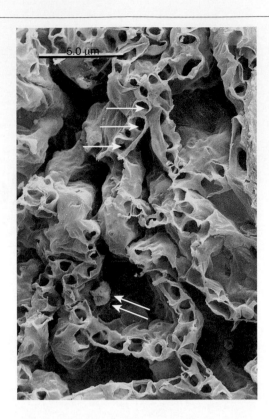

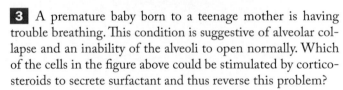

3 A premature baby born to a teenage mother is having trouble breathing. This condition is suggestive of alveolar collapse and an inability of the alveoli to open normally. Which of the cells in the figure above could be stimulated by corticosteroids to secrete surfactant and thus reverse this problem?

4 Where does a second cell type that makes a component of surfactant reside?
- ☐ A. Alveolar ducts
- ☐ B. Bronchi
- ☐ C. Bronchioles
- ☐ D. Capillaries
- ☐ E. Trachea

5 Because of their constant exposure to the environment, pulmonary epithelial cells have a fairly rapid turnover. Which cells in the bronchioles act as stem cells, replacing damaged cells in the bronchiolar epithelium?
- ☐ A. Basal cells
- ☐ B. Ciliated cells
- ☐ C. Clara cells
- ☐ D. Goblet cells
- ☐ E. Type II pneumocytes

Use the figure above to answer the next two questions.

6 In the micrograph above, what are the many small round spaces indicated by the *arrows* in the top of the figure?
- ☐ A. Adipose cells with the fat removed
- ☐ B. Areas occupied by elastic bands in the living lung
- ☐ C. Capillaries
- ☐ D. Empty secretion granules
- ☐ E. Lymphatic drainage channels

7 What is indicated by the *double arrow* in the bottom of the figure?
- ☐ A. Clara cell
- ☐ B. Goblet cell
- ☐ C. Macrophage
- ☐ D. Type I pneumocyte
- ☐ E. Type II pneumocyte

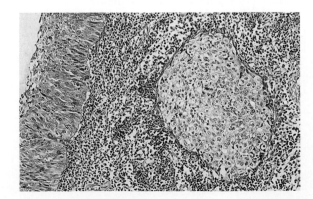

8 A 45-year-old man presents with a mass in the nasopharynx. A biopsy was performed, and a diagnosis of nasopharyngeal carcinoma was made based on the biopsy findings as shown in the figure on the previous page. This tumor is most commonly associated with which of the following oncogenic viruses?

☐ A. Epstein-Barr virus
☐ B. Hepatitis B virus
☐ C. Human herpesvirus 8
☐ D. Human papillomavirus
☐ E. Human T-cell lymphotropic virus

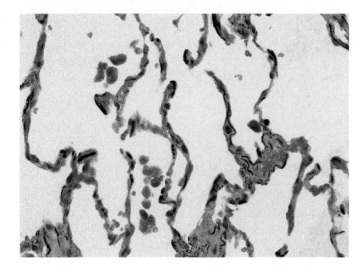

9 What is caused by digestion of the black-staining elastic fibers shown in the figure above?

☐ A. Bronchial inflammation
☐ B. Dilated alveoli
☐ C. Fluid in alveoli
☐ D. Interstitial fibrosis
☐ E. Mucous plugging

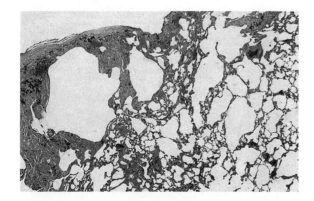

Use the figure above to answer the next two questions.

10 A 55-year-old man with a history of smoking one pack of cigarettes per day for 30 years presents with a cough and shortness of breath. Thoracotomy was performed, and a portion of his right upper lobe was removed. A microscopic section from the resected portion of the lobe is shown in the figure above. What is this pathologic condition?

☐ A. Asthma
☐ B. Bronchitis
☐ C. Bronchopneumonia
☐ D. Emphysema
☐ E. Pulmonary edema

11 Which is a most likely complication of the pathology shown at bottom left?

☐ A. Bronchitis
☐ B. Bronchopneumonia
☐ C. Lung carcinoma
☐ D. Pneumothorax
☐ E. Pulmonary edema

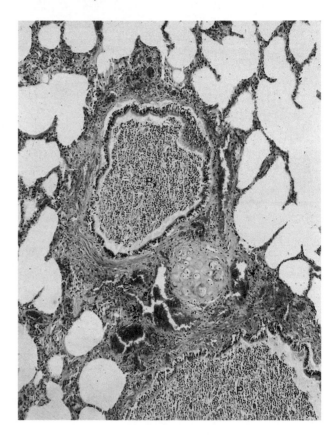

12 A 53-year-old male smoker was admitted to an emergency room with a fever and shortness of breath. A biopsy of lung tissue from this patient is shown above. What is this pathologic condition?

☐ A. Acute bronchitis
☐ B. Chronic asthma
☐ C. Emphysema
☐ D. Pulmonary edema
☐ E. Silicosis

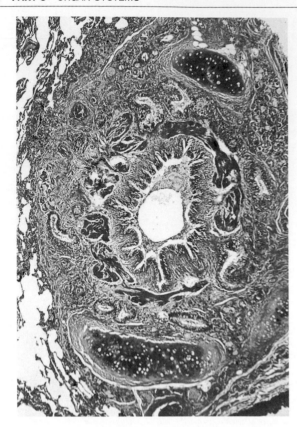

Use the figure above to answer the next two questions.

13 A bronchial biopsy performed in a 22-year-old man is shown in the figure above. What is the cause of the structural abnormalities apparent in this figure?
☐ A. Acute bronchitis
☐ B. Chronic asthma
☐ C. Emphysema
☐ D. Pulmonary edema
☐ E. Silicosis

14 The above patient most likely presented with which of the following symptoms?
☐ A. Chest pain
☐ B. Hemoptysis
☐ C. High-grade fever
☐ D. Marked weight loss
☐ E. Wheezing

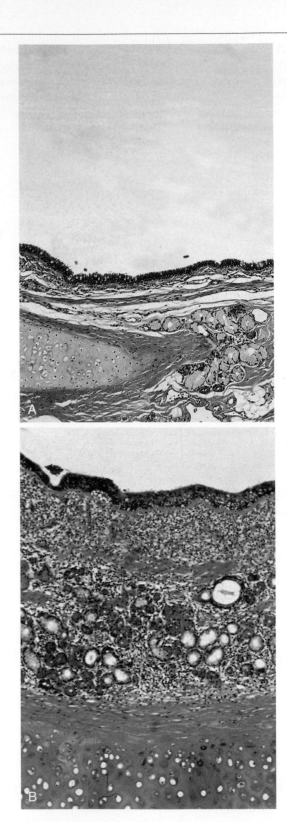

The next four questions refer to the figure above.

A 30-year-old man comes to the doctor complaining that he had been coughing up mucus over the past few weeks. When asked, he admitted to having begun smoking again at about the time his coughing episodes started. Two years ago, he had had a lung biopsy for another problem, and a section was made. The section from this biopsy is shown in part A. To examine the basis of his current symptoms, a second biopsy was taken from a similar area. The section from this later biopsy is shown in part B.

15 What normal structure is shown in part A?
☐ A. Alveolar duct
☐ B. Bronchus
☐ C. Respiratory bronchiole
☐ D. Terminal bronchiole

16 What is the pathologic condition shown in part B?
☐ A. Bronchopneumonia
☐ B. Chronic bronchitis
☐ C. Emphysema
☐ D. Pulmonary fibrosis
☐ E. Silicosis

17 What is a direct consequence of the pathology shown in part B?
☐ A. Accumulation of pus in alveolar ducts
☐ B. Blockage of the pores of Kohn
☐ C. Decreased surface area for oxygen exchange
☐ D. Decreased size of alveoli
☐ E. Increased airway resistance

18 What can result from prolonged damage to the bronchial mucosa as shown in part B?
☐ A. Carbon dioxide movement to alveoli
☐ B. Cystic fibrosis
☐ C. Hyperoxia
☐ D. Lack of surfactant
☐ E. Squamous cell metaplasia

19 A microscopic section of a lung biopsy from a 59-year-old woman is shown in the figure at bottom left. Which of the following is the most likely cause of the pathology depicted?
☐ A. Asbestos exposure
☐ B. Bacterial pneumonia
☐ C. Cigarette smoking
☐ D. Congestive heart failure
☐ E. IgE-mediated hypersensitivity reaction

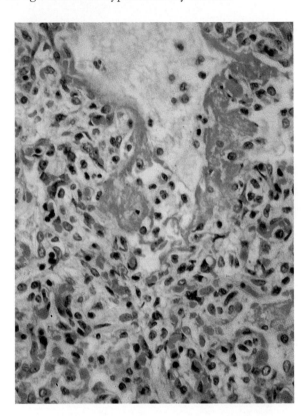

20 A 28-year-old woman was admitted to the hospital in labor pain at 30 weeks' gestation. She gave birth to a boy weighing 5 pounds, 6 ounces. Soon after birth, the newborn was found to have severe shortness of breath with grunting respiration, nasal flaring, and cyanosis. Despite resuscitation, the newborn expired. Autopsy examination was performed, and a microscopic section of the lungs is shown in the figure above. Which of the following is a most likely etiology of the pathology shown?
☐ A. Bacterial pneumonia
☐ B. Cocaine exposure in utero
☐ C. Lack of surfactant
☐ D. Left heart failure
☐ E. Maternal diabetes mellitus

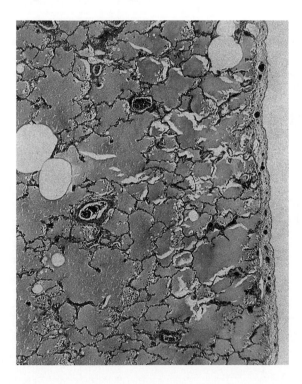

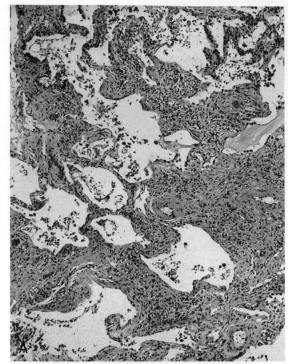

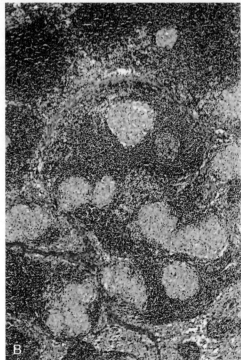

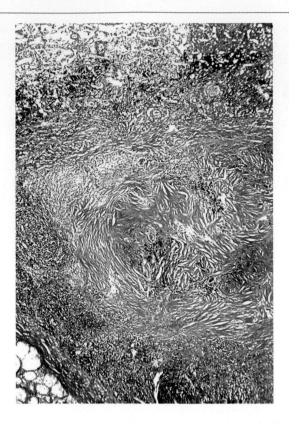

Use the figure above to answer the next two questions.

22 A 67-year-old man presents with shortness of breath of 1 year's duration. Chest radiograph reveals a lung nodule. A biopsy of the lung nodule was performed, and a microscopic section is shown in the figure above. Which of the following is the most likely diagnosis?
- ☐ A. Asbestosis
- ☐ B. Bronchial asthma
- ☐ C. Hyaline membrane disease
- ☐ D. Sarcoidosis
- ☐ E. Silicosis

23 Which of the following is a most likely complication in the above patient?
- ☐ A. Bronchiectasis
- ☐ B. Emphysema
- ☐ C. Pulmonary edema
- ☐ D. Pulmonary hypertension
- ☐ E. Squamous cell carcinoma

21 A 38-year-old woman has a history of shortness of breath of 1 year's duration. Workup of the patient reveals abnormal lung function tests and mediastinal lymphadenopathy. Thoracotomy, with resection of a segment of the right middle lobe (A) and mediastinal lymph node biopsy (B) were performed, and the findings are shown in the above images. Which of the following is the most likely diagnosis?
- ☐ A. Bronchiectasis
- ☐ B. Hyaline membrane disease
- ☐ C. Mesothelioma
- ☐ D. Sarcoidosis
- ☐ E. Silicosis

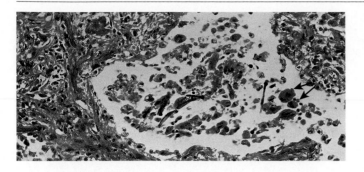

Use the figure above to answer the next two questions.

A 68-year-old man has a long-standing history of shortness of breath. A lung biopsy was performed and is shown in the figure above.

24 What are indicated by the *arrows*?
☐ A. Basophils
☐ B. Giant cells
☐ C. Lymphocytes
☐ D. Megakaryocytes
☐ E. Neutrophils

25 Based on the figure shown above, this patient has an increased risk for what pathology?
☐ A. Bacterial pneumonia
☐ B. Emphysema
☐ C. Left heart failure
☐ D. Mesothelioma
☐ E. Tuberculosis

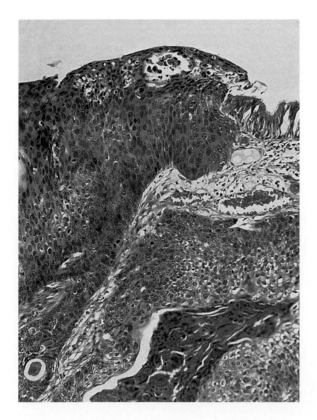

Use the figure at bottom left to answer the next two questions.

26 A 56-year-old man with a long-standing history of smoking presents with shortness of breath. A lung mass was visible on chest radiograph. A biopsy of the mass was performed and shown in the figure. What pathological condition is shown?
☐ A. Acute bronchitis
☐ B. Adenocarcinoma
☐ C. Asbestosis
☐ D. Kaposi sarcoma
☐ E. Squamous cell carcinoma

27 Which of the following is the most likely origin of the pathology shown in the figure?
☐ A. Alveoli
☐ B. Interstitium
☐ C. Bronchi
☐ D. Pleura
☐ E. Pulmonary vessels

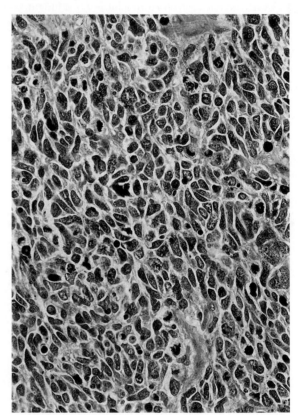

28 A 50-year-old woman presents with shortness of breath and weight loss. A chest radiograph shows a lung mass. A biopsy of the mass was performed and shown in the figure above. This patient has an increased risk for the development of what condition?
☐ A. Cushing syndrome
☐ B. Emphysema
☐ C. Left heart failure
☐ D. Mesothelioma
☐ E. Tuberculosis

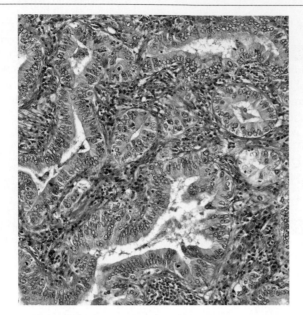

29 A microscopic section from a biopsy of a lung mass in a 62-year-old male is shown in the figure above. Which of the following is the most likely diagnosis?

- [ ] A. Adenocarcinoma
- [ ] B. Bronchioloalveolar carcinoma
- [ ] C. Mesothelioma
- [ ] D. Small cell carcinoma
- [ ] E. Squamous cell carcinoma

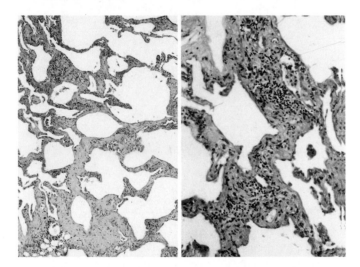

30 A 60-year-old man comes to the physician complaining of breathlessness. This problem had been developing slowly over time. Noting some clubbing of the fingers, the physician orders a biopsy of the lung. Sections of the biopsy are shown above. Based on these images, what is the cause of the patient's signs and symptoms?

- [ ] A. Decreased size of alveoli
- [ ] B. Decreased surfactant production in the alveoli
- [ ] C. Increased distance between air spaces and capillaries
- [ ] D. Increased elastin content of alveolar connective tissue
- [ ] E. Replacement of alveoli by terminal bronchioles

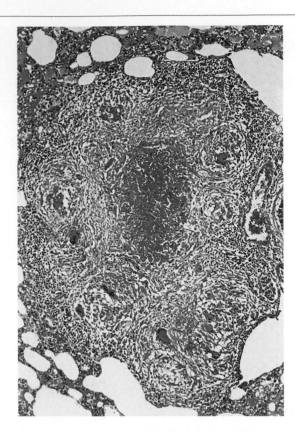

31 A 45-year-old immigrant farmer from West Africa develops fever, night sweats, and weight loss. Chest radiograph reveals a nodule in his left lower lobe. A biopsy of the nodule was performed and a microscopic section shown in the figure above. Which of the following is a most likely diagnosis?

- [ ] A. Bronchiectasis
- [ ] B. Bronchitis
- [ ] C. Pulmonary fibrosis
- [ ] D. Silicosis
- [ ] E. Tuberculosis

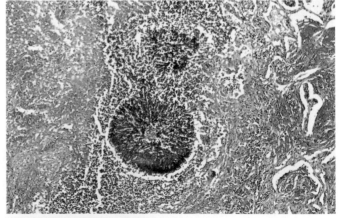

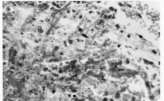

32 A 33-year-old HIV-positive man develops a cough and chest pain. A chest radiograph shows a nodule in the right upper lobe of his lung. A biopsy of the nodule was performed, and microscopic sections are shown in the images at the bottom of the previous page. What is the most likely etiologic agent?

- ☐ A. *Aspergillus*
- ☐ B. *Candida*
- ☐ C. *Cryptococcus*
- ☐ D. *Cytomegalovirus*
- ☐ E. *Pneumocystis*

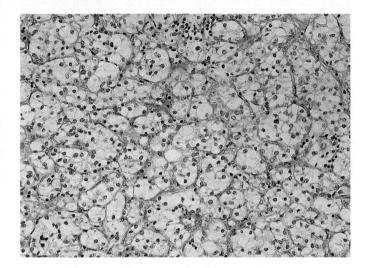

33 A 59-year-old woman presents with cough and a 20-lb weight loss. A computed tomography scan shows multiple nodules in both lungs and the left pleura, consistent with metastatic tumors. A thoracotomy with biopsy of one of the lung nodules was performed, and a histologic section is shown in the figure above. Which of the following is the most likely origin of the metastatic tumor?

- ☐ A. Breast
- ☐ B. Colon
- ☐ C. Kidney
- ☐ D. Pancreas
- ☐ E. Thyroid

ANSWERS

1. C The figure shows a section through the nasal cavities. The nasal mucosa is richly supplied with blood vessels, which function to warm the inspired air. The epithelium is ciliated, pseudostratified columnar and is supported by bone or cartilage. Although elastic fibers are present, the lamina propria is not heavily elasticized, as is seen in the trachea and bronchi. **FH pp. 234-236**

2. B The vocal fold, which contains the elastic vocal ligament, was removed in this specimen. The muscle in the vocal fold is skeletal, not smooth. Mixed mucosal glands are seen in the vestibular fold, above, not in the vocal fold. Cartilage and accumulations of lymphoid cells are normally absent from the vocal fold. **FH p. 237**

3. A This is a type II pneumocyte, recognizable by its characteristic lamellar bodies containing surfactant. When secreted, surfactant decreases surface tension in the alveolar spaces, which decreases the energy necessary for the alveoli to expand normally. The type I pneumocyte (B) and the endothelial cell (C) form the thin alveolar walls. The condensed RBC with its characteristic biconcave shape (D) and the small, granular platelet (E) are located within the capillary space. **FH pp. 243-245**

4. C Clara cells are found only in the bronchiolar epithelium. These cells secrete proteins, which form part of the surfactant. **FH p. 242**

5. C Clara cells are nonciliated cells found only in the bronchioles. They act as stem cells in the bronchiolar epithelium. Ciliated cells are the only other cell type in the bronchioles, and they develop from the Clara cells. **FH p. 241**

6. C The figure shows a scanning electron micrograph of the lung. The large spaces are the alveoli, and the small spaces are the many capillaries that surround the alveoli. From the magnification marker, these spaces cannot be adipose cells, secretion granules, or lymphatic channels. Elastic bands would appear solid, not hollow. **FH p. 242**

7. C This cell is in the alveolar lumen. This is the location of the alveolar macrophages, which clean off the surfaces of the alveoli. Clara cells and goblet cells are not found in the alveoli and the type I and type II pneumocytes are an integral part of the alveolar wall. **FH pp. 242, 247**

8. A Nasopharyngeal carcinoma is strongly associated with the presence of Epstein-Barr virus in the tumor cells. All the other viruses listed are also oncogenic viruses associated with the development of a variety of human cancers. Hepatitis B is associated with hepatocellular carcinoma, human herpesvirus 8 (HHV-8) with Kaposi sarcoma, human papillomavirus (HPV) with squamous cell carcinoma, and human T-cell lymphotropic virus (HTLV-1) is associated with adult T-cell lymphoma/leukemia. **BH p. 126**

9. B Destruction of the elastin results in loss of elastic recoil, which is an important force for expiration. When the recoil capacity of alveoli is lost due to loss of elastin, inspired air is trapped, which leads to expansion and dilation of the alveoli. Loss of elastic fibers would not directly cause the other conditions listed. **FH pp. 245-246**

10. D The figure shows dilated alveolar spaces due to permanent destruction of the alveolar walls. This is a characteristic finding in emphysema where the elastic fibers between alveoli are degraded, most commonly due to cigarette smoking. This leads to loss of the elastic recoil of the lung, trapping of inspired air, and subsequent dilation of alveoli. Breathing becomes labored as the chest muscles have to contract to drive the air from the lungs. Each of the other choices listed have unique histologic findings based on the pathogenic mechanism. In bronchopneumonia, neutrophils and microorganisms fill the alveoli, whereas clear fluid occupies the alveolar spaces in pulmonary edema. In chronic asthma, there is smooth muscle hypertrophy of the bronchi and an inflammatory infiltrate in the bronchial mucosa composed of eosinophils. In chronic bronchitis, there is a lymphocytic inflammation of the bronchial epithelium with excess mucus production and destruction of the mucosa. **FH p. 241, BH p. 129**

11. D The figure shows two small subpleural bullae, which are commonly caused by emphysema. These may rupture into the pleural space, giving rise to a pneumothorax. Chronic bronchitis and bronchopneumonia are also a cause, but not a complication of subpleural bullae. Pulmonary edema most commonly occurs as a consequence of congestive heart failure and is not directly associated with subpleural bullae. **BH p. 129, FH p. 241**

12. A This is acute bronchitis caused by a bacterial infection of the bronchi. This can be recognized by the accumulations of neutrophils and fluid within the lumens of bronchi (purulent exudate (P) in the image). Like acute bronchitis, the pathology in chronic asthma is also centered in the bronchi; however, the two diseases have different histologic (and clinical) findings. Histologically, the distinguishing features of chronic asthma are the mixed inflammatory infiltrates predominated by eosinophils in the submucosa rather than the lumen of the bronchi; this is accompanied by a significant smooth muscle hypertrophy. Emphysema and pulmonary edema are both alveolar rather than bronchial pathologies, characterized by dilated alveoli and fluid within the alveolar spaces, respectively. The histologic hallmark of silicosis is fibrosis in the interstitium (between alveoli) of the lung. **FH p. 240, BH p. 128**

13. B In response to numerous episodes of asthma, the wall of this bronchus has thickened, and mucus has accumulated in the lumen. Emphysema and edema primarily affect the structures of alveoli rather than bronchi; silicosis provokes the appearance of fibrotic nodules in the interstitium of the lung. **FH p. 240, BH p. 130**

14. E The image of the bronchus shows narrowing of the bronchial lumen due to hypertrophy of mucous glands and smooth muscle, with mucus in the bronchial lumen. This leads to wheezing, cough, and shortness of breath. Chest pain can be a manifestation of a variety of pulmonary disorders. Patients with bronchial asthma may present with chest pain; however, if present, it is usually accompanied by wheezing and shortness of the breath. Hemoptysis may occur as a presenting symptom of a number of lung diseases ranging from infectious to neoplastic but is not a manifestation of asthma. High-grade fever is unusual in uncomplicated asthma, unless the patient

has a superimposed infection, and marked weight loss is also not a typical feature of this disease. **BH p. 130, FH p. 240**

15. B This section shows a section through a bronchus. Note the hyaline cartilage, which is seen only in the bronchi in the lungs. **FH p. 239**

16. B This is chronic bronchitis. In this condition, continual irritation of bronchial cells promotes inflammation and enlargement of the lamina propria and of mucus-secreting glands. In emphysema, the alveoli are dilated. In silicosis and pulmonary fibrosis, large amounts of collagen are seen, primarily between alveoli. In bronchopneumonia, neutrophils and cellular debris would be present in the bronchiolar and alveolar lumens. **FH p. 239, BH p. 129**

17. E As the walls of the bronchi are thickened, the diameter of the lumen shrinks, leading to increased airway resistance. The bronchi and bronchioles are the main contributors to airway resistance in the lungs. Alveolar dilation may occur secondary to the increased airway resistance. **BH p. 129, FH p. 241**

18. E Repeated damage to the bronchial mucosa can result in replacement of the pseudostratified columnar epithelium by stratified squamous epithelium. Cystic fibrosis, a disease caused by an inherited mutation in the chloride ion transport gene, leads to, but is not caused by, chronic bronchitis. Surfactant production and carbon dioxide movement to the alveoli are functions of the alveolar epithelia and capillaries and are not directly affected by chronic bronchitis. In severe cases of chronic bronchitis, the thick bronchial wall and narrow lumen can reduce the amount of oxygen entering the lungs, resulting in hypoxia, not hyperoxia. **FH p. 241**

19. D Pulmonary edema, as seen in the figure, is characterized by transudation of clear plasma fluid into the alveolar spaces. This is most commonly caused by left ventricular failure that leads to increased pulmonary venous pressure and escape of fluid into the alveolar spaces. Asbestos exposure is characterized by interstitial fibrosis and pleural thickening, not pulmonary edema. In bacterial pneumonia, fluid may accumulate in the alveolar spaces. However, because the fluid in bacterial pneumonia is caused by inflammation (not increased venous pressure), it would be rich in neutrophils and cell debris. Cigarette smoking causes inflammation, edema, and mucus buildup in the bronchi, whereas in the alveoli, it causes destruction of elastin with minimal inflammation. IgE-mediated hypersensitivity, as in bronchial asthma, causes muscle spasm and inflammation of the bronchi. **BH p. 130**

20. C The pink protein-rich exudate on the alveolar wall is characteristic of hyaline membrane disease. In the neonatal period, this disease is seen most commonly in premature infants and is caused by a lack of pulmonary surfactant. In bacterial pneumonia, the alveoli are filled with neutrophils and cell debris rather than hyaline membrane. Cocaine exposure in utero may result in developmental abnormalities, but it has not been associated with hyaline membrane disease. In left heart failure, the increased pulmonary venous pressure causes clear fluid that is low in protein content (transudate) to leak into the alveoli. Maternal diabetes causes hyperinsulinemia in the fetus that results in increased body fat, muscle mass, and enlarged organs. It is not associated with hyaline membrane disease. **BH p. 131**

21. D The figure shows pulmonary interstitial fibrosis (A) and multiple noncaseating granulomas (B) in the lymph node, which are characteristic findings in sarcoidosis. Granulomas are typically seen only in sarcoidosis and rarely in silicosis. Except for mesothelioma and silicosis, the other pathologies do not involve the mediastinal lymph nodes. In bronchiectasis, there is bronchial fibrosis and dilation due to inflammatory-mediated tissue destruction of the bronchi. Hyaline membrane disease is characterized by a protein-rich exudate and cell debris in the alveoli. Mesothelioma is a malignant tumor of the pleura and may cause mediastinal lymphadenopathy when it metastasizes to the mediastinal lymph nodes. Microscopically, it shows a biphasic (spindle cell and glandular) proliferation of tumor cells. Silicosis, like sarcoidosis, causes interstitial fibrosis in the lung and may involve mediastinal lymph nodes; however, granulomas are rare. **BH pp. 131, 134**

22. E The figure shows hyalinized, fibrotic nodules of collagenous tissue that are characteristically seen in silicosis. This is the most common of the pneumoconioses, which are occupational lung diseases caused by the inhalation of dust particles. Fibrosis is rare in bronchial asthma and hyaline membrane disease. Fibrosis occurs in the other pathologies listed; however, the location and the type of fibrosis help distinguish them. In asbestosis, large fibrotic plaques are seen but are characteristically in the pleura, not in the interstitium of the lung. In sarcoidosis, there may be a diffuse interstitial inflammation in the lung; however, thick hyalinized fibrotic nodules do not occur. **BH p. 132**

23. D Progressive fibrosis of the lung interstitium, as occurs in silicosis, causes disruption of the pulmonary microvasculature and leads to pulmonary hypertension. Bronchiectasis is caused by diseases that cause inflammation and destruction of the bronchi. Silicosis is a fibrosing disease of the interstitium of the lung and does not significantly involve the bronchi. The dilation of alveoli seen in emphysema is caused by destruction of elastin due to smoking-induced increase in neutrophil elastase activity, not by silicosis. Squamous cell carcinoma is not associated with silicosis. **BH p. 132**

24. B These cells are foreign-body giant cells, characterized by their large size, multinucleation, and phagocytic function, as evidenced by the encapsulated asbestos fibers. Encapsulation of the asbestos fibers prevents them from damaging the pneumocytes. Giant cells and megakaryocytes are the only cells among the ones listed that are large with abundant cytoplasm and multiple nuclei. However, megakaryocytes are

neither present in the lung nor phagocytic. They are normally found in the bone marrow, and their function is production of platelets. **FH p. 247, BH p. 132**

25. D The material ingested by the giant cells is identified as an asbestos body based on its linear, beaded appearance and brown color. Exposure to asbestos increases the risk for the development of mesothelioma, which is a malignant tumor of the pleura. There is no increased risk for developing the other diseases listed. **BH p. 132**

26. E The normal respiratory epithelium has been replaced with a highly dysplastic, stratified squamous epithelium. This dysplastic epithelium has invaded the submucosa with evidence of keratin formation, characteristic of squamous cell carcinoma. Asbestosis is characterized by marked thickening and fibrosis of the pleura along with asbestos bodies engulfed by alveolar macrophages. Malignant tumors that arise in the setting of asbestosis are mesotheliomas, which show a biphasic pattern with spindle cell proliferation and gland formation, but not the stratified squamous cells and keratin formation of squamous cell carcinomas. In acute bronchitis, the bronchial wall is thickened by inflammation, and the respiratory epithelium can be undergoing metaplasia to squamous epithelium. However, the metaplastic epithelium is either normal stratified squamous epithelium or would show minimal dysplasia. Adenocarcinomas are also common malignant tumors seen in the lung, but microscopically, they show evidence of gland formation, not stratified squamous cells or keratin formation. Kaposi sarcoma is a common neoplasm affecting immuno-compromised persons and can also involve the lungs, but it is a vascular, not epithelial, tumor and is characterized by spindle cell proliferation. **FH p. 240, BH p. 135**

27. C The figure shows squamous cell carcinoma, as evidenced by keratin formation by the tumor cells. It is the most common primary malignancy of the lung and frequently arises from the main bronchi or their larger branches. Squamous cell carcinomas do not arise from the other structures listed. **BH p. 135**

28. A The figure shows the characteristic histologic appearance of small cell carcinoma, that is, sheets of densely packed, dark-staining small cells, with scant cytoplasm and nuclear molding. These tumors have a tendency to secrete peptide hormones (e.g., adrenocorticotropic hormone) and give rise to tumor-related endocrine syndromes, such as Cushing syndrome. Small cell carcinomas are not directly associated with the other pathologies listed. **BH p. 134**

29. A The figure shows invasion and destruction of the lung tissue by a malignant neoplasm with formation of glands and acini by the tumor cells. This is characteristic of adenocarcinomas. Bronchioloalveolar carcinoma is a subtype of adenocarcinoma that has a unique pattern in which the tumor cells grow along the alveolar wall, without causing invasion or destruction of the lung tissue. Because of their growth pattern, a distinct lung mass may not be evident clinically. Mesothelioma, a neoplasm derived from the lining cells of the pleura, can show evidence of gland formation. However, the tumor is located in the pleura, not the lung parenchyma, and the cells show a biphasic pattern with spindle cell proliferation and gland formation. Gland formation is not a feature of either small cell or squamous cell carcinoma. **BH p. 136**

30. C   The figure shows interstitial fibrosis with thick walls of the alveoli resulting in increased distances between capillary endothelia and type I pneumocytes. Because the efficiency of oxygen diffusion from the airways to the capillaries decreases with the distance between them, thickening results in hypoxia. Finger clubbing is an indication of hypoxia. The fibrosis destroys the elastin in the alveoli and distorts the alveolar walls leading to distention and dilation of alveoli. The fibrosis is predominantly interstitial and may be accompanied by proliferation of pneumocytes, so the production of surfactant is not affected. When the alveoli are damaged, they are replaced by fibrosis, not by terminal bronchioles. **FH p. 245, BH p. 32**

31. E   The characteristic histologic hallmark in tuberculosis is a caseating granuloma. It is characterized by a nodular collection of macrophages and lymphocytes with scattered multinucleated giant cells and the central area of the nodule showing necrosis (caseation). Granulomas are not seen in any of the other conditions, with the exception of silicosis, in which the granulomas are rare, are usually less well defined, and almost never show caseation. **BH p. 38-39**

32. A   All the organisms listed cause opportunistic infections in immunocompromised hosts. They are differentiated by their clinical presentation and morphologic appearance. *Aspergillus, Candida, Cryptococcus,* and *Pneumocystis* are fungi that typically cause cavitary lung lesions, esophagitis, meningitis, and pneumonia, respectively. *Aspergillus* hyphae are characteristically septated and branch at an acute angle (see figure); *Candida* appears as budding yeast and pseudohyphae; and *Cryptococcus* is an encapsulated yeast with no hyphae. *Pneumocystis* appears as very small spherical cysts embedded in frothy alveolar exudates. *Cytomegalovirus* is a herpesvirus that infects a variety of tissues. It causes characteristic enlargement of the infected cell with a prominent intranuclear inclusion, surrounded by a clear halo. **BH p. 48-49**

33. C   The figure shows sheets of malignant cells that are large and polygonal with abundant clear cytoplasm. These features are characteristic of clear cell renal cell carcinoma. The multiple and bilateral distribution of the lung tumors is suggestive of a metastatic lesion and the biopsy findings are consistent with metastasis from the kidney. Although all the other tumors often metastasize to the lungs, none of them show the microscopic features that characterize renal cell carcinomas. **BH pp. 192-193**

FH5 Chapter 5: Epithelial Tissues
FH5 Chapter 13: Oral Tissues
BH5 Chapter 4: Infections of Histological Importance
BH5 Chapter 13: Gastrointestinal System

13

Oral Tissue

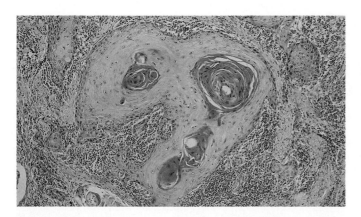

1 A 47-year-old woman is admitted complaining of difficulty in swallowing and a feeling of pain at the back of her tongue. She has a history of chronic alcoholism and heavy smoking. A biopsy of her tongue is shown above. From what is this patient is suffering?
☐ A. Acid reflux
☐ B. Hypotonia
☐ C. Progressive bulbar palsy
☐ D. Ranula of the tongue
☐ E. Squamous cell carcinoma

2 In which portion of the oral cavity would the presence of a keratinized or parakeratinized epithelium be abnormal?
☐ A. Dorsal surface of tongue
☐ B. Gingiva
☐ C. Hard palate
☐ D. Soft palate
☐ E. Vermillion border of the lip

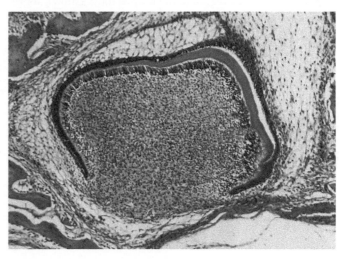

3 What is shown in the figure above?
☐ A. Inflamed hair follicle of the lip
☐ B. Inflamed lingual tonsil
☐ C. Obstructed duct of a salivary gland
☐ D. Pleomorphic adenoma of a salivary gland
☐ E. Tooth bud

4 A young woman comes to the dentist complaining about discolored teeth. Examination shows banding of the enamel. This appearance is consistent with a genetic abnormality in which cells?
☐ A. Ameloblasts
☐ B. Cementoblasts
☐ C. Fibroblasts
☐ D. Myofibroblasts
☐ E. Odontoblasts

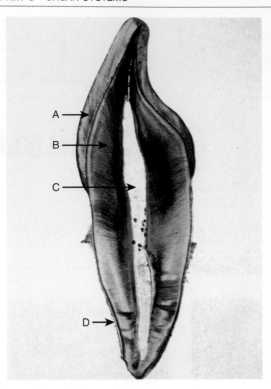

5 Which lettered region of the normal tooth (shown above) has no capacity for repair?

6 Why is having one's teeth cleaned potentially dangerous for patients with compromised immune systems?
- ☐ A. Oral tissues are poorly vascularized and do not heal well after injury.
- ☐ B. Saliva normally contains large numbers of pathogens.
- ☐ C. The nonkeratinized oral epithelium is readily damaged.
- ☐ D. The oral epithelium is interrupted at the gingival crevice.
- ☐ E. The turnover rate of the oral epithelium is slow, so injured areas heal slowly.

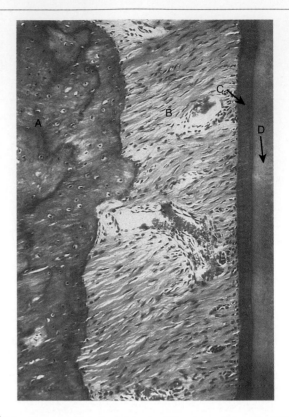

7 The figure above shows part of the root of a tooth. Which labeled structure is most likely to undergo lytic changes when exposed to constant pressure?

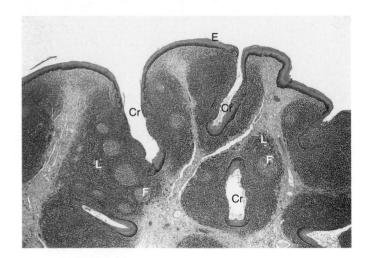

8 In the figure of the posterior tongue (shown above), what do the dark-blue–staining masses of cells represent?
- ☐ A. Carcinoma of minor salivary glands
- ☐ B. Foliate papillae
- ☐ C. Inflammation due to a blockage of a salivary duct
- ☐ D. Lingual tonsils
- ☐ E. Persistent thyroglossal duct tissue

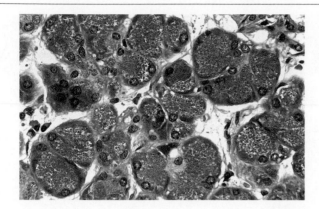

9 A young man comes to the physician complaining of facial pain occurring during meals. Recognizing that these symptoms could be associated with the salivary glands, a biopsy is taken from the affected area and sectioned. In what gland does the imaged section (above) suggest a problem?

☐ A. Labial gland
☐ B. Parotid gland
☐ C. Submandibular gland
☐ D. Sublingual gland

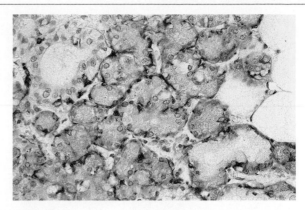

11 The figure above shows a portion of a salivary gland stained using immunocytochemistry to demonstrate actin (brown chromogen). What does this brown stain demonstrate?

☐ A. Intercalated ducts
☐ B. Myoepithelial cells
☐ C. Plasma cells
☐ D. Serous demilunes
☐ E. Skeletal muscle

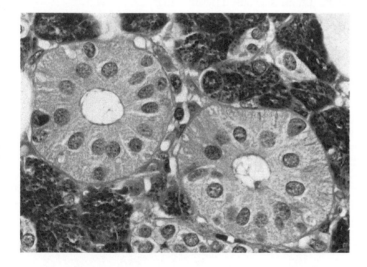

10 How is saliva modified by the ducts shown in the figure above?

☐ A. Calcium will be added
☐ B. Immunoglobulins will be added
☐ C. It will become markedly acidic
☐ D. Some proteins will be removed
☐ E. The saliva will have a reduced concentration of electrolytes

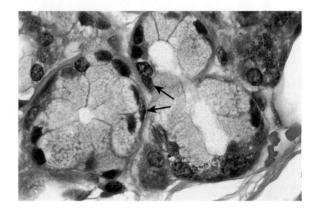

12 What is the function of the cells indicated by the *arrows* in the figure above?

☐ A. Expel saliva
☐ B. Make saliva hypotonic
☐ C. Secrete lysozyme
☐ D. Secrete mucus
☐ E. Synthesize type I collagen

13 A 40-year-old woman has come to her doctor complaining of a chronically dry mouth, reduced flow of saliva, and a recent increase in dental caries. A biopsy of her lip is taken to examine minor salivary glands. Histologic findings indicate focal lymphocytic sialadenitis. This patient is likely to be experiencing which pathologic condition?

☐ A. Bell palsy
☐ B. Mumps
☐ C. Pleomorphic adenoma
☐ D. Sjögren syndrome
☐ E. Warthin tumor

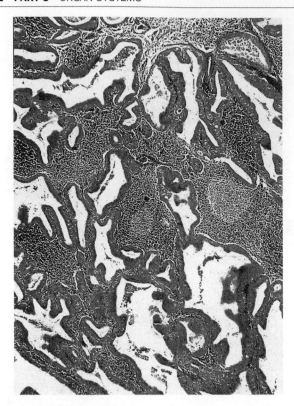

Use the figure above to answer the next two questions.

14 A 57-year-old male smoker presents with a mass in the parotid region. The mass was removed, and a microscopic section is shown in the figure above. In addition to the large glandular acini, which other structures are present?
☐ A. Bone
☐ B. Cartilage
☐ C. Large ganglia
☐ D. Nodular lymphoid tissue
☐ E. Skeletal muscle

15 Based on these microscopic findings, which of the following is the most likely diagnosis?
☐ A. Adenoma
☐ B. Adenocarcinoma
☐ C. Adenoid cystic carcinoma
☐ D. Adenolymphoma
☐ E. Ameloblastoma

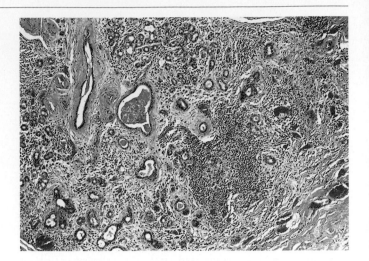

16 A 43-year-old man presents with pain and swelling in the left submandibular area. Physical examination shows a mass, which was removed. A microscopic section of the mass is shown in the figure above. What is the most likely cause of the pathology shown?
☐ A. Chronic inflammation due to obstruction
☐ B. Dysplasia caused by smoking
☐ C. Neoplastic transformation by a virus
☐ D. Ulceration due to *Candida*

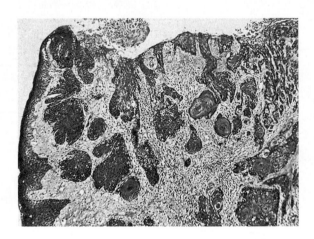

17 A 63-year-old man presents with inability to chew because of pain. Physical examination shows a mass in the floor of the mouth, which underwent biopsy. A microscopic section of the mass is shown in the figure above. What is the most likely origin of the lesion?
☐ A. Dental pulp
☐ B. Facial nerve
☐ C. Minor salivary glands
☐ D. Skeletal muscle
☐ E. Surface epithelium

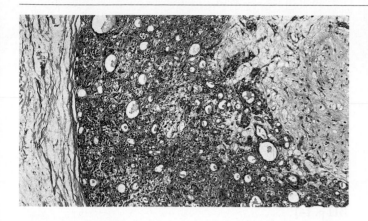

18 A microscopic section of a salivary gland tumor is shown. Which of the following is the most common location of this tumor?
- ☐ A. Minor salivary gland
- ☐ B. Parotid gland
- ☐ C. Sublingual
- ☐ D. Submental gland
- ☐ E. Submandibular gland

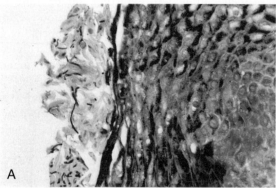

A

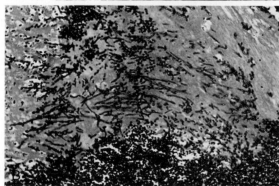

19 A 29-year-old woman presented with recurrent oral pain. Physical examination revealed multiple whitish areas on the soft palate. The patient had similar lesions in the past. A biopsy of one of the lesions was performed, and a microscopic section is shown in the figure above. Which of the following laboratory tests would be most useful in this patient?
- ☐ A. C-reactive protein
- ☐ B. Erythrocyte sedimentation rate
- ☐ C. Hepatitis C virus antibody
- ☐ D. T-lymphocyte count and subset quantitation
- ☐ E. Serum vitamin B$_{12}$ level

ANSWERS

1. E The presence of squamous cell carcinoma is demonstrated by the accumulation of keratinized cells organized into keratin pearls. In ranula of the tongue, a painless swelling filled with salivary mucus develops. If her difficulty in swallowing were related to an abnormality in the neural control of the esophagus, as in hypotonia or progressive bulbar palsy, numerous other neurologic symptoms would be present. In acid reflux, the lower esophagus is inflamed owing to exposure of the epithelium to acid. This results in indigestion (heartburn) and epigastric pain rather than difficulty in swallowing and oral pain. **FH pp. 86-87, BH p. 72**

2. D The soft palate is normally covered by a nonkeratinized stratified squamous epithelium, whereas the other structures may be lined by a keratinized or parakeratinized stratified squamous epithelium. The soft palate may keratinize in response to irritation or chronic inflammation. **FH pp. 251-252**

3. E The multiple layers of cells surrounding the eosinophilic layer of dentin are characteristic of a developing tooth. Only the developing tooth will have the uniform eosinophilic extracellular layer of dentin. The tonsil would have extensive areas of diffuse and nodular lymphatic tissue. Glands will have distinct ducts or acini. A hair follicle can be identified by its central core of keratinocytes. **FH p. 254**

4. A Only ameloblasts produce enamel. The banding described is seen in an X-linked form of amelogenesis imperfecta. **FH p. 255**

5. A This region is the enamel. The enamel is formed before tooth eruption, at which time ameloblasts are lost. Although the saliva can affect the degree of mineralization of the enamel after the teeth emerge, the absence of ameloblasts prevents additional synthesis of amelogenin or enamelin, proteins that create the environment for the mineralization of enamel. In contrast, the dentin, cementum, and pulp retain their cellular elements and thus have some capacity for repair. **FH pp. 253-255**

6. D The oral epithelium is interrupted at the gingival crevice after the teeth erupt. There are hemidesmosomes in the oral epithelium, which bind to a basal lamina that is pressed against the enamel at this location. This arrangement normally keeps pathogens out of the oral mucosa. However, the gingival crevice is a potential route for pathogens to enter the body whenever this region is compromised. Oral tissues are well vascularized and have a high turnover rate. Consequently, they heal rapidly. Saliva contains a variety of antimicrobial substances, so in a normal individual, the number of pathogens in the saliva is limited. The stratified squamous epithelium in the oral cavity is thick and protects well against abrasion. **FH p. 257**

7. A This is the alveolar bone (A) of the tooth socket. Both alveolar bone and the cementum (C) will undergo osteoclastic resorption if put under constant pressure, but the cementum is more resistant than the bone. This is the basis for orthodontic tooth movements. The periodontal ligament (B) is designed to withstand the forces of chewing and under orthodontic pressure remodels to accommodate the changes in the cementum and alveolar bone. **FH p. 257**

8. D These are lingual tonsils. They are recognized by the crypts (Cr) and by organized mucosal lymphoid tissue (L,F) beneath the stratified squamous epithelium (E), as seen here. Foliate papillae possess numerous light-staining taste buds in the epithelium, not present here. A carcinoma of minor salivary glands would be composed of gland-forming abnormal epithelial cells. A persistent thyroglossal duct is characterized by an epithelial-lined cyst containing thyroid tissue in its wall. An inflamed salivary gland duct would show infiltration by neutrophils and lymphocytes surrounding a duct with a simple or stratified columnar epithelium. **FH p. 259**

9. B The presence of only serous acini in the section suggests the problem is in the parotid gland. Labial glands contain mucous acini only, whereas the submandibular and sublingual glands are mixed with different proportions of serous and mucous acini. **FH p. 261**

10. E The figure shows a striated duct, which reabsorbs sodium and chloride. Although some potassium is secreted into the ducts, there is a net removal of electrolytes. Immunoglobulins are transcytosed into the luminal secretion across the acinar epithelium. The ducts do not modify salivary calcium or pH. They do secrete some proteins. **FH p. 262**

11. B The darkly stained cells are myoepithelial cells. They form a basal cell layer around secretory acini and small ducts and use actin in the process of contraction. Therefore, they stain positively for actin. Larger-diameter skeletal muscle cells, which also possess actin, are not present here. The other epithelial cells of the intercalated ducts and demilunes possess relatively small amounts of actin and are not stained. Plasma cells lie within the loose connective tissue surrounding the lobules. They are not contractile and thus contain little actin. **FH p. 262**

12. A The nuclei labeled with the arrows belong to myoepithelial cells, recognized by their peripheral location in the acinus and flattened shape. These cells contract when stimulated and push the saliva into the duct system. Striated ducts remove ions from saliva. The section shows mucus acini with serous demilunes. These acinar cells secrete an isotonic saliva containing lysozyme and mucins. Fibroblasts secrete type I and type III collagen. **FH p. 262**

13. D Sjögren syndrome is a common autoimmune disorder in which salivary and lacrymal glands are damaged by the immune system and accumulations of lymphocytes are seen among salivary acini. The clinical presentation and the histologic findings are consistent with this disease. Reduced saliva

production and dry mouth may also occur in Bell palsy, but this is due to inflammation of the facial nerve and not the salivary glands. These patients characteristically present with unilateral facial drooping and inability to close the eye. Mumps is a viral inflammation of the salivary glands, and patients typically present with fever, headache, swelling, and pain of the affected gland, most often the parotid. Because mumps is a self-limited disease, chronic dry mouth and increased incidence of caries are not usually seen. Both pleomorphic adenoma and Warthin tumor are benign salivary gland tumors, most commonly seen in the parotid gland. They present with a mass in the parotid area and chronic dry mouth is not a feature of either disease. **BH p. 141**

14. D This gland is infiltrated with diffuse and nodular lymphoid tissue recognizable by the masses of purple-staining lymphocytes. The latter have distinct pale germinal centers. Bone and cartilage would have large amounts of pink-staining extracellular matrix. Ganglia are composed of large neurons with large pale nuclei. Skeletal muscle is composed of very large eosinophilic cells. **BH p. 142**

15. D Adenolymphomas (Warthin tumor) are benign tumors that occur almost exclusively in the parotid region and show a unique histologic appearance. The proliferating glands are lined by tall columnar epithelium with a deeply eosinophilic cytoplasm, and the glands are embedded in nodules of dense lymphoid tissue. In adenoma, adenocarcinoma, and adenoid cystic carcinoma, there is a proliferation of glands; however, none of these shows the diffuse and nodular lymphoid tissue characteristic of adenolymphomas. Ameloblastoma is a tumor of odontogenic epithelium and occurs in the mandible or maxilla, not the parotid gland. **BH p. 142**

16. A The figure shows features of chronic sialadenitis with inflammation, acinar atrophy, and fibrosis of the submandibular gland. Obstruction of a duct by a stone is a common cause of chronic sialadenitis. Smoking can cause epithelial dysplasia; however, the epithelium in this figure shows no evidence of dysplasia or neoplastic transformation (i.e., enlarged cells with pleomorphic nuclei and architectural disorganization). *Candida* infections of the lining epithelium of the oral cavity and esophagus are commonly encountered. However, the salivary glands are rarely affected because most infections tend to be superficial. *Candida* ulcers would be characterized by necrotic tissue with numerous fungal pseudohyphae. **BH p. 140**

17. E The figure shows a well-differentiated squamous cell carcinoma with formation of keratin pearls. These tumors arise from the stratified squamous epithelium that lines the oral cavity. Tumors arising from odontogenic epithelium found in the dental pulp are called *ameloblastomas*. Although there may be focal areas of stratified squamous differentiation in ameloblastomas, most of the tumor is characterized by a proliferation of columnar cells palisading around a cystic space. Tumors derived from nerve show a spindle cell, not epithelial, proliferation—hence keratin pearls would not be seen.

Most neoplasms arising from salivary glands are adenomas or adenocarcinomas, which show gland formation, not keratin pearls. Primary squamous cell carcinomas of the salivary glands are extremely rare. Skeletal muscle–derived tumors show proliferation of cells that resemble striated skeletal muscle. **BH p. 140**

18. B The figure shows the characteristic histology of a pleomorphic adenoma (i.e., a mixture of glandular epithelial proliferation and mesenchymal components composed of various elements of connective tissue). Although pleomorphic adenomas can be seen in any of the salivary glands, most of these tumors occur in the parotid gland. **BH p. 141**

19. D The figure shows evidence of fungal infection with pseudohyphae and yeast forms of *Candida*. Because T cells play a major role in immunity against fungal infections, recurrent infections by *Candida* are suggestive of immunosuppression and a defect in T-lymphocyte function. Therefore, a total T-lymphocyte count with CD4 and CD8 quantitation would be useful to screen for HIV or other immunodeficiency disorders. C-reactive protein is a plasma protein that increases in inflammation. Serum levels of this protein are measured clinically as a marker of inflammation and as an indicator of risk for the development of a myocardial infarction. The erythrocyte sedimentation rate is also measured clinically as a marker of inflammation because the rate of sedimentation is affected by an increase in plasma proteins, as occurs in inflammation. Recurrent fungal infections are not a feature of hepatitis C infection; therefore, measuring antibody to hepatitis C virus would not be indicated in this setting, unless the person has risk factors for developing this disease (e.g., intravenous drug use). Measurement of the serum vitamin B_{12} level is useful in investigating patients with anemia but is not indicated in the workup of a patient with recurrent infection because it has no direct effect on the immune system. **BH p. 47**

14

Gastrointestinal Tract

The next four questions refer to the same patient.

1 A 53-year-old man presents with recurrent heartburn and dysphagia. He is discovered to have Barrett esophagus. This means that his normal esophageal epithelium has undergone metaplasia to which type of epithelium?
☐ A. Pseudostratified columnar
☐ B. Stratified columnar
☐ C. Simple columnar
☐ D. Stratified squamous keratinized
☐ E. Transitional

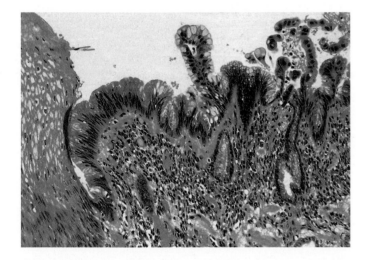

2 The same patient was referred to a gastroenterologist for evaluation. Upper GI endoscopy revealed a reddish area in the lower esophagus. A biopsy was performed, and a microscopic section is shown in the figure above. Which of the following is the most likely cause of this pathology?
☐ A. Acid reflux
☐ B. *Candida* infection
☐ C. Congenital disorder
☐ D. Dilation of veins
☐ E. High-fat diet

3 You recommend regular, frequent screening of the same patient because he has an increased risk for developing what?
☐ A. Adenocarcinoma
☐ B. Carcinoid tumor
☐ C. Gastrointestinal stromal tumor
☐ D. MALT lymphoma
☐ E. Squamous cell carcinoma

4 The same patient was told that the metaplastic epithelium is unusual in this location but is not in itself dangerous. The production of what is its primary function?
☐ A. Acid mucus
☐ B. Bicarbonate-rich mucus
☐ C. Defensin-rich mucus
☐ D. Gastric intrinsic factor
☐ E. Gastric pepsinogen

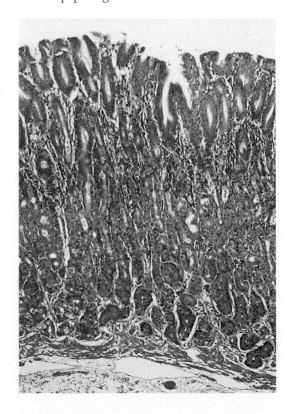

5 Based on its morphology, this section on page 107 was taken from a biopsy of what structure?
☐ A. Appendix
☐ B. Esophagus
☐ C. Stomach
☐ D. Small intestine
☐ E. Large intestine

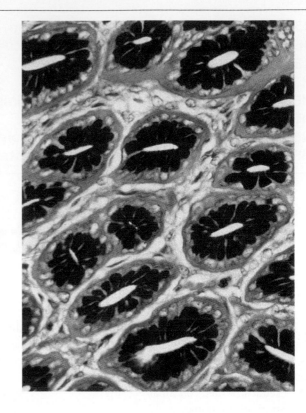

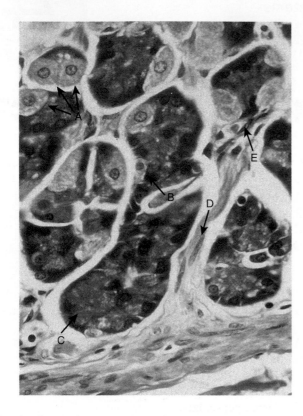

Use the figure above to answer the next two questions.

6 Which labeled cell in the figure above secretes pepsin?

7 Which labeled cell in the figure above secretes serotonin?

8 Which cell in the gastric mucosa synthesizes the IgA that is found in the stomach lumen?
☐ A. Chief cell
☐ B. Neuroendocrine cell
☐ C. Parietal cell
☐ D. Plasma cell
☐ E. Surface mucus cell

9 The figure above is a PAS-stained section of which region?
☐ A. Brunner glands in the duodenum
☐ B. Crypts in the jejunum
☐ C. Crypts in the colon
☐ D. Esophageal glands
☐ E. Gastric pits

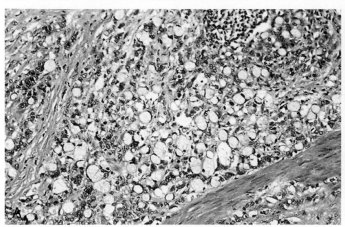

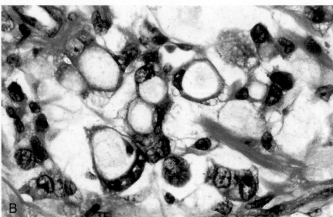

10 A 55-year-old man underwent endoscopy examination for a long-standing complaint of chronic indigestion and heartburn. A biopsy of his stomach is displayed in the figure above. What does this biopsy indicate?

☐ A. Acid reflux
☐ B. Celiac disease
☐ C. Crohn disease
☐ D. Gastric carcinoma
☐ E. Peptic ulcer

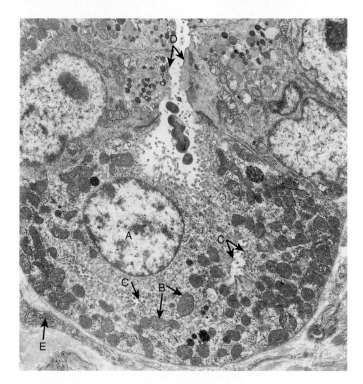

Use the figure above to answer the next two questions.

12 A 54-year-old woman underwent surgery to remove a peptic ulcer. As a result of the surgery, a large number of the cells of the type shown in the center of the figure above (labeled *A* to *C*) are lost. The loss of these cells, in turn, causes a decrease in absorption of what molecule?

☐ A. Gastrin
☐ B. Glycerol
☐ C. Secretin
☐ D. Vitamin B_{12}
☐ E. Vitamin D

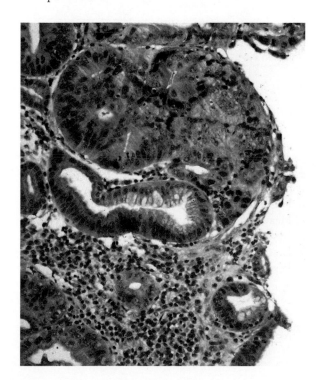

11 An 68-year-old woman comes to a gastroenterologist after a long-standing history of chronic gastritis. What does the biopsy of her stomach (shown in the figure above) indicate?

☐ A. Gastric atrophy
☐ B. Gastric dysplasia
☐ C. Intestinal metaplasia
☐ D. Lymphoma
☐ E. Peptic ulcer

13 Before the surgery described above, this patient was diagnosed with a gastrinoma, which was continuously producing stomach acid. An H^+/K^+-ATPase inhibitor was used to decrease acid production. Which letter in the figure indicates the location of the pumps that produce the stomach acid?

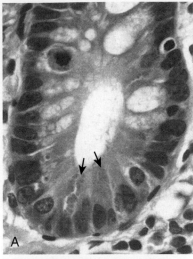

Use the figure above to answer the next two questions.

14 A 20-year-old woman with a long-standing history of abdominal pain undergoes an endoscopic biopsy of the jejunum. The findings are shown in the above photomicrograph. Which of the following is the most likely clinical presentation of this patient?

☐ A. Bloody diarrhea
☐ B. Dysphagia
☐ C. Hematemesis
☐ D. Melena
☐ E. Steatorrhea

15 Which of the following is the best treatment for the above patient?

☐ A. Antiprotozoal drugs
☐ B. Chemotherapy
☐ C. Gluten-free diet
☐ D. Intestinal resection
☐ E. Vitamin B_{12} injections

16 A 32-year-old woman complains of bloating and abdominal cramps after eating dairy products. You diagnose lactose intolerance. Where is the location of the defective lactase enzymes?

☐ A. In digestive organelles of hepatocytes
☐ B. In digestive organelles within the intestinal absorptive cell
☐ C. In the glycocalyx on the intestinal absorptive cell microvilli
☐ D. In the intestinal lumen
☐ E. In the stomach lumen

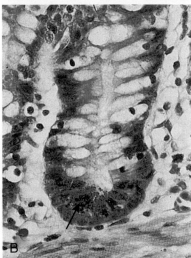

17 What is secreted by the cells that are indicated by the *arrows* in the figure above?

☐ A. Digestive enzymes
☐ B. Heavily glycosylated proteins
☐ C. Lysosomal enzymes
☐ D. Lysozyme and defensins
☐ E. Peptide hormones

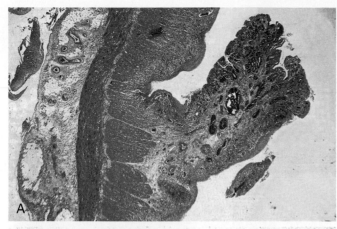

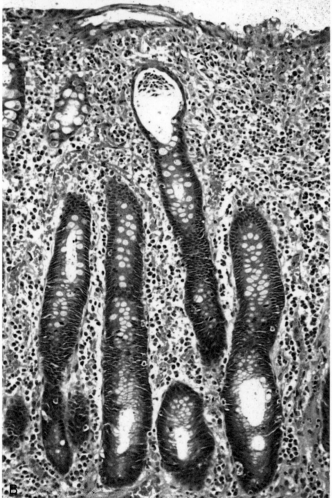

Use the figure above to answer the next two questions.

18 A 20-year-old man was admitted to the hospital following several weeks of diarrhea of increasing severity. Stool samples show the presence of blood and mucus. Based on a colonoscopy and biopsy findings shown in the figure, what is the diagnosis of his condition?

☐ A. Adenocarcinoma of the colon
☐ B. Collagenous colitis
☐ C. Diverticulitis
☐ D. Polyposis coli
☐ E. Ulcerative colitis

19 Which of the following is characteristic of this disease?

☐ A. Formation of fistulas
☐ B. Marked involvement of ileum
☐ C. Skip lesions
☐ D. Superficial ulcers
☐ E. Transmural inflammation

20 What is the mechanism used to expose oral vaccines to the immune system?

☐ A. Endocytosis by intestinal absorptive cells
☐ B. Paracellular transport across the intestinal epithelium
☐ C. Transcytosis by absorptive cells
☐ D. Transcytosis by endothelial cells
☐ E. Transcytosis by M cells

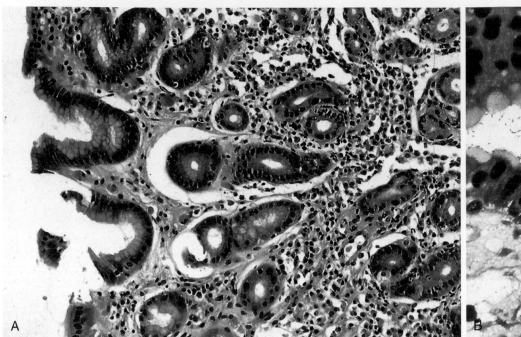

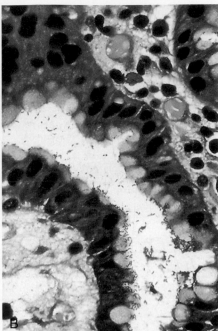

21 A 37-year-old underwent upper GI endoscopic examination for evaluation of abdominal pain, nausea, and vomiting. A biopsy of the gastric antrum was performed, and microscopic sections are shown in the figure above. This patient has an increased risk for developing what?

☐ A. Carcinoid tumor
☐ B. Gastrointestinal stromal tumor
☐ C. Lipoma
☐ D. MALT lymphoma
☐ E. Squamous cell carcinoma

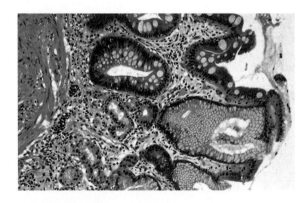

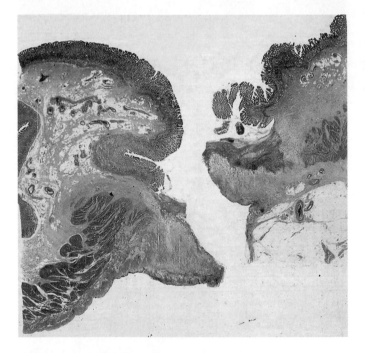

22 A 50-year-old woman complains of fatigue and abdominal pain. Upper GI endoscopy was performed, and a biopsy of the body of the stomach was obtained. Based on the microscopic finding of the biopsy shown in the figure above, which of the following is most likely to be present in this patient?

☐ A. Carcinoid tumor
☐ B. Celiac disease
☐ C. Gastric adenoma
☐ D. Pernicious anemia
☐ E. Stromal tumor

23 A 42-year-old man presented to the emergency room with severe abdominal pain. An exploratory laparotomy was performed, and a segment of the stomach was removed and sectioned for microscopy. Which of the following is a most likely consequence of the pathology shown in the above photomicrograph?

☐ A. Gastric carcinoma
☐ B. Hypoalbuminemia
☐ C. Malabsorption
☐ D. Megaloblastic anemia
☐ E. Peritonitis

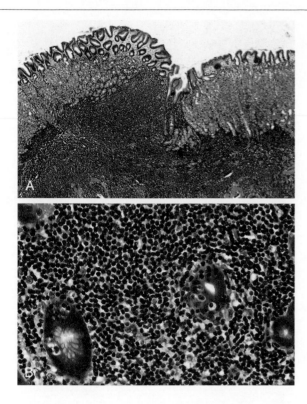

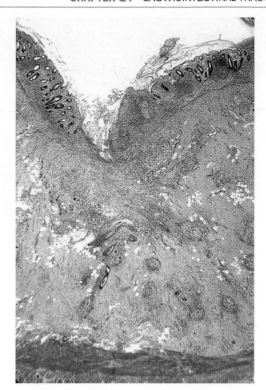

24 Upper GI endoscopy performed in a 49-year-old woman complaining of nausea and abdominal pain reveals a mass in the gastric antrum. The patient had been previously treated for *Helicobacter pylori* infection, with no response. A biopsy of the mass was performed, and microscopic sections revealed a lymphoma as shown in the figure above. Which of the following is a characteristic histologic finding in this tumor?

☐ A. Lymphoepithelial lesions
☐ B. Numerous follicles
☐ C. Pautrier microabscess
☐ D. Reed-Sternberg cells
☐ E. Starry-sky pattern

25 A 23-year-old woman with a history of diarrhea and weight loss presented to the emergency room with severe abdominal pain. An exploratory laparotomy was performed, and an abscess was found near the cecum, with a fistula tract between the small and large bowel. A segment of the ileum and cecum was removed, and a section of the affected segment is shown in the photomicrograph at top right. Which of the following is characteristic of this disease?

☐ A. Chronic inflammation with scattered granulomas
☐ B. Diffuse involvement of the intestine
☐ C. Inflammation limited to the mucosa
☐ D. Marked thinning of the intestinal wall
☐ E. Pseudomembrane formation

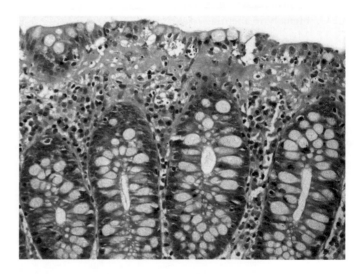

26 A 53-year-old woman underwent colonoscopy with biopsy of the colon. A microscopic section of her biopsy is shown in the figure above. Which of the following would most likely be present in this patient?

☐ A. Bright-red blood in stool
☐ B. Constipation
☐ C. Melena
☐ D. Steatorrhea
☐ E. Watery diarrhea

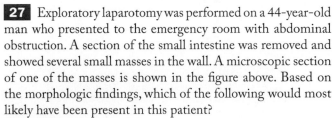

27 Exploratory laparotomy was performed on a 44-year-old man who presented to the emergency room with abdominal obstruction. A section of the small intestine was removed and showed several small masses in the wall. A microscopic section of one of the masses is shown in the figure above. Based on the morphologic findings, which of the following would most likely have been present in this patient?

☐ A. Flushing of the face
☐ B. Hematemesis
☐ C. Hemolytic anemia
☐ D. Myocardial infarction
☐ E. Sustained hypertension

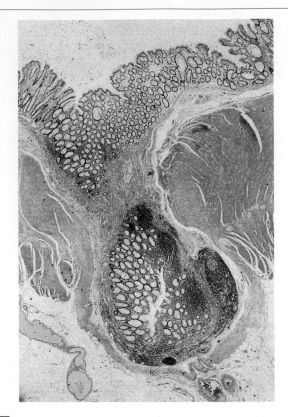

29 Examination of the colon in a 66-year-old woman reveals the pathology shown in the figure above. Which of the following is the most likely cause?

☐ A. Autoimmune destruction
☐ B. Bacterial inflammation
☐ C. Excess aspirin intake
☐ D. Low-fiber diet
☐ E. Sensitivity to gluten

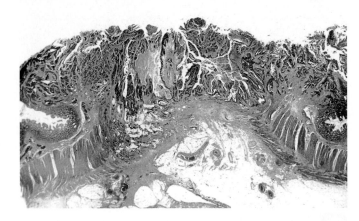

28 A 63-year-old man presented with abdominal pain. Exploratory laparotomy with total colectomy was performed. A microscopic section of the colon is shown in the figure above. Which of the following was most likely present in the patient before development of the lesion shown?

☐ A. Diverticula
☐ B. Hyperplastic polyp
☐ C. Inflammatory polyp
☐ D. Pseudomembranous colitis
☐ E. Villous adenoma

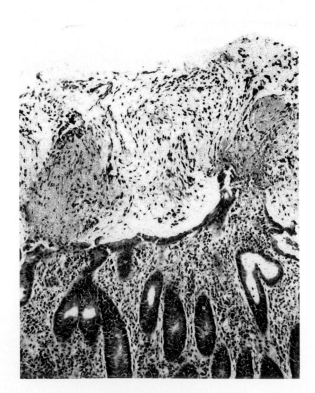

30 A 71-year-old man who is hospitalized for a chronic illness develops diarrhea. He underwent colonoscopy examination with biopsy of the colon. A microscopic section of his colon is shown in the figure at the bottom of the previous page. What organism most likely caused the infection resulting in his diarrhea?

☐ A. *Escherichia coli*
☐ B. *Clostridium difficile*
☐ C. *Salmonella enteritidis*
☐ D. *Shigella flexneri*
☐ E. *Staphylococcus aureus*

☐ A. *Clostridium difficile*
☐ B. *Entamoeba histolytica*
☐ C. *Escherichia coli*
☐ D. *Giardia lamblia*
☐ E. *Schistosomia haematobium*

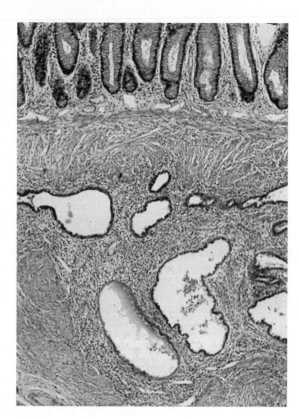

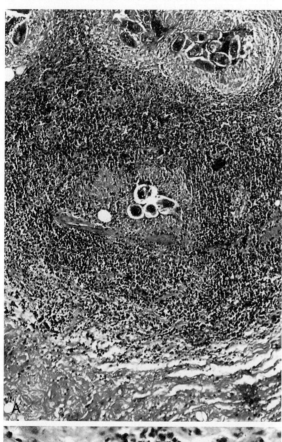

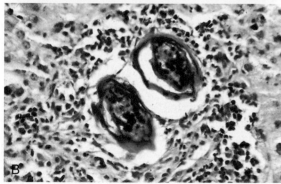

31 A 46-year-old man presented to his primary care physician with complaints of abdominal pain. He immigrated to the United States from Egypt, where he had worked as a farmer near the Nile River. He was referred to a gastroenterologist, who performed a colonoscopy and biopsy of his colon. A microscopic section of his colon in the figure above shows infection by which of the following organisms?

32 A 35-year-old woman presented to the emergency room with severe abdominal pain. She underwent exploratory laparotomy with segmental resection of her colon. A microscopic examination revealed the pathology shown in the figure above. In addition, numerous hemosiderin-laden macrophages were present. Which of the following is the most likely cause of her abdominal pain?

☐ A. Carcinoid tumor
☐ B. Crohn disease
☐ C. Diverticula
☐ D. Intestinal adhesions
☐ E. Pseudomembranous colitis

ANSWERS

1. C The simple columnar esophageal epithelium in Barrett esophagus resembles that of the intestine or the stomach. The typical epithelial lining of the esophagus is stratified squamous epithelium. Pseudostratified epithelium is characteristic of the larynx, trachea, and bronchi. Stratified columnar epithelium is limited to excretory ducts of salivary glands. Transitional epithelium lines part of the urinary system.
FH p. 268, BH pp. 143-144

2. A The normal squamous epithelium of the esophagus has undergone metaplasia to glandular (simple columnar) epithelium. This is seen in Barrett esophagus, which is caused by long-standing acid reflux. Dilation of veins occurs as a result of portal hypertension in patients with cirrhosis. In such cases, the veins in the submucosa of the lower esophagus are distended and cause ulceration (not metaplasia) of the overlying mucosa. *Candida* infection of the esophagus results in whitish plaques on the epithelium that are composed of necrotic squamous epithelium with embedded fungi. A high-fat diet by itself does not cause Barrett esophagus. If a patient consuming a high-fat diet becomes obese, the elevated abdominal pressure may cause acid reflux and Barrett esophagus. The epithelial metaplasia is an acquired disease and not a congenital disorder. **FH p. 268, BH pp. 143-144**

3. A Patients with Barrett esophagus have an increased risk for developing adenocarcinoma, a malignancy arising in the metaplastic epithelium. Hence, the esophageal epithelium must be monitored regularly by endoscopic examinations with biopsies. Because the metaplastic epithelium is a columnar epithelium, the neoplasm would be an adenocarcinoma, not a squamous cell carcinoma. The other tumors listed occur primarily in the stomach or small intestine and are not associated with Barrett esophagus. **FH p. 268, BH pp. 143-144**

4. B The cells formed by this metaplastic transformation produce a bicarbonate-rich secretion that protects the stratified squamous epithelium against the effects of stomach acid. Acid, defeasins, and gastric intrinsic factor are all secreted in the stomach by gastric parietal cells. These are concentrated in the upper parts of the glands in the fundus of the stomach. Chief cells produce pepsinogen, which is cleaved to pepsin. **FH p. 268, BH pp. 143-144**

5. C The presence of the gastric pits and the lamina propria filled with glands are identifying features of the stomach mucosa. Crypts (intestinal glands) would be found in the appendix and large intestine, whereas villi would be present as well in the small intestine. Normal stratified squamous nonkeratinized epithelium characteristic of the esophagus is not present in the figure. **FH pp. 269-270, BH p. 146**

6. C The cell at C is a gastric chief cell which secretes pepsin and can be identified as the main cell type at the base of the gastric glands. **FH p. 272**

7. B Neuroendocrine cells in the gastric glands secrete serotonin and other peptides. Neuroendocrine cells are recognized as pale-staining cells in the gastric glands. **FH p. 269, 272**

8. D Only plasma cells in the lamina propria synthesize IgA. IgA is then transcytosed into the lumen by the gastric epithelial cells. The other cell types listed are part of the gastric glands and surface epithelium. The chief cells produce enzymes; the neuroendocrine, or enteroendocrine, cells secrete various local-acting hormones; parietal cells secrete the stomach acid and gastric intrinsic factor, and export bicarbonate to the lamina propria; surface epithelial cells produce a protective mucus, which incorporates this bicarbonate from the parietal cells. **FH pp. 208-209, 226, BH p. 28**

9. E The figure shows a transverse section of the upper gastric mucosa with cross sections of the gastric pits, lined by a continuous layer of mucus-secreting epithelial cells. The regular appearance of the epithelium differentiates this from the esophageal or duodenal glands. The crypts of the jejunum or colon have scattered mucus-secreting cells distributed among columnar cells. **FH p. 270**

10. D The figure shows a diffuse infiltration of the stomach wall by neoplastic cells. The cells exhibit cytoplasmic mucin-filled vacuoles pushing the nuclei to the periphery of the cells and are therefore referred to as *signet ring cells*. This is characteristic of the diffuse type of gastric carcinoma. Because these tumors infiltrate the wall of the stomach diffusely, they result in a marked thickening of the stomach wall, which resembles a leather bottle (linitis plastica). Acid reflux causes metaplasia of the squamous epithelium in the esophagus. Celiac disease is an inflammatory disorder of the small intestine characterized by inflammation and atrophy of the small intestinal mucosa. Crohn disease is also an inflammatory disease that most commonly affects the small intestine mucosa and deeper layers. Peptic ulcer occurs in the stomach and small bowel. The affected epithelium would show ulceration with a necrotic mucosa. **FH p. 270, BH p. 149**

11. B The figure shows dysplasia of the gastric epithelium characterized by irregular glands with enlarged, hyperchromatic, crowded nuclei. The cells exhibit loss of polarity. Dysplasia may arise in patients with long-standing chronic gastritis. Gastric atrophy and intestinal metaplasia are also caused by chronic gastritis. The chronic inflammation leads to atrophy and loss of gastric glands, which are replaced either by fibrosis or intestinal-type metaplastic epithelium. The latter is characterized by goblet cells and Paneth cells but does not show evidence of dysplasia. In lymphoma, the gastric glands would be replaced by infiltrating lymphocytes, and a peptic ulcer would show necrosis and ulceration of the normal mucosa, **FH p. 270, BH p. 148**

12. D The figure shows a parietal cell, recognized by its intracellular canaliculi and many mitochondria. These cells produce the gastric intrinsic factor needed for absorption of vitamin B_{12} in the ileum. Gastrin and secretin are produced by enteroendocrine cells. Vitamin D can be made by the skin or acquired from the diet. **FH p. 271**

13. C The acid pumps are located in the membranes of the canaliculi, which form an open channel to the outside of the cell. **FH p. 271**

14. E The figure shows villous atrophy and infiltration of the mucosa by lymphocytes. This is a characteristic histologic finding in celiac disease, which results in malabsorption. As a result, the stool contains increased amounts of unabsorbed fat (steatorrhea), and the stool is bulky and foul smelling. A small amount of blood may be present in the stool as a result of the inflammation; however, it is usually too small to cause a bloody diarrhea or a black discoloration of the stool (melena). Dysphasia (difficulty swallowing) is caused by diseases of the oropharynx or esophagus, but not the small bowel. Vomiting with or without blood is not a feature of celiac disease. **FH p. 275, BH p. 151**

15. C Long-standing malabsorption with villous atrophy, diarrhea, and steatorrhea is characteristic of celiac disease, which is caused by hypersensitivity to gluten. This disease can be easily managed by strict adherence to a gluten-free diet, which results in a restitution of the normal mucosa. Surgery and drug therapy are not treatment modalities. Vitamin B_{12} injections may be useful to treat megaloblastic anemia, if the malabsorption has resulted in a deficiency of this vitamin; however, administration of this vitamin does not treat the disease. **BH p. 151, FH p. 275**

16. C Lactase is a membrane protein, which forms part of the glycocalyx lining the microvilli of the intestinal absorptive cells. **FH pp. 4-5, 276**

17. D The cells indicated are Paneth cells, which reside at the base of the crypts of Lieberkühn. They secrete a variety of antimicrobial substances such as lysozyme and defensins. Digestive enzymes are synthesized by the epithelial absorptive cells on the villi and by the pancreas. Peptide hormones are synthesized by neuroendocrine cells in the intestinal epithelium. Heavily glycosylated proteins (mucins) are secreted by goblet cells. Most cells synthesize lysosomal enzymes, but they generally are used internally and are not secreted. **FH p. 282**

18. E The figure shows acute and chronic inflammation with a crypt abscess, mucosal inflammation, ulceration and an inflammatory pseudopolyp. These features are characteristic of ulcerative colitis. Patients with ulcerative colitis have an increased risk for developing adenocarcinoma of the colon, but the glands in these images do not show evidence of dysplasia. In polyposis coli (familial adenomatous polyposis), caused by a mutation in the *APC* gene, there is a formation of numerous adenomatous polyps throughout the colon. These polyps are neoplastic, not inflammatory. Diverticulitis occurs when a segment of colonic mucosa that has herniated through the wall gets inflamed. This condition is common in older individuals and is rare before the age of 40 years. Moreover, the inflammation is limited to the herniated segment of the colon. In collagenous colitis, there is a thickened band of collagen in the lamina propria, which may be accompanied by lymphocytic infiltration of the epithelium. The inflammation is evident only microscopically, with no disruption or ulceration of the mucosa. This latter disease affects older individuals. **FH p. 283, BH p. 156**

19. D Ulcerative colitis is characterized by involvement of the rectum, with inflammation that extends proximally in a continuous fashion to involve the remaining colon. The inflammation is limited to the mucosa with superficial ulcers. Crohn disease and ulcerative colitis are closely related inflammatory bowel diseases that are distinguished based on the location, extent of inflammation, and types of complications that develop. The other choices listed are characteristic of Crohn disease, not ulcerative colitis. **BH pp. 156-157**

20. E M cells are found in the intestinal epithelium covering lymphoid nodules. They transcytose whole antigens from the intestinal lumen and deliver them to immune cells in the lamina propria. Endocytosis of the oral vaccine by absorptive cells would result in its digestion and loss of function. Little paracellular transport occurs in the intestinal epithelium. Absorptive cells transcytose IgA into the lumen, but do not bring material into the mucosa that way. Immunoglobulins may be transcytosed by endothelial cells, but these molecules would only reach the endothelial cells after being exposed to the immune cells while passing though the lamina propria. **FH p. 228, 285**

21. D The figure shows *Helicobacter pylori*–induced chronic gastritis as evidenced by the presence of bacilli on the surface of the epithelium. There is an increased risk for developing MALT lymphoma and adenocarcinoma of the stomach in this setting. The other tumors listed have no association with *Helicobacter pylori*. **BH pp. 146-147**

22. D The figure shows atrophy of the gastric glands, loss of parietal cells, and intestinal metaplasia, which are features of chronic atrophic gastritis. This entity is associated with autoantibodies to gastric parietal cells. The subsequent deficiency of intrinsic factor results in pernicious anemia. The other choices listed are more common in the small intestine and the colon and have no association with atrophic gastritis. **FH p. 269, 271, BH p. 146**

23. E The figure shows a perforated gastric ulcer. Discharge of gastric contents in the peritoneal cavity would result in peritonitis. Gastric ulcers caused by inflammation do not undergo malignant transformation; therefore, carcinoma is not a complication. The stomach produces intrinsic factor necessary for absorption of vitamin B_{12}; a deficiency of the latter results in megaloblastic anemia. Diseases that affect a large area of the stomach such as chronic gastritis (not a single ulcer) would result in a deficiency of intrinsic factor. Absorption of protein and other nutrients occurs in the small intestines and is not affected by a gastric ulcer. **BH p. 147**

24. A Lymphoepithelial lesions are characterized by intraepithelial infiltration by clusters of lymphocytes and subsequent destruction of the epithelium. These lesions are typically seen in MALT lymphomas. The other histologic findings are characteristically seen in other types of lymphomas:

numerous follicles in follicular lymphomas; Pautrier micro-abscess in mycoses fungoides; Reed-Sternberg cells in Hodg-kin lymphoma, and starry-sky pattern in Burkitt lymphoma. **BH p. 145, 204**

25. A The clinical presentation and the microscopic find-ings are consistent with Crohn disease, which is character-ized by a transmural chronic inflammation and scattered granulomas. Pseudomembrane formation is due to a bacterial infection. The other choices listed are more commonly seen in ulcerative colitis. **BH p. 154**

26. E The figure shows features of collagenous colitis characterized by a thick band of collagen below the base-ment membrane and an increased number of intraepithelial lymphocytes. In this disease, the inflammation in the colon is microscopic, with no ulceration of the mucosa; therefore, these patients present with chronic nonbloody, watery diar-rhea. Bright-red blood in the stool is more commonly seen in hemorrhoids or rectal cancer. Constipation is a nonspe-cific symptom that may be seen in a variety of colon dis-orders, but is not a feature of collagenous colitis. Melena or black, tarry stool occurs when the blood in the GI tract has been there long enough for red blood cells to be bro-ken down and the hemoglobin to become oxidized. There-fore, it is associated with bleeding from the upper GI tract (stomach or duodenum). Steatorrhea or increased fat in the stool occurs in malabsorption diseases of the small intestine. **BH p. 155**

27. A The figure shows a nesting and trabecular pattern of small uniform cells. These are characteristic features of carci-noid tumors of neuroendocrine origin. These tumors secrete a variety of hormone products, such as serotonin, which may cause the carcinoid syndrome, characterized by flushing, abdominal cramps, diarrhea, and wheezing. Hematemesis is not a usual symptom of carcinoid syndrome. If the small intestine is significantly involved by carcinoid tumor, mal-absorption of vitamin B_{12} may result in a megaloblastic, not hemolytic, anemia. Carcinoid syndrome may affect the heart, with fibrosis of the cardiac valves resulting in valvular dys-function and subsequent congestive heart failure, not myo-cardial infarction. The flushing seen in carcinoid syndrome is due to vasodilation, which usually results in hypotension. **BH p. 149**

28. E The figure shows adenocarcinoma of the colon. Ade-nomas, both tubular and villous, have the potential to undergo malignant transformation, and most adenocarcinomas of the

colon arise from adenomas. The other choices listed are nei-ther neoplastic nor predisposed to the development of adeno-carcinomas. **BH pp. 158-161**

29. D The diverticula shown in the figure are herniations of colonic mucosa caused by the increased intraluminal pres-sure associated with a low-fiber diet. Sensitivity to gluten with subsequent autoimmune destruction of the intestinal mucosa leads to villous atrophy, not diverticula. Excessive aspirin intake results in inflammation and damage to the gastric mucosa, and bacterial inflammation causes mucosal damage in the infected segment of the GI tract; neither condition results in the for-mation of diverticula. **BH p. 157**

30. B The figure shows an inflammatory exudate com-posed of necrotic epithelium and fibrin that overlies the colonic mucosa. This is characteristic of pseudomembranous colitis, which is caused by the bacteria *Clostridium difficile*. The bacteria produce a toxin that causes necrosis of the epithelium. Elderly patients who are being treated by some antibiotics are at risk for developing this condition because the antibiotics eliminate the normal bacterial flora, allowing uncontrolled multiplication of the *C. difficile*. The other organisms listed are common causes of infectious diarrhea. However, they are not associated with pseudomembrane formation or antibiotic usage. **BH p. 37**

31. E The figure shows eggs of *Schistosomia haematobium*, which are characterized by their terminally located spine. Schistosomes are parasitic trematodes that are endemic to the Nile delta. This organism infects people when they bathe in contaminated water. The larvae enter through the skin and travel to the liver, where they mature. The eggs produced by the adults are excreted in feces or urine. They may also enter the gut and lodge in the intestinal epithelium. All the other organisms listed can cause infections of the colon, but the eggs, characteristic of schistosomes, are not seen in infections caused by these organisms. **BH p. 52**

32. D In the figure, uterine endometrial glands and stroma are seen embedded in the muscular layer of the colon. The pres-ence of endometrial glands and stroma outside of the uterus is termed *endometriosis*. These glands undergo cyclical changes in response to estrogen and progesterone and often show evidence of hemorrhage. An inflammatory reaction leads to fibrosis, adhesions, and obstruction of the organs involved by endometriosis. The other choices listed can all cause intestinal obstruction; however, endometrial tissue would not be present in the wall of the intestine in these cases. **BH p. 223**

FH5 Chapter 1: Cell Structure and Function
FH5 Chapter 15: Liver and Pancreas
BH5 Chapter 7: Neoplasia
BH5 Chapter 14: Hepatobiliary System

15

Liver and Pancreas

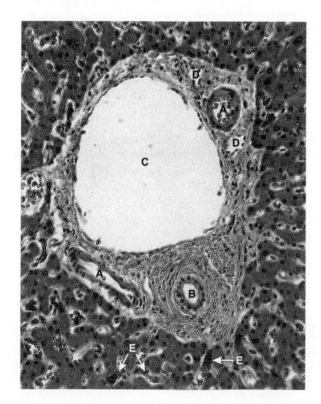

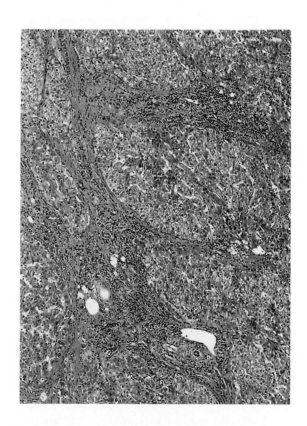

Use the figure above to answer the next two questions.

1 Which structure shown in the figure above conveys exocrine secretions?

2 Which structure contains the most poorly oxygenated blood?

Use the figure above to answer the next three questions.

3 A liver biopsy performed in a 55-year-old man with abdominal pain and hepatomegaly is shown in the figure above. What would be a direct consequence of this pathologic change?

☐ A. Cardiomegaly
☐ B. Hepatic vein thrombosis
☐ C. Portal hypertension
☐ D. Splenic atrophy
☐ E. Varices in the legs

4 Based on the biopsy findings, which hormonal abnormality may be present in this patient?
☐ A. Acromegaly
☐ B. Cushing syndrome
☐ C. Gynecomastia
☐ D. Hyperaldosteronism
☐ E. Hyperparathyroidism

5 Which of the following would most likely be present on physical examination of the same patient?
☐ A. Ascites
☐ B. Cyanosis of the fingers
☐ C. Elevated jugular venous pressure
☐ D. Plethora of the face
☐ E. Silvery-white scaly lesions on the elbow

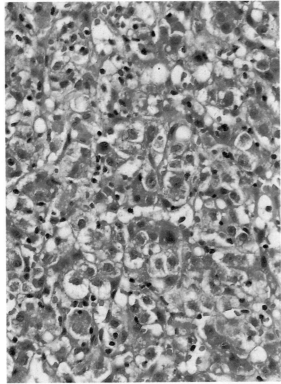

Use the figure above to answer the next two questions.

6 A 32-year-old woman presented to her primary care physician with nausea, vomiting, and abdominal pain. She had recently returned from vacationing in Central America. Her liver was enlarged and tender on examination. A liver biopsy was performed, and a microscopic section is shown in the figure above. Based on the biopsy finding, serologic testing for hepatitis was requested and showed the presence of antibody to hepatitis A virus. Through what means did the patient most likely acquire the infection?
☐ A. Air droplets
☐ B. Blood transfusion
☐ C. Contaminated food or water
☐ D. Needle sharing
☐ E. Sexual intercourse

7 What is the most likely outcome in this patient?
☐ A. Carrier state
☐ B. Complete resolution
☐ C. Development of cirrhosis
☐ D. Prolonged chronic inflammation
☐ E. Rapid progression to chronic hepatitis

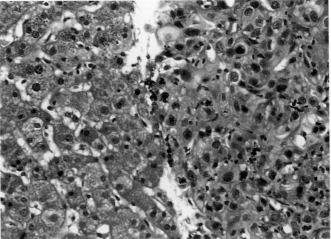

Use the figure above to answer the next three questions.

8 A 52-year-old man is admitted to the hospital with abdominal pain and general malaise. He had taken analgesics to relieve the pain. Past medical history is positive for chronic hepatitis. A CT scan of the abdomen shows a 5-cm nodular lesion in the right lobe of the liver. A biopsy of his liver is shown in the figure above. What pathology is depicted?
☐ A. Biliary cirrhosis
☐ B. Cholestasis
☐ C. Chronic unresolved hepatitis
☐ D. Hepatocellular carcinoma
☐ E. Massive liver necrosis

9 Which of the following is a most likely predisposing factor?
☐ A. Acetaminophen toxicity
☐ B. Alcohol abuse
☐ C. Gallstones
☐ D. Hepatitis A virus
☐ E. Smoking

10 In the same patient, laboratory studies would show elevated serum levels of what?
☐ A. Alpha-fetoprotein
☐ B. Carcinoembryonic antigen
☐ C. CA 19.5
☐ D. CA 125
☐ E. Human chorionic gonadotropin

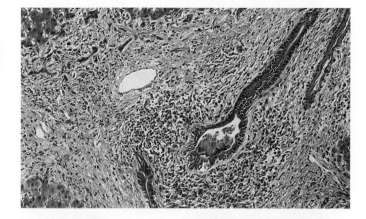

11 A 45-year-old woman presented with chronic complaints of itching. She had icteric sclera on physical examination. Laboratory studies showed elevated bilirubin, and the liver was found to be enlarged on a CT scan. A liver biopsy was performed, and a microscopic section is shown in the figure above. What is the most likely cause of the pathology depicted?
☐ A. Acute viral hepatitis
☐ B. Alcohol-induced hepatocyte injury
☐ C. Inflammatory destruction of bile ducts
☐ D. Iron overload
☐ E. Metabolic derangement

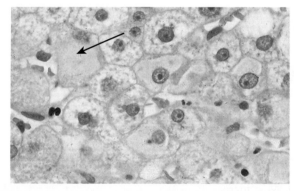

12 A 41-year-old man presented with nausea and abdominal pain of several months' duration. On physical examination, the liver was palpable below the costal margin. A liver biopsy was performed, and a microscopic section is shown in the figure above. Based on the cell indicated by the *arrow*, measurement of the serum levels of which of the following would be most useful?
☐ A. Alcohol
☐ B. Alpha-1 antitrypsin
☐ C. Copper
☐ D. Hepatitis B antigen
☐ E. Insulin

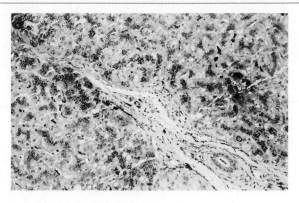

Use the figure above to answer the next three questions.

13 A 35-year-old man has come to his physician complaining of fatigue, weight gain, and a depressed libido. He is a smoker and drinks one cocktail each night after returning home from work. He noted that his grandfather had suffered from liver disease. A biopsy of his liver, shown in the figure above, stains intensely blue after exposure to the histochemical reagents used for the Perl reaction. From what is this patient likely suffering?
☐ A. Alcoholic cirrhosis with fatty change
☐ B. Cholestasis
☐ C. Chronic hepatitis
☐ D. Hemochromatosis
☐ E. Hepatocellular carcinoma

14 What is the most likely cause of the pathology described above?
☐ A. Bone marrow suppression
☐ B. Chronic GI bleeding
☐ C. Drug toxicity
☐ D. Gallstones
☐ E. Genetic defect

15 Which of the following abnormalities also may be present in the same patient?
☐ A. Acromegaly
☐ B. Conn syndrome
☐ C. Cushing syndrome
☐ D. Diabetes mellitus
☐ E. Hypoparathyroidism

16 The specialized capillaries between rows of hepatocytes have which unique characteristic?
☐ A. Adjacent endothelial cells are bound together by extensive tight junctions
☐ B. The endothelial cells have fenestrae covered by fine filaments
☐ C. The endothelial cells possess numerous pinocytic vesicles
☐ D. The endothelial cells secrete a discontinuous basal lamina

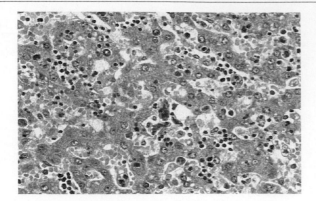

Use the figure above to answer the next two questions.

17 A 35-year-old woman was examined by a physician after complaining of chronic fatigue. Physical examination revealed hepatosplenomegaly. A liver biopsy was obtained and is shown in the figure above. What is this abnormal condition?
- [ ] A. Dysplasia of Kupffer cells
- [ ] B. Excessive blood levels of bilirubin
- [ ] C. Excessive transport of iron to the liver
- [ ] D. Hepatocellular carcinoma
- [ ] E. Intrahepatic hematopoiesis

18 The above abnormality may be seen in which of the following diseases?
- [ ] A. Aplastic anemia
- [ ] B. Iron deficiency anemia
- [ ] C. Megaloblastic anemia
- [ ] D. Sideroblastic anemia
- [ ] E. Thalassemia major

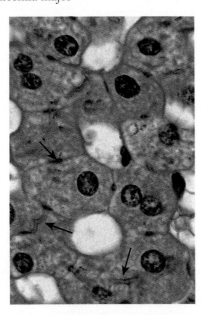

19 This preparation has been stained to show the structures indicated by the *arrows*. What are they?
- [ ] A. Communicating (gap) junctions
- [ ] B. Dilated cisternae of the endoplasmic reticulum
- [ ] C. Extracellular channels
- [ ] D. Glycogen storage deposits
- [ ] E. Intracellular channels

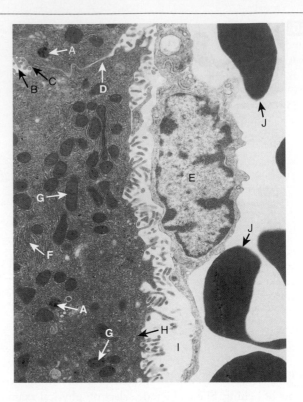

Use the figure above to answer the next four questions. Match the descriptions with the letters on the figure.

20 This figure shows a transmission electron micrograph of a small fragment of the liver. Identify the site where albumin is synthesized.

21 Alkaline phosphatase is localized here.

22 Oxidation of fatty acids occurs here.

23 The escape of bile from which labeled location will result in jaundice?

24 The figure at top left of the next page shows a section of a biopsy of the gallbladder from a 45-year-old man with chronic cholecystitis. Which layer in the organ, shown in the figure, is abnormally thickened?
- [ ] A. Adventitia
- [ ] B. Lamina propria
- [ ] C. Luminal epithelium
- [ ] D. Muscularis

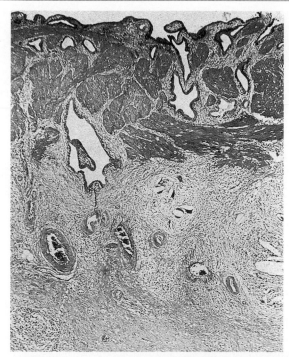

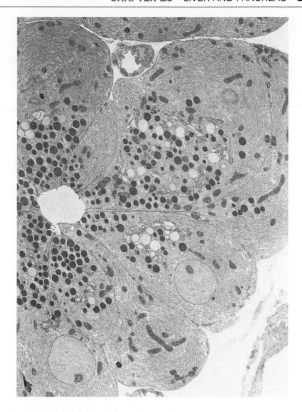

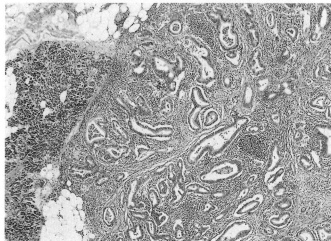

27 This electron micrograph depicts cells found where?
- ☐ A. Bile ducts
- ☐ B. Endocrine pancreas
- ☐ C. Exocrine pancreas
- ☐ D. Gallbladder
- ☐ E. Liver parenchyma

Use the figure above to answer the next two questions.

25 A 58-year-old woman complaining of abdominal pain and weight loss was found to have a mass in the head of the pancreas. A biopsy of the mass was performed and a microscopic section is shown in the figure above. What is the most likely origin of the lesion?
- ☐ A. Islets of Langerhans
- ☐ B. Pancreatic acini
- ☐ C. Pancreatic ducts
- ☐ D. Scattered neuroendocrine cells
- ☐ E. Supporting connective tissue

26 Which of the following would most likely be present in the above patient?
- ☐ A. Diabetes mellitus
- ☐ B. Fat necrosis
- ☐ C. Gallstones
- ☐ D. GI hemorrhage
- ☐ E. Jaundice

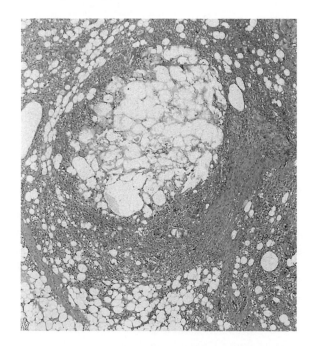

Use the figure above to answer the next two questions.

28 A 37-year-old man presented to the emergency room with severe abdominal pain and expired shortly afterward. An autopsy showed that numerous chalky-white spots were present on the omentum and peripancreatic tissue. A microscopic section of one of these areas is shown in the figure. What is the cause of this pathology?

☐ A. Autoimmune destruction
☐ B. Bacterial inflammation
☐ C. Enzymatic digestion
☐ D. Malignant cell infiltration
☐ E. Vascular occlusion

29 Which of the following is a most likely predisposing factor for the development of the above condition?

☐ A. Alcohol abuse
☐ B. Atherosclerosis
☐ C. Gluten sensitivity
☐ D. Hepatitis
☐ E. Obesity

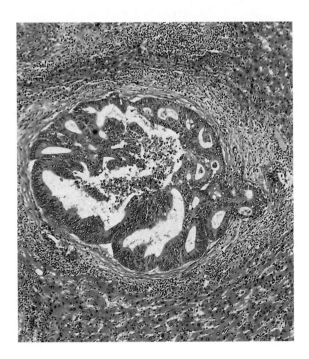

30 A 60-year-old woman presented to her physician with a history of constipation and a 25-pound unintentional weight loss. On physical examination, she appeared cachectic, and her sclera was icteric. Her liver was palpable 5 cm below the right costal margin. A guaiac test is positive for blood in the stool, and serum bilirubin is elevated. A liver biopsy was performed, and a microscopic image is shown in the figure above. Which of the following is the most likely diagnosis?

☐ A. Carcinoid tumor
☐ B. Hepatocellular carcinoma
☐ C. Metastatic adenocarcinoma
☐ D. Small cell carcinoma
☐ E. Squamous cell carcinoma

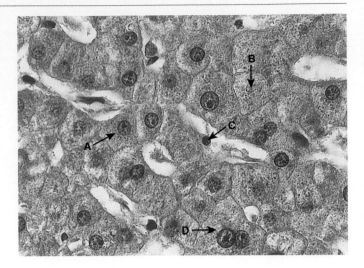

31 A 56-year-old man visits his physician as a follow-up to a car accident. A portion of his liver had been damaged. The physician took a biopsy and had it sectioned. The image is shown in the figure above. Which lettered structure provides evidence for liver growth and regeneration?

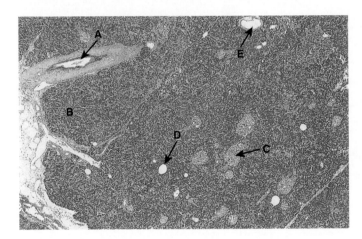

32 Blockage of the pancreatic duct can cause release of pancreatic lipase and destruction of nearby adipose tissue. The cells in which lettered area synthesize the pancreatic enzymes?

ANSWERS

1. B This is a bile duct in the portal tract of the liver. It conveys bile, which will pass to the gallbladder to be concentrated and stored. The other hollow structures are blood vessels and have a simple squamous epithelium, unlike the simple cuboidal epithelium characteristic of bile ducts. **FH pp. 290, 295**

2. C This is a branch of the portal vein that carries nutrients to the hepatocytes. This blood is collected from the digestive tract, where it is partially depleted of oxygen. Blood in the sinusoids (E) also contains portal blood, but because it is mixed with oxygenated blood from branches of the hepatic artery (A), it would contain more oxygen than that of the portal vein. **FH pp. 288-290**

3. C The figure shows cirrhosis of the liver with disruption of the lobular architecture by bands of fibrous tissue and regenerating nodules. This architectural disruption results in alteration of blood flow in the liver with subsequent development of portal hypertension. The portal hypertension in turn leads to congestion and enlargement of the spleen (not atrophy). The portal hypertension can cause anastomoses between the portal and venous circulation leading to the formation of varices in various areas. However, varices in the legs are due to incompetence of the valves within the legs, not to portal hypertension. When cardiomegaly leads to chronic congestive heart failure, the liver may be damaged secondary to congestion, and hence, cardiomegaly would be a cause, not a consequence of cirrhosis. Hepatic vein thrombosis (Budd-Chiari syndrome) is idiopathic or associated with thrombotic disorders, but usually is not caused by cirrhosis. If the thrombosis involves many branches of the portal vein, it can lead to cirrhosis. **BH pp. 169-171, FH pp. 288-289**

4. C In cirrhosis, failure to metabolize endogenous estrogens leads to stimulation and enlargement of the breast in males (i.e., gynecomastia). The levels of other endocrine hormones are not increased in liver cirrhosis. Therefore acromegaly (due to elevated GH), hyperaldosteronism, or hyperparathyroidism would not be expected in this patient. **BH pp. 164, 169-171, FH pp. 288-289**

5. A In cirrhosis, low serum albumin and portal hypertension result in ascites and edema of the lower extremities. The other conditions listed are not associated with liver cirrhosis. Cyanosis of the extremities results from localized vasoconstriction or the presence of deoxygenated blood in the arterial circulation. Elevated jugular venous pressure occurs as a result of congestion of the superior vena cava due to obstruction or heart failure. Plethora of the face occurs in persons with elevated hemoglobin and hematocrit (polycythemia). Silvery-white scaly lesions on the elbow are seen in patients with psoriasis. **BH pp. 164, 169-171, FH pp. 288-289**

6. C Hepatitis A virus is transmitted by the fecal-oral route through contaminated food or water. Hepatitis B and C viruses are both transmitted parenterally through blood transfusion, needle sharing, or sexual intercourse. None of the hepatitis viruses are transmitted by air droplets. **BH p. 165-168, FH p. 290**

7. B Hepatitis A virus causes acute viral hepatitis that is usually mild and self-limited with complete recovery. Carrier state and chronic hepatitis with development of cirrhosis are seen in hepatitis B and C viral infections, but are not caused by hepatitis A. **BH p. 165, 167, FH p. 290**

8. D The mass of small, rapidly dividing hepatocytes with loss of the orderly architecture of the liver seen in the right half of this figure is characteristic of hepatocellular carcinoma. In biliary cirrhosis, there is an inflammatory destruction of bile ducts, with granuloma and fibrosis. Chronic hepatitis is characterized by inflammation with lymphocytic infiltration of the liver. Obstruction of bile flow leads to cholestasis, which would be manifested clinically as jaundice. Histologically, yellow bile pigment would be present within the sinusoids and hepatocytes. In massive liver necrosis, the sinusoids would be collapsed, and the liver cells would be necrotic, with eosinophilic cytoplasm and loss of their nuclei. **FH p. 290, BH p. 172**

9. B Alcohol abuse and chronic viral infections with hepatitis B and C viruses are major predisposing factors for hepatocellular carcinoma. The other choices listed are not associated with an increased risk for developing hepatocellular carcinoma. Acetaminophen toxicity results in massive hepatic necrosis. Gallstones may cause biliary obstruction and jaundice. Hepatitis A virus causes an acute, self-limited hepatitis. Cigarette smoking has not been significantly associated with hepatocellular carcinoma. **BH p. 172**

10. A Alpha-fetoprotein is secreted into the serum by the cancer cells in hepatocellular carcinoma and is a useful diagnostic marker for this tumor. It is also used as a marker for germ cell tumors. The other choices listed are serum markers that are useful in diagnosing or monitoring a variety of tumors; carcinoembryonic antigen for colon cancer; CA 19.5 for pancreatic cancer; CA 125 for ovarian cancer; and human chorionic gonadotropin for gestational trophoblastic and germ cell tumors. **BH p. 172**

11. C The figure shows chronic inflammation and destruction of bile ducts, with proliferation of small bile ducts and fibrosis of portal tracts. These features are characteristic of primary biliary cirrhosis, a chronic disease of the liver with inflammatory destruction of bile ducts. Alcohol, iron overload, and metabolic derangement such as obesity, diabetes, and Wilson disease are all associated with the development of cirrhosis. In these cases, unlike primary biliary cirrhosis, selective inflammation and destruction of the bile ducts does not occur. Acute viral hepatitis is not associated with the development of cirrhosis, unless it progresses to chronic hepatitis. **BH p. 169, FH p. 290**

12. D In chronic hepatitis caused by the hepatitis B virus, the cytoplasm of hepatocytes stains pink with a ground-glass appearance caused by accumulation of viral particles. The viral particles (antigens) are found in the serum and can be identified to confirm the diagnosis. Excess of alcohol and copper and deficiencies of alpha-1 antitrypsin and insulin can all lead to liver damage with cirrhosis. However, the characteristic ground-glass appearance of hepatocytes is not seen in these cases. **BH p. 168, FH p. 290**

13. D The figure shows excessive amounts of iron deposited within hepatocytes as demonstrated by the Perl stain.

Accumulation of iron in liver hepatocytes is most likely due to hemochromatosis, a disorder of iron metabolism that can damage the liver and pituitary gland, leading to liver dysfunction and reduced pituitary hormone secretion. Alcohol, viruses, and other toxins can cause chronic hepatitis and lead to liver cirrhosis. In these cases, iron can accumulate in the damaged hepatocytes. However, in such cases, the iron accumulation in the liver is not usually this extensive, and evidence of damage to other organs is not seen. In cholestasis, bile, not iron, accumulates in the liver, and bile does not stain with the Perl reaction. **FH p. 294, BH p. 171**

14. E Excess iron deposition in the liver that occurs in hemochromatosis is due to an inherited defect in a protein regulating iron absorption. Bone marrow suppression may lead to an inability of marrow cells to use iron. In this case, iron accumulates in the marrow, not in the liver. Chronic GI bleeding causes loss of iron, not excess deposition. Drug toxicity can damage the liver; however, it is usually acute, and iron deposition is unlikely. Gallstones may cause accumulation of bile, not iron. **BH p. 171**

15. D In hemochromatosis, excess iron may be deposited in the pancreas. This causes destruction of the islet cells and leads to diabetes mellitus. Also, deposition of iron in the pituitary can impair hormone secretion, which would lead to growth hormone deficiency, not acromegaly, and to decreased ACTH, rather than to an increase in ACTH and Cushing syndrome. The excess iron does not deposit in significant amounts in the adrenal glands. If it did, it would lead to a deficiency, not an increase of adrenocortical hormones, which is seen in Conn syndrome. Likewise, the excess iron does not deposit in the parathyroid in significant amounts to cause hypoparathyroidism. **BH p. 171**

16. D Although both fenestrated capillaries and sinusoids have fenestrations, only the sinusoids have a discontinuous basal lamina and spaces (gaps) between adjacent endothelial cells. This arrangement allows hepatocytes to have easy access to the blood in the sinusoids. **FH p. 294, 297**

17. E The figure shows intrahepatic hematopoiesis. In disorders involving the bone marrow, extramedullary hematopoiesis may be stimulated in organs such as the kidney or liver. The appearance of megakaryocytes and normoblasts in the liver is thus a compensation for impaired marrow function. These normal cells do not resemble abnormal Kupffer cells or cancerous hepatocytes. **FH p. 295**

18. E Thalassemia major is a genetic disorder of hemoglobin resulting in severe hemolytic anemia. The marrow is unable to keep up with the excess destruction of RBCs, and the liver and spleen become sites of extramedullary hematopoiesis. All the other anemias listed are hypoproliferative anemias characterized by a decreased production of RBCs. Extramedullary hematopoiesis does not occur in these types of anemias. **FH p. 295**

19. C These cells are hepatocytes, and they have been stained to show the bile canaliculi, which are extracellular channels running between adjacent hepatocytes. Gap junctions are too small to be visualized with light microscopy, whereas the other choices in this question are located within the cell cytoplasm rather than being associated with the cell membrane. **FH p. 295**

20. F This is the rough endoplasmic reticulum. Albumin is a secreted protein and is thus synthesized on the rough endoplasmic reticulum of the hepatocyte. **FH pp. 296-297**

21. B Alkaline phosphatase is found on the bile canaliculus membrane. If abnormal levels are detected in the blood, it can mean a blockage in the bile transport system. **FH pp. 295-297**

22. G These are mitochondria. One of their functions is the beta-oxidation of fatty acids. **FH pp. 21, 297**

23. C This is a tight junction that seals off the bile canalicular space. In the event of a stone in the gallbladder, increased bile pressure may cause bile to traverse the tight junctions of the junctional complexes binding hepatocytes to one another. This allows bile to escape into the space of Disse and into the bloodstream, causing jaundice. **FH p. 297**

24. D The muscularis shows marked hypertrophy. In the normal gallbladder, the muscularis is quite thin and forms a discontinuous layer. **FH p. 298, BH p. 173**

25. C The figure shows a moderately differentiated adenocarcinoma of the pancreas. These tumors almost always arise from the pancreatic ductal epithelium. Only 1% of pancreatic adenocarcinomas arise from the pancreatic acini. Tumors arising from islets of Langerhans or neuroendocrine cells would show the growth pattern of neuroendocrine tumors. Gland formation by tumor cells, as seen here, would not be present in tumors arising from either neuroendocrine cells or supporting connective tissue. **BH p. 175**

26. E Most pancreatic adenocarcinomas arise in the head of the pancreas with compression and obstruction of the common bile duct. Hence, the patients usually present with jaundice. Because most of the bile backs up in to the liver and the systemic circulation, gallstones do not usually form. The islets of Langerhans are distributed throughout the pancreas, especially in the tail. Therefore, in carcinoma of the head of the pancreas, diabetes mellitus is uncommon because the islets are usually spared. Fat necrosis is most commonly seen with acute pancreatitis. Pancreatic adenocarcinoma causes GI obstruction, not hemorrhage. **BH p. 175**

27. C Cells in pancreatic acini are highly polarized and possess large secretory granules. Endocrine cells are nonpolarized and have small secretory granules. Secretory granules are lacking from cells of the gallbladder, bile ducts, or liver parenchyma. **FH pp. 301-301**

28. C The figure shows foci of fat necrosis. Acute pancreatitis causes release of pancreatic enzymes in the pancreas and surrounding tissue, with subsequent necrosis and digestion of adipose tissue. In inflammation, autoimmune destruction, or malignant cell infiltration, accumulations of inflammatory cells or malignant cells would be apparent that are not visible in the figure. **BH p. 175**

29. A The two most important predisposing factors for the development of acute pancreatitis with fat necrosis are alcohol abuse and biliary tract disease. Atherosclerosis does not especially impair liver or pancreatic function, and gluten sensitivity results in malabsorption. Hepatitis and obesity can affect liver function but do not directly contribute to pancreatitis. **BH p. 175**

30. C The figure shows a moderately differentiated adenocarcinoma with evidence of gland formation. The clinical presentation is suggestive of a possible metastasis from a colon carcinoma. Gland formation is not characteristic of any of the other tumors listed. **BH p. 83**

31. D Binucleate hepatocytes or hepatocytes with very large nuclei are formed when cells undergo mitosis without cytokinesis. Both cell types indicate tissue growth. Normal-appearing endothelial cell nuclei are not diagnostic of a regenerative response. **FH p. 290**

32. B The pancreatic acinar tissue, which synthesizes digestive enzymes, is located here. **FH p. 299**

Urinary System

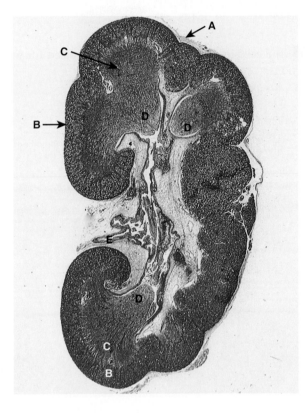

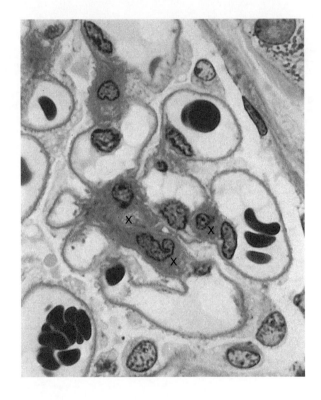

The figure above shows a section through a fetal kidney. Use this figure to answer the next two questions.

1 Where are both the afferent and efferent arterioles of the kidney's portal system located?

2 Where does the maximal ion concentration in the tissue fluid surrounding the nephron occur?

3 In the micrograph of a renal corpuscle shown in the figure on the right, what are the cells labeled X?
- ☐ A. Cells of the parietal layer of Bowman capsule
- ☐ B. Endothelial cells
- ☐ C. Juxtaglomerular cells
- ☐ D. Mesangial cells
- ☐ E. Podocytes

Use these answer choices for the next four questions.

- ☐ A. Afferent arteriole
- ☐ B. Ascending limb of the loop of Henle
- ☐ C. Collecting duct
- ☐ D. Descending limb of the loop of Henle
- ☐ E. Distal convoluted tubule
- ☐ F. Glomerular basement membrane
- ☐ G. Glomerular capillary
- ☐ H. Mesangium
- ☐ I. Parietal layer of Bowman capsule
- ☐ J. Vasa recta
- ☐ K. Visceral layer of Bowman capsule

4 This structure contains phagocytic cells.

5 This structure contains the macula densa.

6 This structure contains renin-secreting cells.

7 This structure is relatively impermeable to H$_2$O at all times.

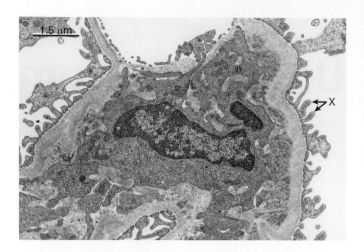

8 In the micrograph of the kidney above, the letter *X* labels portions of which type of cell?
- ☐ A. Capillary endothelial cell
- ☐ B. Juxtaglomerular cell
- ☐ C. Fibroblast
- ☐ D. Mesangial cell
- ☐ E. Podocyte

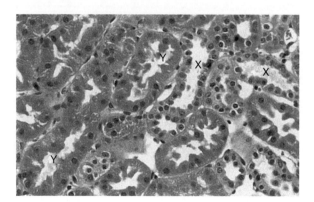

9 In the absence of antidiuretic hormone (ADH; vasopressin), the concentration of which of the following is higher in structure *X* than it is in structure *Y* in the figure above.
- ☐ A. Amino acids
- ☐ B. Calcium ions
- ☐ C. Glucose
- ☐ D. Sodium ions
- ☐ E. Water

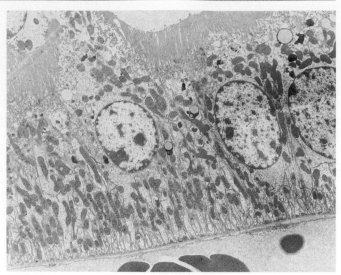

10 The cells in the figure above are specialized for which functions?
- ☐ A. Absorption and ion transport
- ☐ B. Detoxification of xenobiotics
- ☐ C. Phagocytosis and digestion
- ☐ D. Protein synthesis and secretion
- ☐ E. Steroid synthesis and secretion

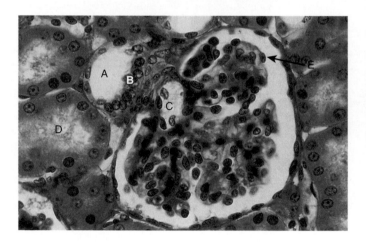

11 Which portion of the nephron, shown in the figure above, promotes secretion by juxtaglomerular smooth muscle cells?

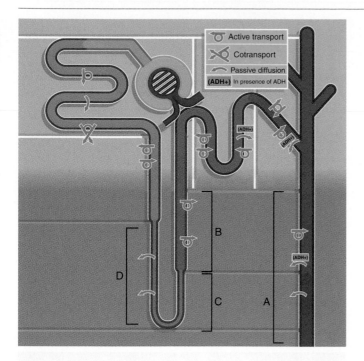

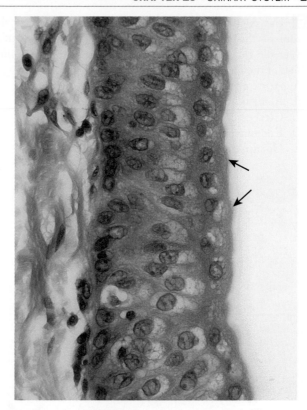

12 In order to treat edema in a patient's legs, a doctor prescribes the diuretic furosemide. Because this drug prevents reabsorption of sodium, potassium, and chloride ions from the urine, it causes more water to be excreted with the urine. Where would this drug have its effect?

13 Researchers have recently found that a familial form of diabetes insipidus is caused by a mutation in the aquaporin 2 gene. Aquaporin 2 is present in locations where water reabsorption in the kidney is regulated by ADH (vasopressin). What do these locations include?
☐ A. Calyx
☐ B. Collecting duct
☐ C. Glomerulus
☐ D. Macula densa
☐ E. Proximal convoluted tubule

14 The ureter can be recognized in microscopic sections by its transitional epithelium and what other characteristic structure?
☐ A. Distinct submucosa
☐ B. Mixture of smooth and skeletal muscle in the muscularis
☐ C. Mucosal glands
☐ D. Star-shaped lumen
☐ E. Very thick muscularis layer

15 The cells indicated by the *arrows* in the figure above are specialized in what way?
☐ A. Large amount of rough endoplasmic reticulum
☐ B. Large amount of smooth endoplasmic reticulum
☐ C. Thickened plasma membrane
☐ D. Very large Golgi complex
☐ E. Well-developed glycocalyx

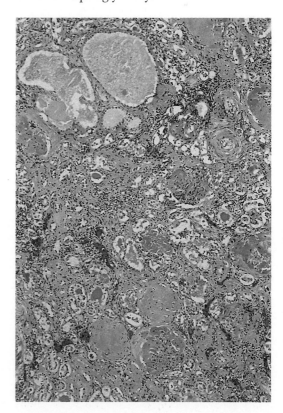

16 The microscopic section shown in the figure at the bottom of the previous page is from a renal biopsy of a 55-year-old woman with elevated BUN and serum creatinine. Which of the following is the most likely diagnosis?

- ☐ A. Acute pyelonephritis
- ☐ B. Acute tubular necrosis
- ☐ C. Clear cell carcinoma
- ☐ D. End-stage renal disease
- ☐ E. Goodpasture syndrome

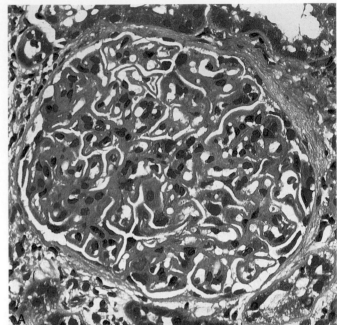

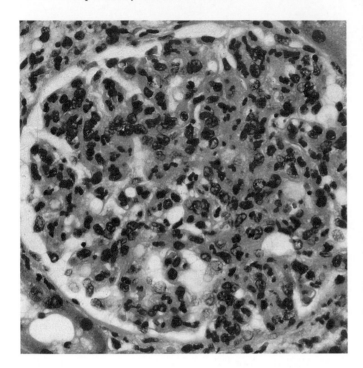

17 A 5-year-old girl was brought to the pediatrician by her mother who noticed that her daughter had reddish urine and puffy eyes. Physical examination showed elevated blood pressure and facial edema. Numerous RBCs were present on urine analysis. A renal biopsy was performed, and a microscopic section is shown in the figure above. Which disorder is suggested by the histologic findings?

- ☐ A. Acute glomerulonephritis
- ☐ B. Diabetic glomerulosclerosis
- ☐ C. Goodpasture syndrome
- ☐ D. Membranous nephropathy
- ☐ E. Rapidly progressive glomerulonephritis

18 Which of the following most likely preceded the pathology shown in the above kidney?

- ☐ A. Gastroenteritis
- ☐ B. Pharyngitis
- ☐ C. Urinary tract infection
- ☐ D. Vasculitis
- ☐ E. Viral pneumonia

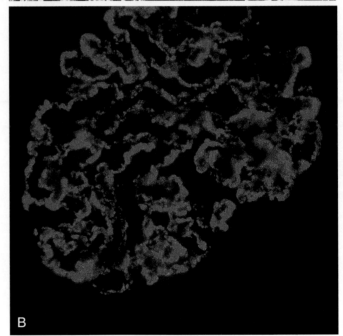

19 A renal biopsy was performed in a 45-year-old man. The biopsy was stained to demonstrate the presence of immunoglobulin deposits in the figure above. Which of the following diseases is the patient most likely to have, that resulted in the renal pathology shown?

- ☐ A. Diabetes
- ☐ B. Hepatitis C
- ☐ C. Hypertension
- ☐ D. Pyelonephritis
- ☐ E. Vasculitis

20 Which of the following is most likely to be present in the urine of the same patient?
☐ A. Increased bilirubin
☐ B. Increased glucose
☐ C. Marked proteinuria
☐ D. Numerous RBCs
☐ E. Numerous WBCs

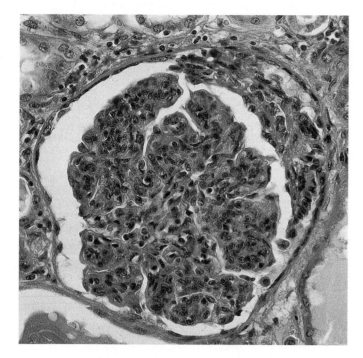

21 A 33-year-old man with complaints of reddish urine and a decreased urine output was found to have hematuria and proteinuria. A renal biopsy was performed and is shown in the figure above. An additional study using antibody against IgG shows a linear pattern of immunofluorescence in the glomerular basement membrane. Which of the following is the most likely diagnosis?
☐ A. Goodpasture syndrome
☐ B. Henoch-Schönlein purpura
☐ C. IgA nephropathy
☐ D. Poststreptococcal glomerulonephritis
☐ E. Systemic lupus erythematosus

22 Which of the following would also be present in this patient?
☐ A. Hemoptysis
☐ B. Myocarditis
☐ C. Pleuritis
☐ D. Skin rash
☐ E. Thrombocytopenia

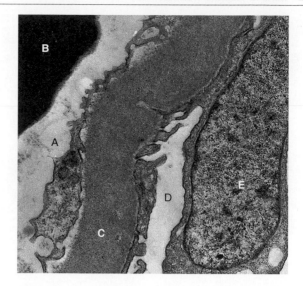

23 A 60-year-old woman has developed proteinuria. A biopsy of her kidney sectioned for electron microscopy is shown in the figure above. What pathology is indicated by the figure?
☐ A. Acute poststreptococcal glomerulonephritis
☐ B. Acute pyelonephritis
☐ C. Diabetes insipidus
☐ D. Diabetes mellitus
☐ E. Preeclampsia

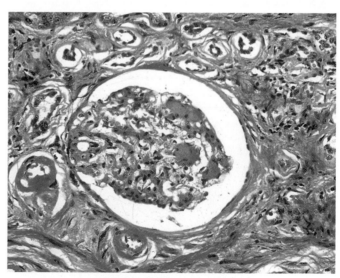

24 A 56-year-old woman was noted to have pedal edema by her primary care physician. Urine analysis showed marked proteinuria. A microscopic section of her renal biopsy is shown in the figure above. Which of the following is the most likely diagnosis?
☐ A. Diabetes mellitus
☐ B. Goodpasture syndrome
☐ C. Henoch-Schönlein purpura
☐ D. Poststreptococcal glomerulonephritis
☐ E. Rapidly progressive glomerulonephritis

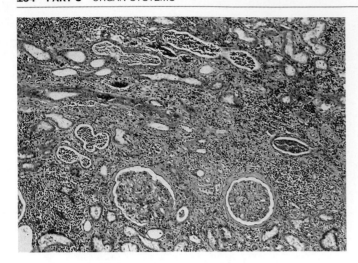

25 A 23-year-old woman is examined by a physician after complaining of flank pain. Her blood pressure is 120/80 mm Hg. A biopsy of her kidney is displayed in the figure above. What is her most likely diagnosis?

☐ A. Acute pyelonephritis
☐ B. Diabetic glomerulosclerosis
☐ C. Hypertensive nephrosclerosis
☐ D. Nephroblastoma
☐ E. Polycystic kidney disease

26 Which of the following would be present in markedly increased amounts in the urine of this patient?

☐ A. Crystals
☐ B. Glucose
☐ C. Protein
☐ D. RBCs
☐ E. WBCs

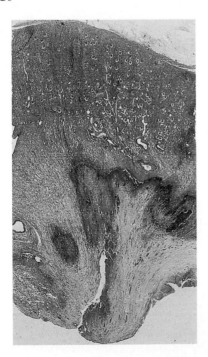

27 A 55-year-old man has chronic back pain after a fall from a ladder 5 years ago. He now presents to his primary care physician with complaints of flank pain and brown urine. A microscopic section of his kidney is shown in the figure below left. Which of the following is the most likely cause?

☐ A. Analgesic abuse
☐ B. Essential hypertension
☐ C. Rapidly progressive glomerulonephritis
☐ D. Systemic lupus erythematosus
☐ E. Infective endocarditis

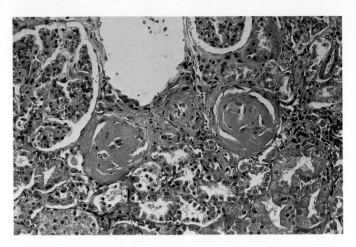

28 The pathology shown in the microscopic section of the kidney in the figure above is most likely to be seen in which of the following patients?

☐ A. A 25-year-old woman with massive bleeding
☐ B. A 28-year-old woman with malar rash and joint pain
☐ C. A 32-year-old man with hemoptysis and hematuria
☐ D. A 45-year-old man with marked hyponatremia
☐ E. A 55-year-old man with chronic hypertension

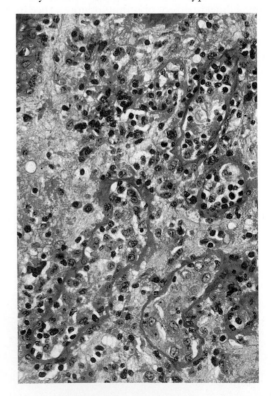

29 A 27-year-old woman with an elevated BUN and creatinine underwent a renal biopsy. A microscopic section of the biopsy is shown in the figure at bottom right of the previous page. Which of the following is the most likely mechanism that caused this pathology?

☐ A. Cardiogenic shock
☐ B. Cell-mediated immunity
☐ C. Immune complex deposition
☐ D. Severe hypertension
☐ E. Syndrome of inappropriate ADH secretion

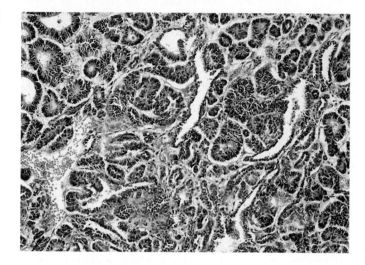

30 A 5-year-old boy was brought to his pediatrician by his mother who felt a swelling in her son's abdomen while bathing him. Physical examination revealed a large abdominal mass. The mass was resected, and a microscopic section is shown in the figure above. Which of the following is the most likely diagnosis?

☐ A. Acute lymphoblastic leukemia
☐ B. Ewing sarcoma
☐ C. Nephroblastoma
☐ D. Oncocytoma
☐ E. Renal cell carcinoma

31 A 65-year-old woman underwent imaging studies for evaluation of abdominal pain. A CT scan showed a solid renal mass. The patient underwent laparotomy, and the mass was resected. On gross examination, the mass was homogeneous and brownish in color with a central scar. A histologic section is shown in the figure at above right. Which of the following is the most likely diagnosis?

☐ A. Acute lymphoblastic leukemia
☐ B. Ewing sarcoma
☐ C. Nephroblastoma
☐ D. Oncocytoma
☐ E. Renal cell carcinoma

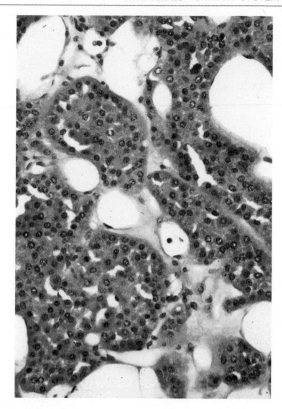

32 What is the cause of the appearance of the cells in the above tumor?

☐ A. Decreased protein synthesis
☐ B. Hydropic degeneration
☐ C. Increased mucin production
☐ D. Increased RNA content
☐ E. Numerous mitochondria

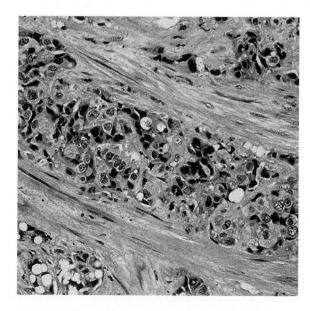

33 A 51-year-old man is examined by his physician after complaining of frequent pain upon urination. Traces of blood are visible in the urine. A biopsy of this patient's urinary bladder is shown in the figure above. What is the diagnosis for this patient?

☐ A. Chronic cystitis
☐ B. Diverticula
☐ C. Malakoplakia
☐ D. Transitional cell papilloma
☐ E. Urothelial carcinoma

34 This pathology is linked to which of the following?
☐ A. Aniline dyes
☐ B. Analgesic abuse
☐ C. Chronic diuretic use
☐ D. High estrogen levels
☐ E. Urinary tract obstruction

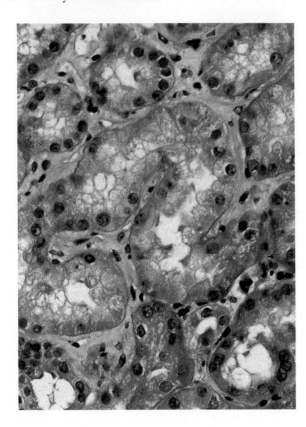

35 The pathology shown in the microscopic section of the kidney in the figure above is most likely to be seen in which of the following patients?
☐ A. A 25-year-old woman with massive bleeding
☐ B. A 28-year-old woman with malar rash and joint pain
☐ C. A 32-year-old man with hemoptysis and hematuria
☐ D. A 45-year-old man with marked hyponatremia
☐ E. A 55-year-old man with chronic hypertension

ANSWERS

1. B Both the afferent and efferent arterioles are located in the cortex, at the vascular pole of each glomerulus. No glomeruli are present in the capsule (A), outer medulla (C), inner medulla (D), or ureter (E). **FH pp. 303-305**

2. D The maximal osmolarity of the tissue fluid occurs in the kidney's inner medulla. This is established through reabsorption of sodium, chloride, and potassium ions from the thick ascending limbs of loops of Henle and urea from medullary collecting ducts. Other regions of the kidney have a relatively normal osmolarity. **FH p. 303, 324**

3. D Mesangial cells are located in the interstitium between glomerular capillaries and represent a special type of pericyte with contractile properties. The parietal layer of Bowman capsule is located outside of the glomerulus (upper right-hand corner of figure). Endothelial cells have flattened nuclei, and podocytes (round, pale cell at top of figure) have paler nuclei and attach to the outer surfaces of capillaries. **FH p. 309**

4. H The intraglomerular mesangial cells are phagocytic and are thought to remove debris from the glomerulus. **FH p. 314**

5. E The macula densa is part of the distal convoluted tubule. **FH p. 319**

6. A The smooth muscle cells of afferent arteriole are modified to secrete the peptide hormone renin. **FH p. 319**

7. B The cells of the ascending limb of the loop of Henle are relatively impermeable to H_2O, which allows the medullary interstitium to become hypertonic. **FH p. 320**

8. E The electron microscopic image shows the branching pedicels of podocytes. These are recognized as relatively thick cytoplasmic processes adjacent to the glomerular basement membrane. Endothelial cells appear similar because of their many fenestrations but are much lower in height. The pedicels form an important part of the filtration barrier between the blood and provisional urine in the kidney. **FH p. 314**

9. E Structure X is a distal convoluted tubule, and structure Y is a proximal convoluted tubule. All the molecules and ions above are reabsorbed in the proximal tubule, but the active transport of ions out of the ascending limb of the loop of Henle results in hypotonic urine in the distal convoluted tubule. **FH pp. 315, 324**

10. A The apical brush border is characteristic of absorptive cells and the basal infoldings with mitochondria are characteristic of ion-transporting cells. Cells that detoxify xenobiotics would be rich in smooth endoplasmic reticulum, which is associated with detoxifying enzymes (cytochrome P-450). Cells synthesizing proteins or steroids have abundant rough and smooth endoplasmic reticulum, respectively. Phagocytic cells would contain many lysosomes and endosomes. **FH pp. 316-317**

11. B The macula densa is a specialized part of the distal convoluted tubule adjacent to the juxtaglomerular apparatus. It reacts to changes in urinary ions and regulates the function of the JG cells. It is recognized as a thickened region in the distal tubule, with closely packed nuclei in the epithelium. **FH pp. 318-319**

12. B Regulation of the reabsorption of sodium, potassium, and chloride ions from the urine occurs in the thick ascending loop of Henle. The drug prevents this reabsorption of the ions. The resulting lower ion content in the interstitium, in turn, reduces the amount of water resorbed from the collecting ducts, and the water is excreted in the urine. **FH pp. 324-325**

13. B Under the influence of ADH, the collecting duct increases its permeability to water by merging subplasmalemmal vesicles containing aquaporin 2 with the plasma membrane. Other renal structures have different isoforms of aquaporin that permit water transport across membranes, but these structures lack the aquaporin 2 isoform and are not sensitive to ADH. **FH p. 325**

14. D The contraction of the muscle in the ureter wall frequently causes the lumen to take on a star shape. None of the other features listed are present in the ureter. **FH p. 326**

15. C The surface cells of this urothelium have a modified, thickened plasma membrane containing plaques that protect the cells from damage during long-term storage of urine. Because these are not secretory cells, they do not possess large amounts of smooth or rough endoplasmic reticulum or Golgi membranes. A well-developed glycocalyx is found on absorptive cells. **FH p. 327**

16. D The figure shows hyalinized glomeruli, atrophic and dilated tubules, and interstitial fibrosis, which are characteristic features of an end-stage kidney. Acute pyelonephritis is characterized by neutrophils within the renal tubules. In acute tubular necrosis, the renal tubular epithelium would be necrotic and devoid of nuclei; some of the dead cells would slough into the lumen. Sheets of large epithelial cells with abundant, clear cytoplasm are characteristic of clear cell carcinoma. In Goodpasture syndrome, antibodies to the glomerular basement membrane would result in damage to the glomeruli and result in crescent formation. **BH p. 178**

17. A The clinical presentation and biopsy findings are characteristic of acute postinfectious glomerulonephritis. This disease is characterized by a hypercellular mesangium with infiltration by neutrophils, as illustrated in the figure. All the other choices are also diseases of the glomeruli, which have diagnostic histopathologies: thickened basement membrane and fibrotic nodules in diabetic glomerulosclerosis; crescents in Goodpasture syndrome and rapidly progressive glomerulonephritis; and thickened basement membrane with subepithelial deposits in membranous nephropathy. **BH p. 180, FH pp. 308-309**

18. B Acute glomerulonephritis occurs most commonly in children, following streptococcal pharyngitis. Glomerulonephritis can also occur following streptococcal skin infections but is not associated with any of the other infections listed. **BH p. 180**

19. B The figure shows features of membranous glomerulonephritis (i.e., a thickened basement membrane and granular immune complex deposits). Most often, membranous glomerulonephritis is idiopathic, but secondary forms may be seen in patients with malignancies and hepatitis B and C infections. Thickening of the glomerular basement membrane also occurs in diabetes; however, granular immune complex deposits are not seen. Hypertension leads to thickening of the vascular basement membrane, and some types of vasculitis cause disruption of the glomerular basement membrane. Pyelonephritis affects the tubules, not the glomeruli. **BH p. 182**

20. C Membranous glomerulonephritis usually presents as nephrotic syndrome with marked proteinuria, owing to a greater permeability of glomerular basement membranes to protein. WBCs in the urine usually result from infections of the urinary tract. Normally, all the glucose that is filtered through the glomeruli is reabsorbed by the proximal renal tubule. Therefore, an elevation in urinary glucose would result from either excess glucose in the blood or a failure of proximal tubule cells to reabsorb glucose, rather than an increased leakage of glucose into the urine at the level of the glomerulus. Increased bilirubin in the urine occurs in patients with hemolytic anemia, liver disorder, or biliary obstruction. Numerous RBCs in the urine occur with glomerular diseases that present as nephritic syndrome (poststreptococcal glomerulonephritis), renal stones, and tumors of the urinary tract. **BH pp. 182-183**

21. A Epithelial cell proliferation in Bowman capsule with formation of crescents (shown in the figure) and a linear pattern of immunofluorescence is characteristic of Goodpasture syndrome. The linear pattern is due to antibodies to the glomerular basement membrane. Systemic lupus erythematosus can also show formation of crescents in the glomeruli; however, immunofluorescence studies would show a granular pattern because the deposits are immune complexes rather than specific antibodies. In both IgA nephropathy and Henoch-Schönlein purpura, there is mesangial thickening with IgA deposition in the mesangium. Although IgA nephropathy is limited to the kidney, patients with Henoch-Schönlein purpura have vasculitis, which manifests as skin rash, abdominal pain, and joint pain. The glomeruli in poststreptoccal glomerulonephritis are hypercellular with a neutrophilic infiltrate. **BH p. 183**

22. A In Goodpasture syndrome, autoantibodies attack the glomerular and pulmonary alveolar basement membranes resulting in hematuria and hemoptysis, respectively. The other findings listed are not commonly seen in patients with Goodpasture syndrome. **BH p. 183**

23. D The unusual thickening of the basement membrane (C) is an indication of diabetes-induced damage to the glomerulus. Acute poststreptococcal glomerulonephritis occurs in younger patients and presents with hematuria in addition to mild proteinuria. The glomeruli show mesangial hypercellularity and infiltration by neutrophils. Diabetes insipidus, caused by a decreased secretion of pituitary ADH, affects the water reabsorption function of collecting tubules rather than glomeruli and would not provoke a proteinuria. Preeclampsia, a complication of pregnancy provoked by placental hypoxia, results in an elevated blood pressure and proteinuria. The glomeruli show endothelial swelling rather than basement membrane thickening. The structure of the podocytes (E), endothelium (A), RBCs (B), and urinary space (D) are normal in diabetes. **BH p. 185, FH p. 314**

24. A The figure shows Kimmelstiel-Wilson nodules in the glomeruli and hyalinization of arterioles, characteristic of diabetes mellitus. All the other choices are also diseases of the glomeruli with diagnostic histopathologic findings: crescents in Goodpasture syndrome and rapidly progressive glomerulonephritis; mesangial IgA deposition in Henoch-Schönlein purpura; and mesangial hypercellularity with neutrophilic infiltrate in poststreptococcal glomerulonephritis. **BH pp. 184-185**

25. A The abundance of leukocytes within tubules and in the renal interstitium is indicative of a bacterial infection, as seen in acute pyelonephritis. Diabetes and hypertension result in thickening of the glomerular and vascular basement membranes, respectively. The absence of large cysts and the normal appearance of glomeruli, plus a normal blood pressure, rule out the other choices. **BH p. 186, FH p. 315**

26. E In acute pyelonephritis, the infection affects mainly the distal portions of the tubules. WBCs migrate across the ductal epithelium and into the urine. In severe cases, the inflammation may extend to the proximal tubules and may result in mild proteinuria and glycosuria; however, marked elevation of urinary protein and glucose usually is not seen. Crystals may be present in the urine in a variety of physiologic and pathologic conditions and may or may not be associated with infections so are not diagnostic for particular infections. Numerous RBCs in the urine occur with glomerular diseases that present as nephritic syndrome (poststreptococcal glomerulonephritis), renal stones, and tumors of the urinary tract. **BH p. 186, 193**

27. A Renal papillary necrosis, shown in the figure, is caused by analgesic abuse, diabetes mellitus, and urinary tract obstruction. Given the history of chronic back pain, analgesic abuse is the most likely cause in this patient. None of the other conditions are associated with renal papillary necrosis. **BH p. 187**

28. E In essential hypertension, there is hyalinization and thickening of arterioles as shown in the figure. This will eventually lead to ischemia and sclerosis of the glomeruli. Massive bleeding may lead to shock and acute tubular necrosis. Malar rash and joint pain are characteristic of systemic lupus erythematosus, and the renal effects of this disease are manifested in the glomeruli, not in the arterioles. Goodpasture syndrome, characterized by hemoptysis and hematuria, is

also a glomerular, not an arteriolar, disease. Hyponatremia is a consequence of a variety of pathologic conditions but is not caused by hyalinization of renal arterioles. **BH pp. 188-189**

29. B The figure shows interstitial lymphocytic infiltrate with lymphocytes attacking the tubular epithelium (tubulitis). This occurs in acute cellular transplant rejection, which is a T-cell–mediated immune response. This patient was a renal transplant recipient. Cardiogenic shock would lead to acute tubular necrosis, which is characterized by necrotic renal epithelial cells with minimal inflammation. Immune complex deposition results in glomerular damage, not inflammation in the interstitium. Severe hypertension is characterized by damage to arterioles. In syndrome of inappropriate ADH secretion, excessive ADH results in excessive reabsorption of water in the distal tubules. Tubular or interstitial inflammation is not seen. **BH p. 190**

30. C Nephroblastoma, or Wilms tumor, is a common childhood tumor composed of undifferentiated cells that show areas resembling primitive renal tubules (shown in figure) and glomeruli (not shown). Acute lymphoblastic leukemia and Ewing sarcoma are also common tumors of childhood; however, renal involvement by these tumors is rare. Moreover, formation of primitive tubules and glomeruli is not seen in either disease. Oncocytoma and renal cell carcinomas are tumors of the kidney that most often occur in older individuals. The former is characterized by cells with eosinophilic cytoplasm, whereas the latter shows cells with clear cytoplasm. **BH p. 191**

31. D Oncocytoma has a characteristic gross appearance, as described previously, and a characteristic microscopic finding, with sheets of cells containing abundant eosinophilic granular cytoplasm (see figure). Renal cell carcinoma, the other renal tumor seen in older patients, shows cells with abundant and clear, but not eosinophilic, cytoplasm. Acute lymphoblastic leukemia and Ewing sarcoma are common tumors of childhood characterized by small, basophilic cells with scant cytoplasm. Nephroblastoma, a renal tumor of children, shows undifferentiated cells with areas resembling primitive renal tubules and glomeruli. **BH p. 191**

32. E The cells in oncocytoma have abundant, granular, eosinophilic cytoplasm due to the presence of a very large number of mitochondria. Decreased protein synthesis does not result in cytoplasmic eosinophilia. In hydropic degeneration, the cells would show cloudy swelling of the cytoplasm. Increased mucin production in a cell would manifest as large, well-defined intracellular vacuoles. Increased RNA content in a cell causes the cells to stain blue with H&E stain because of the affinity of RNA for basic dyes. **BH p. 191**

33. E This biopsy has the features of invasive high-grade urothelial (transitional cell) carcinoma. The tumor cells are large, with hyperchromatic nuclei, abundant mitotic figures, and invasion of the smooth muscle bundles. Transitional cell papillomas are characterized by elongated, frondlike outgrowths of the epithelium. The thickness of the epithelium is increased, but the cells do not show evidence of dysplasia. In cystitis or malakoplakia, a bacterial infection provokes accumulations of neutrophils or macrophages, absent here. In diverticula, there is outpouching of the bladder mucosa through the muscular wall. The epithelial cells would not show evidence of malignancy. **BH p. 195, FH p. 327**

34. A These tumors are associated with exposure to industrial chemicals, such as aniline dyes. The other conditions listed are not linked to the development of urothelial carcinoma. **BH p. 195**

35. A The figure shows early signs of acute tubular necrosis, with hydropic degeneration and loss of nuclei caused by ischemia. Massive blood loss would lead to hypotension and ischemic damage of renal tubules. Malar rash and joint pain are characteristic of systemic lupus erythematosus, and the renal effects of this disease are manifested in the glomeruli, not in the tubules. Goodpasture syndrome, characterized by hemoptysis and hematuria, is also a glomerular, not a tubular, disease. Hyponatremia is a consequence of a variety of pathologic conditions but is not caused by massive bleeding. In essential hypertension, there is hyalinization and thickening of arterioles. **BH pp. 6-7, 185**

Endocrine System

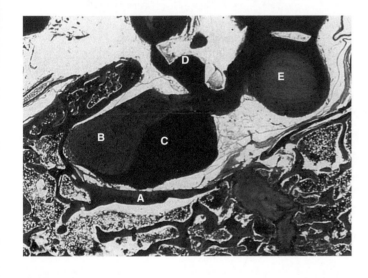

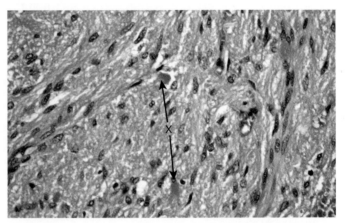

1 If in situ hybridization histochemistry were performed on the structures shown in the figure above in order to localize messenger RNA for antidiuretic hormone, which region would be expected to stain the most heavily?

2 Which region in the above figure would be expected to stain most heavily with antibodies to type I collagen?

3 A 37-year-old woman presented to her physician with palpitations and heat intolerance. The woman was found to have a pituitary adenoma. A biopsy showed a monomorphic population of basophils. Antibodies against which of the following molecules would be useful in establishing the diagnosis?
- ☐ A. Melatonin
- ☐ B. Oxytocin
- ☐ C. Secretin
- ☐ D. Thyrotropin (thyroid-stimulating hormone, TSH)
- ☐ E. Vasopressin

4 What is the function of the structure in the posterior pituitary labeled *X* in the figure above?
- ☐ A. ATP production
- ☐ B. Electrical conduction
- ☐ C. Hormone storage
- ☐ D. Protein synthesis
- ☐ E. Regulation of hypothalamic function

5 Basophils that are located in the pars intermedia of the pituitary mostly secrete what?
- ☐ A. Follicle-stimulating hormone (FSH)
- ☐ B. Luteinizing hormone (LH)
- ☐ C. Prolactin
- ☐ D. Pro-opiomelanocortin (POMC)
- ☐ E. Thyrotropin (TSH)

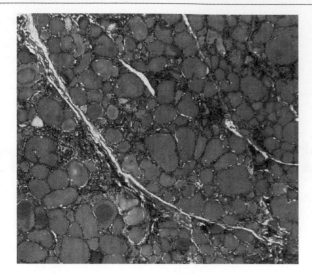

6 A 15-year-old girl is in for a routine physical examination, and you notice a small pink mass on the back of her tongue. Biopsy of the mass yielded the section shown in the figure above. What is the correct diagnosis of her condition?

- ☐ A. Metastatic thyroid tumor
- ☐ B. Normal lingual thyroid
- ☐ C. Thyroid adenoma
- ☐ D. Thyroid carcinoma
- ☐ E. Thyroid hyperplasia

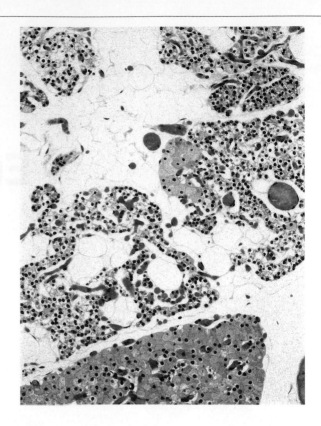

10 The micrograph above illustrates a parathyroid gland recovered from a 76-year-old man. The cells seen at the bottom of the figure are an accumulation of what?

- ☐ A. Brown fat cells
- ☐ B. Chromophobe cells
- ☐ C. Lymphocytes
- ☐ D. Oxyphil cells
- ☐ E. White fat cells

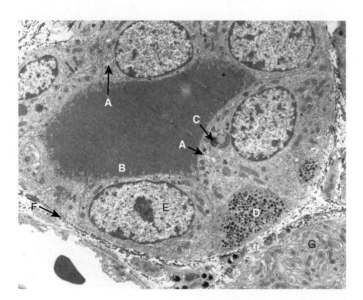

7 Which letter in the figure above indicates the site where iodine is added to thyroglobulin?

8 Which letter indicates the site where thyroglobulin is converted into T_3 and T_4?

9 Which letter indicates the location of calcitonin?

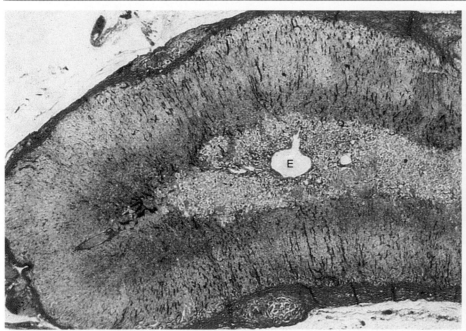
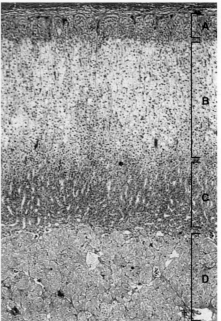

Use the figure above to answer the next three questions.

11 A 40-year-old man presents with excess sweating, a moon face, and central obesity. High levels of cortisol are seen in his blood. ACTH levels are very low. From which area of the organ shown in the figure above would a tumor develop that would cause these symptoms?

12 A 50-year-old woman presents with high blood pressure and hypernatremia. From which area of the organ shown in the figure above would a tumor develop that would cause these symptoms?

13 Which ultrastructural feature is common to the cells in the areas labeled *A, B*, and *C* in the right-hand figure above?
☐ A. Large amounts of rough endoplasmic reticulum
☐ B. Large perinuclear Golgi
☐ C. Mitochondria with tubular cristae
☐ D. Unilocular accumulations of lipid
☐ E. Zymogen granules

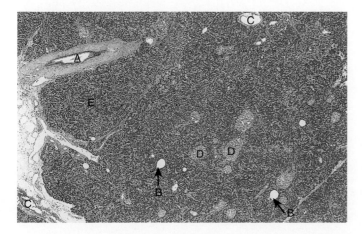

14 A 10-year-old boy presents with polyuria, polydipsia, hyperglycemia, and ketoacidosis. A biopsy through the pancreas (shown in the figure below left) would be expected to show damage primarily in which labeled area?

15 A 49-year-old woman is admitted to the hospital after losing consciousness at work. She has a history of hyperglycemia and obesity and lately has developed abdominal pain, intermittent diarrhea, and feelings of bloating after eating. Among the tests proposed for her was a biopsy of her pancreas. The biopsy showed accumulations of extracellular amyloid among the cells of the islets of Langerhans. From what is she most likely suffering?
☐ A. Obstruction of the pancreatic duct
☐ B. Pancreatic carcinoma
☐ C. Pancreatitis
☐ D. Type I diabetes mellitus
☐ E. Type II diabetes mellitus

16 A 39-year-old man was found to have multiple nodules in his pancreas. A biopsy of one of the nodules was performed. The morphologic finding is shown in part A of the figure at the top of the next page. The nodule showed diffuse and intense staining for glucagon, shown in part B. This patient is most likely to present with which of the following signs and symptoms?
☐ A. Fat malabsorption
☐ B. Hyperglycemia
☐ C. Hypertension
☐ D. Multiple gastric ulcers
☐ E. Obstructive jaundice

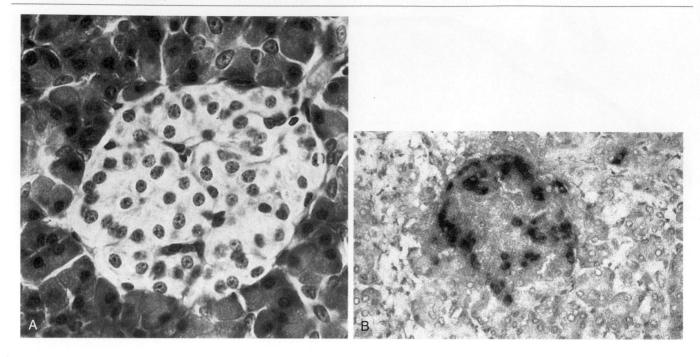

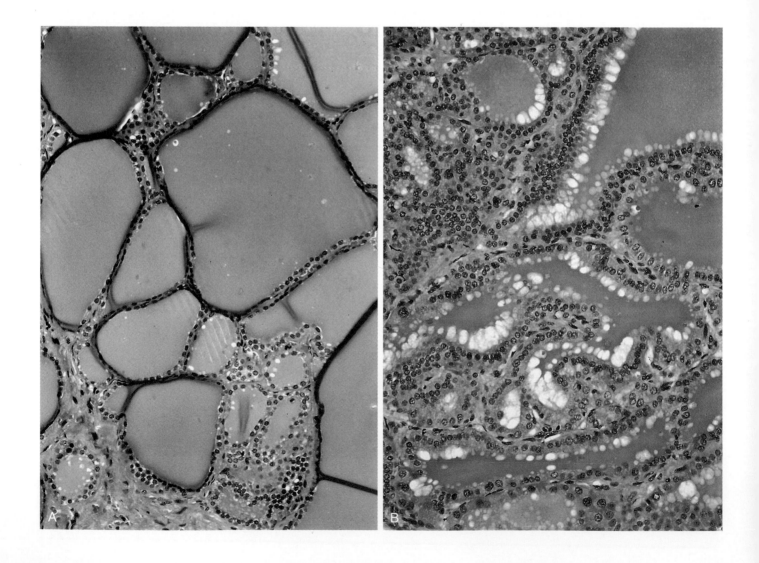

17 Part A of the figure at the bottom of the previous page illustrates the normal appearance of an organ, and part B shows a pathologic condition of the same organ. What disease process accounts for the transformation shown in part B?

☐ A. Adrenal cortical tumor
☐ B. Parathyroid carcinoma
☐ C. Pituitary adenoma
☐ D. Thyroid papillary adenocarcinoma
☐ E. Thyroid hyperplasia

18 A 27-year-old woman presented to her primary care physician with complaints of amenorrhea and partial loss of vision in one visual field. She stated that she has started a new job that is very tiring and demanding. Vital signs were within normal limits. A whitish fluid was expressed from the nipples on breast examination. Which of the following is the most likely cause of the patient's symptoms?

☐ A. Endometrial polyps
☐ B. Excessive stress
☐ C. Pituitary adenoma
☐ D. Polycystic ovary syndrome
☐ E. Turner syndrome

☐ A. Hashimoto thyroiditis
☐ B. Sheehan syndrome
☐ C. Thyroid adenoma
☐ D. Thyroid carcinoma
☐ E. Toxic goiter

20 Which of the following is the most likely cause of the pathology shown in the same patient?

☐ A. Autoimmune destruction
☐ B. Iodine deficiency
☐ C. Sclerosing fibrosis
☐ D. Stimulating antibody
☐ E. Viral inflammation

21 What pathology is this patient at increased risk for developing?

☐ A. Benign adenoma
☐ B. Follicular carcinoma
☐ C. MALT lymphoma
☐ D. Medullary carcinoma
☐ E. Multinodular goiter

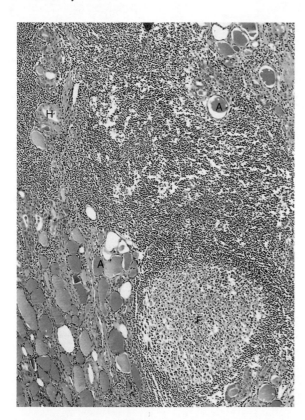

Use the figure above to answer the next three questions.

19 A 38-year-old woman with a history of chronic fatigue and weight gain is examined by her physician. Blood levels of thyroxine are low, and TSH levels are elevated. A biopsy of her thyroid gland is shown in the figure above. From what is this patient probably suffering?

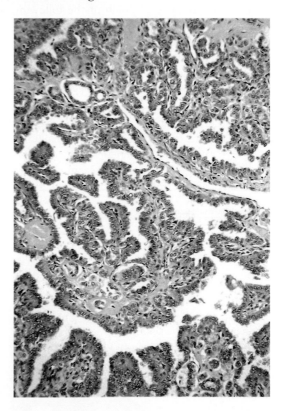

22 A 56-year-old woman was noted by her primary care physician to have a small nodule in her thyroid gland. She underwent surgical removal of the nodule, and a microscopic section is shown in the figure above. Which of the following is the most likely diagnosis?

☐ A. Anaplastic carcinoma
☐ B. Follicular carcinoma
☐ C. Medullary carcinoma
☐ D. Papillary carcinoma
☐ E. Small cell carcinoma

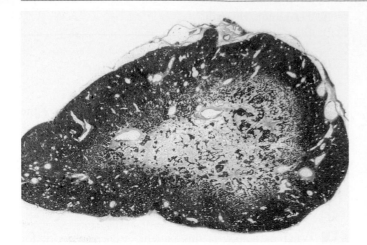

A. Headache and hypertension
B. Hypernatremia and hypokalemia
C. Hyperpigmentation and hypotension
D. Oliguria and hyperphosphatemia

23 A 47-year-old man was being evaluated for complaints of abdominal pain, recurrent renal stones, and hypercalcemia. Surgical removal of two parathyroid glands was performed. Both parathyroid glands showed the same pathology as depicted in the figure above. Which of the following is the most likely cause of the patient's symptoms?

A. Chronic renal failure
B. Excess intake of vitamin D
C. Hypophosphatemia
D. Osteoporosis
E. Parathyroid adenoma

24 A 47-year-old woman, who was on a long-term steroid therapy for systemic lupus erythematosus, died as a result of complications of her illness. Autopsy examination was performed. A microscopic image of her adrenal gland (B) is shown compared with a normal adrenal gland (A). Which of the following signs and symptoms would have been present in this patient?

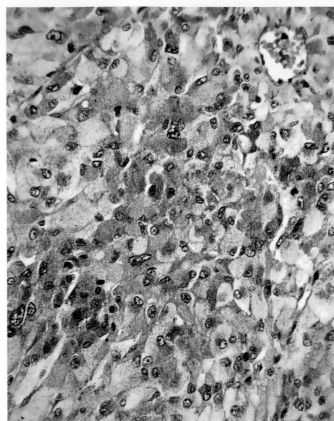

Use the figure above to answer the next three questions.

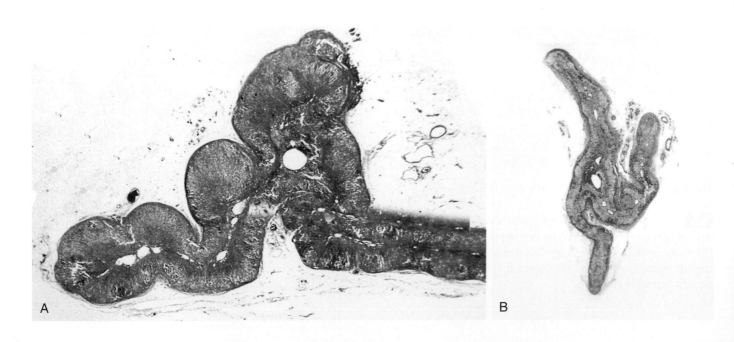

A

B

25 A 37-year-old man underwent surgical removal of a mass in the adrenal gland. On gross examination, a 3-cm, well-circumscribed nodule was present in the adrenal medulla. A microscopic section of the mass is shown in the figure on the previous page. Which of the following is the most likely diagnosis?
☐ A. Addison disease
☐ B. Conn syndrome
☐ C. Cushing syndrome
☐ D. Pheochromocytoma
☐ E. Pituitary adenoma

26 Which of the following signs and symptoms was most likely present in this patient?
☐ A. Headache and hypertension
☐ B. Hypernatremia and hypokalemia
☐ C. Hyperpigmentation and hypotension
☐ D. Oliguria and hyperphosphatemia
☐ E. Weight gain and hyperglycemia

27 Measurement of which of the following would be most useful in diagnosing the same patient?
☐ A. ACTH
☐ B. Aldosterone
☐ C. Cortisol
☐ D. Testosterone
☐ E. Vanillylmandelic acid

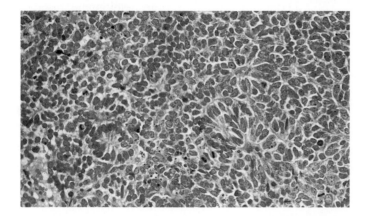

28 A 1-year-old boy was brought to the hospital by his mother who felt a mass in his abdomen while bathing him. A CT scan of the abdomen shows a mass in the right adrenal gland. The mass was resected and showed the morphologic pattern depicted in the microscopic section in the figure above. Which of the following is the most likely diagnosis?
☐ A. Adrenocortical adenoma
☐ B. Ewing sarcoma
☐ C. Neuroblastoma
☐ D. Rhabdomyosarcoma
☐ E. Wilms tumor

ANSWERS

1. D ADH is synthesized in the hypothalamus, identified by its location above the pituitary gland. It passes down neurons to the posterior lobe of the pituitary gland, where it is stored and then secreted into the bloodstream. The posterior pituitary contains the peptide form of ADH, but not the messenger RNA, because it is not synthesized there. **FH pp. 330-332**

2. A The pituitary gland sits in a bony cavity called the sella turcica (A). Bone contains abundant type I collagen, whereas neural and endocrine tissues contain very little. **FH pp. 196, 330**

3. D TSH, gonadotropins, and corticotropins are produced by pituitary basophils. Because the patient showed signs of hyperthyroidism, the best way to confirm that these are basophils that secrete TSH is through staining with an antibody to TSH. Oxytocin and vasopressin are present only in the posterior pituitary, whereas melatonin is found in the pineal gland and secretin in the gut. **FH pp. 330-331**

4. C These are Herring bodies, which contain accumulations of hormones that are transported down the axons from the hypothalamus. **FH p. 332**

5. D The basophils in the pars intermedia are mostly corticotrophs that secrete POMC. Basophils in the pars distalis secrete a variety of molecules, including FSH, LH, TSH, and POMC. Prolactin is secreted by acidophils. **FH p. 331**

6. B The thyroid gland develops from a down-growth at the back of the fetal tongue and migrates to its ultimate position in the neck. Occasionally, cells remain in the lingual position and develop into normal thyroid tissue. The normal appearance of the thyroid follicles and their lining cells rules out conditions of hyperplasia or cancer. **FH p. 333**

7. B Iodination of thyroglobulin occurs in the follicular lumen. This reaction is catalyzed by enzymes, which are attached to the apical membranes of the follicular cells. **FH p. 335**

8. C Thyroglobulin is endocytosed from the follicular lumen and partially digested in lysosomes. This releases the T_3 and T_4 from the thyroglobulin, and the hormones are secreted from the basal surface of the cell. **FH p. 335**

9. D The only cells in the thyroid gland that have small dense granules are parafollicular cells. The granules in these cells contain calcitonin. **FH p. 335**

10. D During aging, some parathyroid chief cells lose their ability to secrete hormone. Instead, they accumulate masses of mitochondria, causing the eosinophilic appearance of the cytoplasm in these oxyphil cells. Lipid droplets would be apparent in the cytoplasm of either brown fat or white fat cells, and lymphocytes would have a small amount of cytoplasm. **FH p. 337**

11. B This is the zona fasciculata, which produces mainly cortisol. A tumor in this location would result in high levels of cortisol and low levels of ACTH in the blood and the symptoms described. Region A, the zona glomerulosa, mainly produces aldosterone, which has little effect on pituitary secretion of ACTH. Region C, the zona reticularis, produces sex steroids that influence the secretion of LH and FSH, but not of ACTH, by the pituitary. **FH pp. 338-339**

12. A These cells produce mineralocorticoids, including aldosterone, which increases retention of sodium by the kidneys, leading to hypertension. Overproduction of this hormone can result in Conn syndrome, with the symptoms described previously. Tumors of the adrenal medulla (D) can cause hypertension due to excess catecholamine secretion, but would not provoke hypernatremia. **FH pp. 338-339**

13. C Specialized mitochondria with tubular cristae and the smooth endoplasmic reticulum metabolize the lipid into various hormones. Lipid is stored as multiple small droplets in the cortical cells. Steroid secretion and synthesis does not require the participation of the rough endoplasmic reticulum, secretion granules, or the Golgi apparatus because these organelles mediate the secretion and synthesis of proteins, but not steroids. **FH p. 299, 340**

14. D The symptoms are those of diabetes type I. This disease is thought to be caused by autoimmune destruction of the islets of Langerhans. Inflammation of the other structures (a fat cell, blood vessel, duct, and exocrine lobule) would not result in type I diabetes. **FH p. 343**

15. E In type II diabetes mellitus, pancreatic beta cells become overactive due to systemic insulin resistance. They secrete increased amounts of protein, including insulin and another peptide called *amylin*. Amylin becomes deposited within islets and forms masses in type II diabetes. They are not found in type I diabetes. The hyperglycemia present in diabetes exerts damaging effects on the enteric nervous system, causing delayed stomach emptying and disturbances in digestion. However, it does not lead to pancreatic inflammation, obstruction, or carcinoma. **FH p. 343**

16. B Patients with glucagon-producing islet cell tumors present with hyperglycemia, weight loss, diarrhea, and skin lesions. Gastrin-producing islet cell tumors cause multiple gastric ulcers. Unlike pancreatic carcinomas, islet cell tumors are usually small and do not obstruct the bile duct; therefore, obstructive jaundice is not associated with these tumors. Islet cell tumors are also not associated with hypertension. An impaired function of the exocrine pancreas, rather than the endocrine pancreas, results in malabsorption. **FH p. 343**

17. E This figure shows the thyroid gland, recognized by the presence of colloid-filled follicles. In thyroid hyperplasia, follicle cells multiply and become taller. Adrenal, parathyroid, or pituitary cells normally do not form fluid-filled epithelial follicles. In papillary adenocarcinoma of the thyroid, the epithelial cells proliferate with little or no colloid production and show abnormal nuclear features. **FH p. 333, BH pp. 257, 259**

18. C Amenorrhea, galactorrhea, and visual disturbances are associated with a prolactin-secreting pituitary adenoma. The latter symptom is due to the tumor pressing on the optic chiasm. Endometrial polyps usually cause bleeding rather than amenorrhea. Irregular menstrual cycles and amenorrhea can be caused by both polycystic ovary syndrome and excessive stress; however, neither condition causes loss of vision or galactorrhea. Patients with Turner syndrome have primary amenorrhea due to failure of the ovaries to develop, but loss of vision and galactorrhea do not occur in this condition. **BH pp. 254-255, FH pp. 328-332**

19. A The infiltration and destruction of the thyroid acini (A) with lymphocytes and formation of lymphoid follicles (F) is a characteristic finding in Hashimoto thyroiditis. The destruction of the thyroid results in diminished thyroxine production with compensatory elevation of TSH. Low levels of thyroxine can also be caused by pituitary insufficiency, as occurs in Sheehan syndrome; however, in this case, the TSH levels would be low rather than elevated. In thyroid adenoma and malignant carcinoma, there is a proliferation of epithelial cells with no or minimal lymphocytic infiltrate. **FH p. 333, BH pp. 256-258**

20. A Hashimoto thyroiditis is an autoimmune disorder characterized by immune destruction of the thyroid gland. Lymphocytic infiltration can be seen in Graves disease, which is also an autoimmune disorder. However, in Graves disease, there is a stimulating antibody, which leads to an increase, rather than a decrease, in thyroid function. A deficiency of iodine results in compensatory enlargement of the thyroid follicles, but lymphocytic infiltration and gland destruction are not seen. Viral inflammation and sclerosing fibrosis would both lead to low thyroxine and high TSH levels, but no germinal centers would be present in these diseases. **BH p. 256, FH pp. 333-334**

21. C Patients with Hashimoto thyroiditis have an increased risk for developing MALT lymphoma in the thyroid gland. Hashimoto thyroiditis is not associated with an increased incidence of developing the other pathologies listed. **BH p. 256**

22. D The figure shows a proliferation of epithelial cells with a papillary growth pattern and a narrow fibrovascular core. This growth pattern is a characteristic morphologic finding of papillary carcinoma of the thyroid. In addition, the malignant cells show unique nuclear features, including nuclear clearing and grooves, and calcified laminated bodies known as *psammoma bodies* are seen scattered in the tumor (not shown). **BH p. 259**

23. A The figure shows a hyperplastic parathyroid gland with a minimal adipose tissue component. Hyperplastic changes affect all parathyroid glands, as evidenced by the changes seen in both glands removed from this patient. The most common cause of parathyroid hyperplasia is chronic renal failure and a loss of calcium in the urine. This overstimulates the parathyroid glands. In contrast, parathyroid adenomas are neoplastic processes that usually involve a single gland without evidence of hyperplasia in the remaining glands. In chronic renal failure, there is failure of the kidneys to excrete phosphate, resulting in hyperphosphatemia. Osteoporosis is a consequence, not a cause of parathyroid hyperplasia. A deficiency, rather than excess intake, of vitamin D would result in parathyroid hyperplasia. **BH p. 260, FH pp. 336-337**

24. C The patient's adrenal gland shows atrophic changes, mostly in the cortex, with reduction in gland size. The ensuing deficiency of adrenocortical hormones results in hypotension and a compensatory increase in ACTH by the pituitary results in skin hyperpigmentation. In this patient, the cause of the atrophy is most likely iatrogenic, given the history of long-term steroid use. Hypernatremia, hypokalemia, and hypertension would result from hyperplasia, rather than atrophy, of the adrenal cortex. Oliguria and hyperphosphatemia are seen in renal failure, not adrenal atrophy. **BH p. 262, FH pp. 338-340**

25. D Pheochromocytomas are tumors of the adrenal medulla that are composed of sheets of cells with abundant pink granular cytoplasm and small, centrally located nuclei. Addison disease, Cushing syndrome, and Conn syndrome all involve the adrenal cortex and not the medulla. A pituitary adenoma that secretes ACTH would likewise affect the adrenal cortex and not the medulla. **BH p. 263, FH pp. 338-340**

26. A Pheochromocytomas secrete excess catecholamines, resulting in headache and episodic hypertension. The other symptoms in this list result from disorders of the adrenal cortex rather than from the adrenal medulla. Consequently, hypernatremia and hypokalemia result from oversecretion of aldosterone, whereas hyperpigmentation and hypotension result from a deficiency of cortisol. Weight gain and hyperglycemia result from oversecretion of cortisol. Oliguria and hyperphosphatemia occur in renal failure. **BH p. 263**

27. E Vanillylmandelic acid is the metabolite of the catecholamine norepinephrine. It is found in the urine in increased amounts in patients with pheochromocytoma. Levels of ACTH, cortisol, testosterone, or aldosterone are useful in diagnosing an abnormal function of the adrenal cortex rather than the medulla. **BH p. 263**

28. C The tumor shown in the figure is composed of small, undifferentiated cells with scant cytoplasm within a fibrillary stroma. These are characteristic features of neuroblastoma, a common childhood tumor. It also shows the formation of Homer-Wright rosettes, with cells arranged around a central zone of neurofibrils. All the other tumors listed, except for adrenocortical adenoma, are commonly seen in children and are distinguished by their locations and morphologic appearance. Wilms tumor shows primitive cells with an attempt at formation of glomeruli and is found in the kidney, not the adrenals. A rhabdomyosarcoma is a tumor of skeletal muscle, with the tumor cells showing evidence of cytoplasmic striation. Ewing sarcoma is composed of sheets of small cells and arises within bone or connective tissue. An adrenocortical adenoma would contain cells filled with lipid droplets. **BH p. 264**

Male Reproductive System

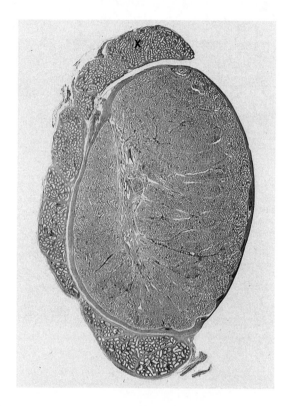

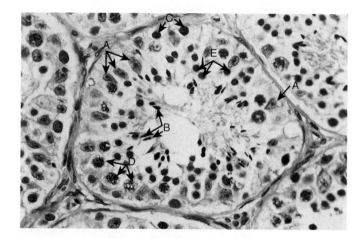

Use the figure above to answer the next two questions.

3 Which labeled cell phagocytoses the discarded cytoplasm of developing sperm?

4 Which labeled cell is the earliest stage that is committed to undergoing spermatogenesis?

1 Which function occurs specifically in the structure labeled *X*?
- ☐ A. Accumulation and storage of sperm
- ☐ B. Meiosis
- ☐ C. Secretion of citrate
- ☐ D. Secretion of fructose and vitamin C
- ☐ E. Secretion of inhibin

2 A 54-year-old man has come to a urologist requesting a reversal of his vasectomy. The operation is performed, but the patient is determined to be infertile owing to an autoimmune reaction caused by leakage of cells out of the vas deferens. Which cells would induce such an autoimmune reaction?
- ☐ A. Primary spermatocytes
- ☐ B Secondary spermatocytes
- ☐ C. Spermatids
- ☐ D. Spermatogonia
- ☐ E. Spermatozoa

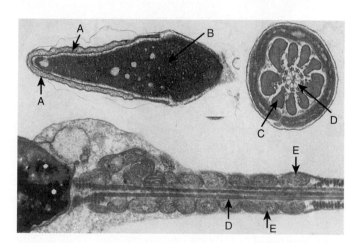

Use the figure at the bottom of the previous page to answer the next three questions.

5 Which structure would be expected to stain well with antibodies to hydrolytic enzymes?

6 Which structure forms a coil when viewed in three dimensions?

7 The fluid-filled, membranous structure labeled *A* in the micrograph on the previous page is derived directly from what?
☐ A. Golgi apparatus
☐ B. Lysosomes
☐ C. Nuclear envelope
☐ D. Rough endoplasmic reticulum
☐ E. Smooth endoplasmic reticulum

8 A 25-year-old man presents with infertility. Further tests reveal that he has Kartagener syndrome. What does this suggest is the cause of his infertility?
☐ A. Deficiency in mitochondrial ATP production
☐ B. Immotile flagellum
☐ C. Inability to penetrate the zona pellucida
☐ D. Incomplete manchette
☐ E. Uncondensed nucleus

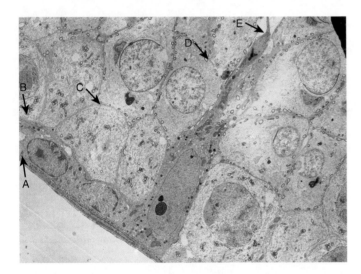

Use the figure above to answer the next two questions.

9 What letter indicates the location of the blood-testis barrier?

10 What is the cell with a very prominent nucleolus?
☐ A. Leydig cell
☐ B. Myoid cell
☐ C. Sertoli cell
☐ D. Spermatid
☐ E. Spermatocyte

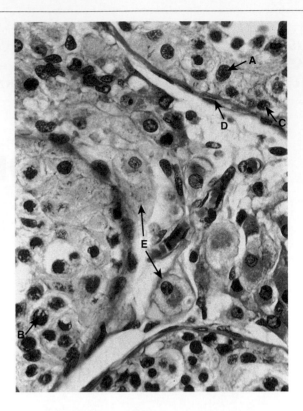

11 A 10-year-old boy presents to the physician with pubic hair and postpubertal changes in his muscle and skeleton. An intratesticular mass is felt on palpitation. Crystals of Reinke are seen in a fine-needle aspirate taken from the mass. Which cells in the figure above are most likely responsible for these results?

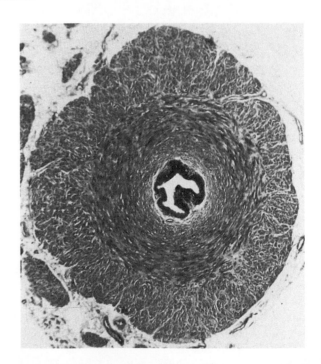

12 What is the structure shown in the figure at the bottom of the previous page?
☐ A. Efferent ductule
☐ B. Epididymis
☐ C. Penile urethra
☐ D. Prostatic urethra
☐ E. Vas deferens

13 In which organ is the connective tissue stroma mixed in with a large number of smooth muscle cells?
☐ A. Corpus cavernosum
☐ B. Corpus spongiosum
☐ C. Epididymis
☐ D. Prostate
☐ E. Seminal vesicle

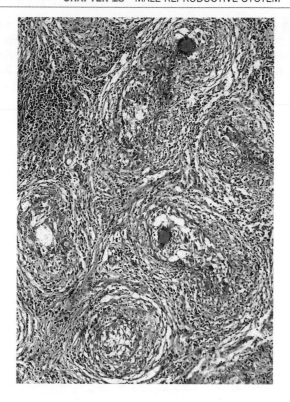

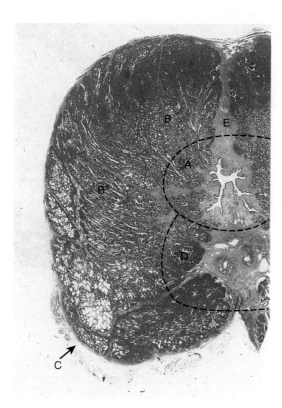

14 A 60-year-old man presents with frequent urination. The most common cause of this is a benign hyperplasia of a specific part of the prostate. From which region of the prostate should the biopsy be taken to confirm this diagnosis?

15 A 32-year-old man presented to his primary care physician with complaints of a mass in his testis. On physical examination, there was a hard, firm mass in the right testis. Orchiectomy was performed, and a microscopic section of the testis is shown in the figure. What is the most likely etiology of the pathology depicted?
☐ A. Hyperplasia of Leydig cells
☐ B. Immotile sperm cells
☐ C. Neoplasia of germ cells
☐ D. Trauma
☐ E. Vascular compromise

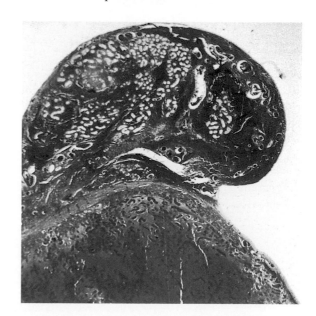

16 A 30-year-old man presented to the emergency room with a sudden onset of severe pain in the inguinal area. On physical examination, the left testis is swollen and painful. Emergency surgery with orchiectomy was performed. Based on the pathologic finding depicted in the figure at bottom of previous page, which of the following is the most likely etiology?

☐ A. Atherosclerosis
☐ B. Arteritis
☐ C. Embolism
☐ D. Thrombosis
☐ E. Vascular torsion

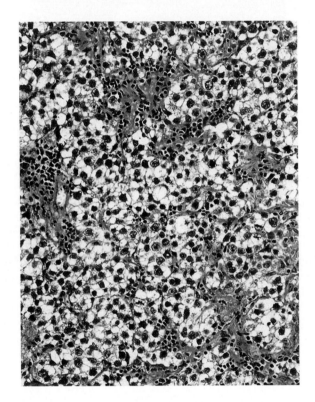

17 A 35-year-old man presented to his primary care physician with swelling of his testis. On physical examination, a mass was felt in the left testis, which was found to be a solid mass on ultrasound imaging. An orchiectomy was performed and a microscopic section is shown in the figure above. Which of the following is the most likely diagnosis?

☐ A. Choriocarcinoma
☐ B. Embryonal carcinoma
☐ C. Seminoma
☐ D. Teratoma
☐ E. Yolk sac tumor

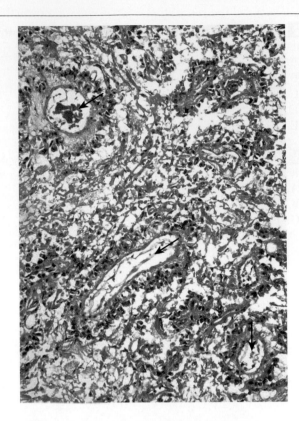

Use the figure above to answer the next two questions.

18 An orchiectomy was performed in a 3-year-old boy, who was found to have a testicular mass. Based on the microscopic appearance, a diagnosis of a yolk sac tumor was made. What are the characteristic structures shown by the *arrows*?

☐ A. Brenner tumors
☐ B. Call-Exner bodies
☐ C. Psammoma bodies
☐ D. Reinke crystals
☐ E. Schiller-Duval bodies

19 Serum measurement of which of the following would be most useful for diagnosis and monitoring of the same patient?

☐ A. Alpha-fetoprotein
☐ B. Human chorionic gonadotropin-beta
☐ C. Carcinoembryonic antigen
☐ D. CA 19.5
☐ E. CA 125

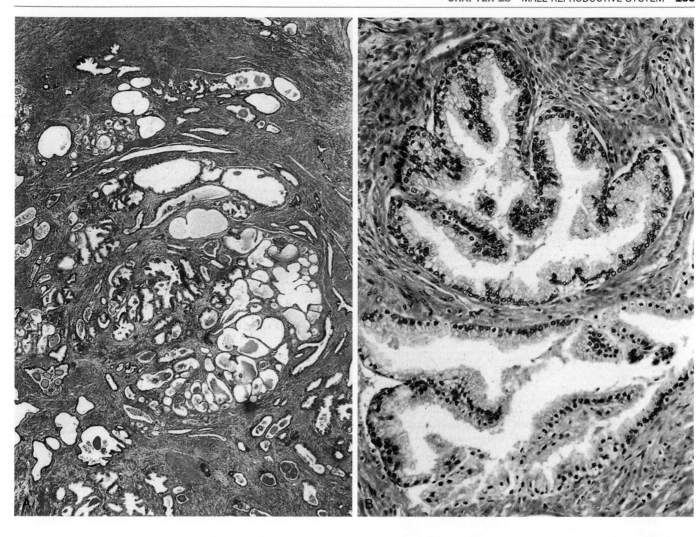

20 A 62-year-old man underwent a transurethral biopsy of the prostate. Based on the microscopic finding shown in the figure above, which of the following is the most likely presenting sign and symptom in this patient?

☐ A. Hard nodules in the periphery of the prostate
☐ B. Markedly elevated prostate specific antigen (PSA)
☐ C. Severe bone pain and pathologic fracture
☐ D. Urinary retention and obstruction

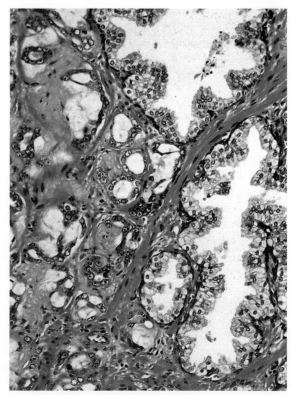

21 A 67-year-old man presents with complaints of straining to pass urine with a weak stream and dribbling. A prostate biopsy was performed, and a microscopic section is shown in the figure at the bottom of the previous page. Which of the following is the most likely diagnosis?

☐ A. Atrophy of the prostate
☐ B. Benign prostatic hyperplasia
☐ C. Chronic inflammation
☐ D. Granulomatous prostatitis
☐ E. Prostatic adenocarcinoma

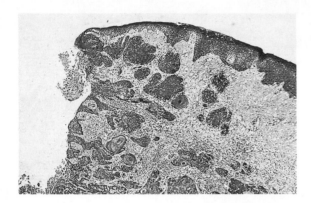

22 A 30-year-old man presents with an ulcerated lesion on the penis. A biopsy of the lesion was performed, and a microscopic section is shown in the figure above. This lesion is associated with which of the following organisms?

☐ A. *Chlamydia trachomatis*
☐ B. Herpes simplex
☐ C. Human papillomavirus
☐ D. *Neisseria gonorrhoeae*
☐ E. *Treponema pallidum*

ANSWERS

1. A This is the epididymis. Sperm from the testes may be stored here for up to a month. In contrast, meiosis and secretion of inhibin occur within the seminiferous tubules, whereas the secretion of citrate or fructose into seminal fluid takes place in accessory organs of the male reproductive system (prostate gland and seminal vesicles). **FH pp. 347, 354**

2. E Only spermatozoa are found in the vas deferens. Sperm trigger an immune response when exposed to the blood because they are normally hidden from the immune system by the blood-testis barrier. The other cells are found in the seminiferous tubules and would not be affected to damage to the vas deferens. **FH pp. 348-352**

3. A The Sertoli cell, recognizable by its pale irregular nucleus, phagocytoses cytoplasm shed during spermiogenesis. The other cells in this figure are stages in the development of sperm cells. **FH pp. 349, 352**

4. D The primary spermatocytes are the earliest stage committed to developing into spermatozoa. They are recognizable as having the largest of the round germ cell nuclei in the seminiferous tubule. Spermatogonia are not committed to differentiating exclusively to spermatocytes. **FH p. 349**

5. A This is the acrosome; it contains digestive enzymes needed for the penetration of the zona pellucida around the oocyte. **FH p. 351**

6. E The mitochondria form a tightly packed spiral around the axoneme and outer dense fibers. They provide the ATP needed for flagellar action. **FH p. 351**

7. A The acrosomal cap of a developing spermatid is constructed from Golgi-derived vesicles that fuse into a single structure. **FH p. 351**

8. B Dynein is attached to flagellar microtubules to generate movement. In Kartagener syndrome, a defect in the dynein gene results in immotile sperm and infertility. This defect does not affect the function of mitochondria, the nucleus, or the acrosome. **FH pp. 92, 351**

9. B The blood-testis barrier, formed by lateral processes from Sertoli cells, lies between the spermatogonia (having smaller, oval nuclei at the base of the seminiferous epithelium) and the primary spermatocytes (having larger, round nuclei above the spermatogonia). **FH p. 352**

10. C An identifying histologic feature of a Sertoli cell is a prominent nucleolus. Spermatocytes, which are undergoing meiosis, have condensed chromosomes and lack nucleoli. Leydig cells are not seen in the figure, and the myoid cell nucleus lacks a nucleolus in this image. **FH p. 352**

11. E The cells most likely forming the tumor are Leydig cells. Leydig cells in the testicular interstitium have abundant pale cytoplasm containing characteristic elongated crystals, named *crystals of Reinke*. Leydig cell tumors, generally benign in young males, produce testosterone, which is responsible for precocious development of the male secondary sex characteristics. **FH. p. 353**

12. E This vas deferens is identifiable by its very thick muscle wall and pseudostratified epithelium (not discernable in this figure). In contrast, the epididymis has a very tall pseudostratified columnar epithelium that is much thicker than the surrounding strands of smooth muscle, and the urethra is lined with a transitional epithelium. **FH p. 354**

13. D The connective tissue surrounding the prostatic acini is unusual in that it contains a large amount of smooth muscle mixed in among the collagen fibers. In most organs, smooth muscle forms a layer separate from the connective tissue layers. **FH p. 356**

14. A The periurethral area of prostatic tissue is most commonly enlarged in benign prostatic hyperplasia. Compression of the urethra results in difficulty emptying the bladder. **FH p. 356**

15. D The figure shows a granulomatous inflammation, which most commonly follows trauma to the testis or surgery to the spermatic cord. None of the other choices listed are associated with a granulomatous inflammation. Hyperplasia of Leydig cells would result in increased secretion of sex hormones and immotile sperm cells are a cause of infertility. Vascular compromise would result in infarction of the testes. Depending on the type of tumor, various histologic findings would be seen in germ cell tumors, but granulomas are not present. **BH p. 246**

16. E The figure shows marked congestion and infarction of the testis. This is most often caused by torsion of the spermatic cord, leading to obstruction of the venous drainage and infarction of the testis. Arteritis, atherosclerosis, and thrombosis of the testicular arteries would result in narrowing of the lumen and diminished blood flow to the testes, but complete occlusion of the vessel and subsequent infarctions are rare. An embolism can occlude a branch of the testicular artery and can lead to infarction of the area supplied by the occluded branch, but infarction of the whole testes is unlikely. **BH p. 246**

17. C The microscopic appearance, consisting of sheets of uniform polygonal cells with clear cytoplasms, which are surrounded by delicate fibrous septae infiltrated by lymphocytes, is characteristic of a seminoma. All the other tumors listed are also germ cell tumors of the testes, and they are distinguished by their characteristic morphologic findings. Hence, in choriocarcinoma, malignant syncytioblasts and cytotrophoblasts are present, whereas embryonal carcinoma is characterized by large atypical cells with areas of gland formation. In teratomas, tissues derived from more than one germ layer are present in the tumor. Yolk sac tumors have structures resembling endodermal sinuses. **BH pp. 246-248**

18. E The *arrows* point to a Schiller-Duval body (i.e., a structure resembling a fetal glomerulus consisting of a central blood vessel surrounded by visceral and parietal layers of embryonal cells). This is a characteristic feature of yolk sac tumors. Reinke's crystals are seen in Leydig cell tumors, and Call-Exner bodies are seen in granulosa cell tumors. Psammoma bodies are seen in papillary serous tumors of the ovary. Brenner tumors are small nests of transitional type epithelia seen in the ovary. **BH p. 249**

19. A Yolk sac tumors secrete alpha-fetoprotein, which is useful for diagnosis and monitoring of patients with these tumors. Human chorionic gonadotropin-beta is used to monitor patients with choriocarcinomas, whereas CEA, CA 19.5, and CA 125 are used to monitor patients with colon, pancreatic, and ovarian carcinomas, respectively. **BH p. 249**

20. D The figure shows a rounded nodule formed by a proliferation of prostatic glands and hypertrophy of the fibromuscular stroma. These findings are characteristic of benign prostatic hyperplasia, which leads to obstruction of the urethra and urinary retention. In benign hyperplasia, the PSA is usually not elevated, and the prostate is rubbery, not hard. A hard nodule in the periphery of the prostate, markedly elevated PSA and severe bone pain with pathologic fractures, are all suggestive of a prostatic adenocarcinoma, rather than a benign hyperplasia. **BH pp. 250-251**

21. E The figure shows small, round prostatic acini lined by a single layer of malignant cells displaying prominent nucleoli. These features are characteristic of prostatic adenocarcinoma. Atrophy of the prostate would show small acini lined by a shrunken, atrophic epithelium with small hyperchromatic nuclei. In benign prostatic hyperplasia, large round nodules formed by a proliferation of prostatic glands and hyperplasia of the fibromuscular stroma are seen. The proliferating glands have large lumens and are lined by more than one cell layer. Infiltration by neutrophils or lymphocytes would be seen in chronic inflammation, and multiple granulomas would be present in granulomatous prostatitis. **BH pp. 250-252**

22. C The figure shows a well-differentiated, keratinizing squamous cell carcinoma of the penis. These tumors are associated with infection by human papillomavirus. The other agents listed are causes of sexually transmitted diseases; however, none is associated with an increased risk for developing squamous cell carcinoma of the penis. **BH p. 253**

Female Reproductive System

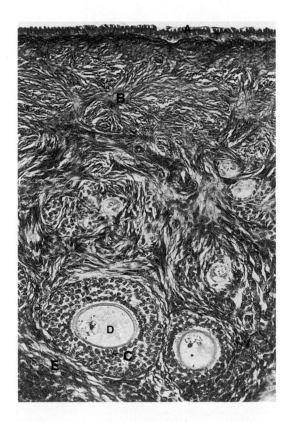

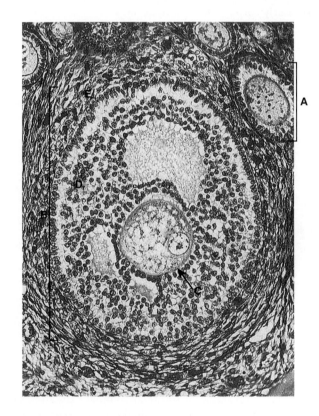

Use the figure above to answer the next two questions.

1 Which labeled region in the figure above is the most common source of tumors in this organ?

2 The cell labeled *D* in the figure above is in which phase of the cell cycle?
- ☐ A. Mitotic interphase
- ☐ B. Prophase of meiosis I
- ☐ C. Between meiosis I and meiosis II
- ☐ D. Prophase of meiosis II
- ☐ E. Meiosis II completed

3 Which labeled region indicates the site of androstenedione synthesis?

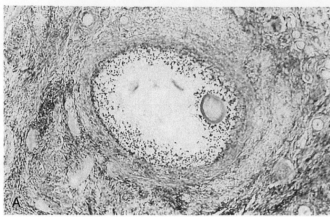

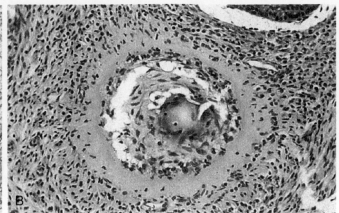

4 An oophorectomy was performed in a 38-year-old woman. The images above, taken from microscopic sections of her ovaries, show indications of what process or condition?
- ☐ A. Benign serous adenoma
- ☐ B. Early corpus luteum formation
- ☐ C. Normal follicular atresia
- ☐ D. Polycystic ovarian disease
- ☐ E. Poor preservation of the specimen

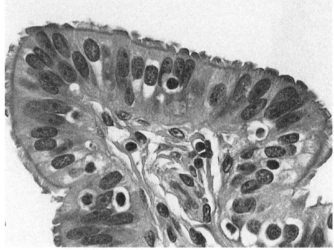

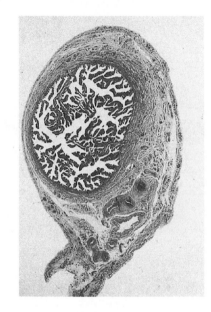

6 What is the major reproductive event that normally occurs in the structure shown in the above figure?
- ☐ A. Capacitation
- ☐ B. Corpus luteum formation
- ☐ C. Fertilization
- ☐ D. Implantation
- ☐ E. Production of the first polar body

5 A 21-year-old woman is admitted to the emergency room after complaining of severe abdominal pain and light-headedness. A diagnosis of a ruptured ectopic pregnancy was made, and the patient was operated on to stop her abdominal bleeding. The surgeon removed the damaged structures, and they were examined by a pathologist. A section adjacent to the rupture is shown in the figure above. Based on this appearance, what was the site of the ectopic implantation?
- ☐ A. Broad ligament
- ☐ B. Fallopian tube
- ☐ C. Ovary
- ☐ D. Rectal pouch
- ☐ E. Uterine cervix

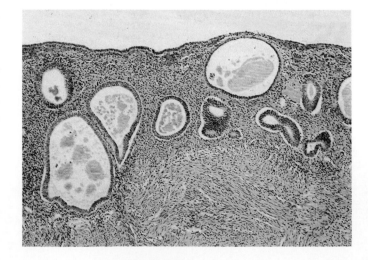

7 A 56-year-old woman comes to her physician complaining of vaginal bleeding. Her last menstrual period occurred 2 years previously. She is obese and has mild diabetes. A dilation and curettage of the endometrium is performed and analyzed histologically. What do the histologic findings in the figure at the bottom of the previous page suggest?

☐ A. Endometrial polyp
☐ B. Endometrioid adenocarcinoma
☐ C. Endometriosis
☐ D. Leiomyoma
☐ E. Simple endometrial hyperplasia

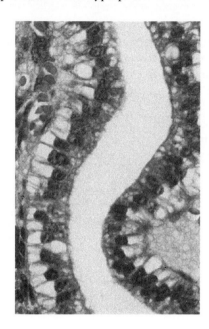

8 The figure above illustrates a biopsy section of the endometrial glands taken during the luteal phase of the cycle. The simple columnar epithelial cells lining these glands have pale-staining regions of cytoplasm. This appearance is due to the presence in these cells of large amounts of what?

☐ A. Glycogen
☐ B. Golgi stacks
☐ C. Lipid
☐ D. Rough endoplasmic reticulum
☐ E. Smooth endoplasmic reticulum

9 A 40-year-old woman was examined by her physician because of a failure to conceive a child following a difficult pregnancy and delivery 3 years earlier. She has a history of irregular menstrual periods. Among other tests, a biopsy of the corpus of the uterus is taken, shown in the figure at the top of the next column at low (A) and high (B) magnifications. What does the histologic analysis shown in the images suggest?

☐ A. Chronic endometritis
☐ B. Hyperplasia of the endometrium
☐ C. Leiomyoma of the myometrium
☐ D. Nabothian cyst
☐ E. Postmenopausal endometrium

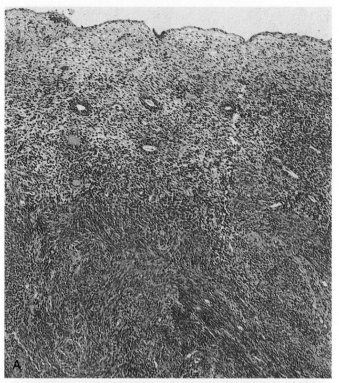

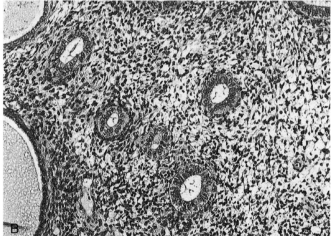

10 The epithelial cells of the vagina, shown in the figure at the top of the next page, have a characteristic appearance due to their high content of what?

☐ A. Actin
☐ B. Glycogen
☐ C. Keratin
☐ D. Lipid
☐ E. Mucins

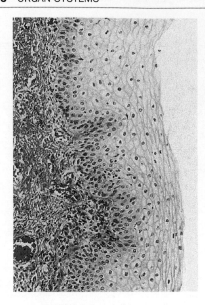

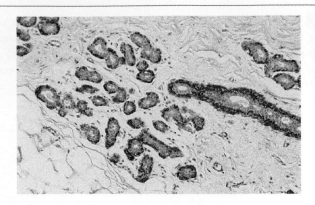

13 The image of breast tissue shown in the figure above was prepared using immunostaining. Use of a primary antibody to which protein would give this appearance?
☐ A. Actin
☐ B. Casein
☐ C. Collagen type IV
☐ D. Keratin
☐ E. Vimentin

11 What is the most likely pathology in an individual with abnormally low levels of vaginal epithelial glycogen?
☐ A. An increased risk for cervical cancer
☐ B. Increased bacterial infections
☐ C. Increased mucus secretion
☐ D. Infertility
☐ E. Pain during intercourse

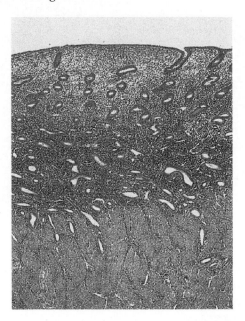

12 Which process normally occurs at the stage of the menstrual cycle shown in the figure above?
☐ A. Implantation of the blastocyst
☐ B. Rapid mitoses among the cells of the glandular epithelium
☐ C. Shedding of the endometrium
☐ D. Synthesis of glycogen in the glandular epithelium

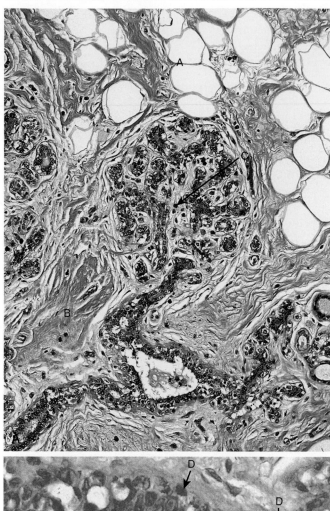

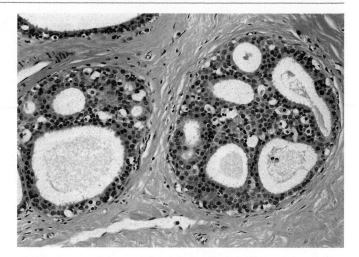

15 A 30-year-old woman is examined by her physician 2 months after the cessation of nursing of her third child. She has noticed a mass in her left breast. A biopsy of the mass is shown in the figure above. What does this histologic analysis suggest?

☐ A. Apoptosis of regressing acinar cells
☐ B. Crinophagy of secretory granules
☐ C. Ductal carcinoma in situ
☐ D. Hyperplasia of myoepithelial cells
☐ E. Inflammation secondary to a bacterial infection

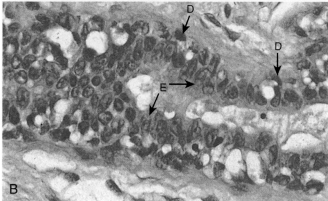

14 Identify the oxytocin-sensitive cells shown in the figure above.

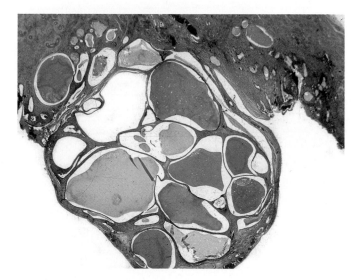

16 A 32-year-old woman was found to have a mass protruding from the cervical os. A microscopic section of the lesion is shown in the figure above. Which of the following most likely would be a presenting symptom in this patient?

☐ A. Anorexia and weight loss
☐ B. Milky vaginal discharge
☐ C. Primary amenorrhea
☐ D. Right lower quadrant pain and fever
☐ E. Vaginal bleeding

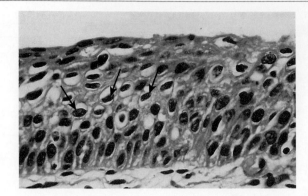

A. Amenorrhea
B. Dysmenorrhea
C. Menorrhagia
D. Postcoital bleeding

17 A biopsy of the cervix was performed in a 30-year-old woman who had an abnormal finding on a Papanicolaou (Pap) test. A microscopic section of her cervix is shown in the figure above. The cells depicted by the *arrows* show changes characteristic of infection with which of the following?

☐ A. *Chlamydia trachomatis*
☐ B. Herpes simplex virus
☐ C. Human papillomavirus
☐ D. *Neisseria gonorrhoeae*
☐ E. *Trichomonas vaginalis*

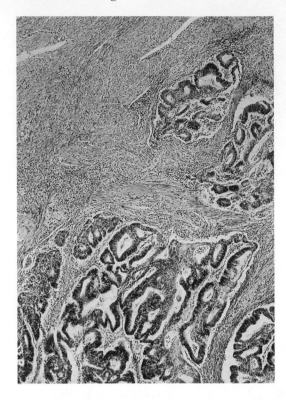

19 A hysterectomy was performed in a 59-year-old woman with postmenopausal bleeding. A microscopic section of her uterus is shown in the figure above. Which of the following lesions most likely preceded the finding shown in the image?

☐ A. Adenomyosis
☐ B. Complex hyperplasia
☐ C. Endometritis
☐ D. Hydatidiform mole
☐ E. Leiomyoma

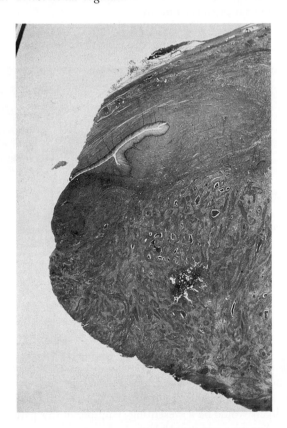

18 A biopsy of the cervix was performed in a 30-year-old woman who had an abnormal finding on a Pap test. A microscopic section of her cervix is shown in the figure above. Which of the following most likely would be a presenting symptom in this patient?

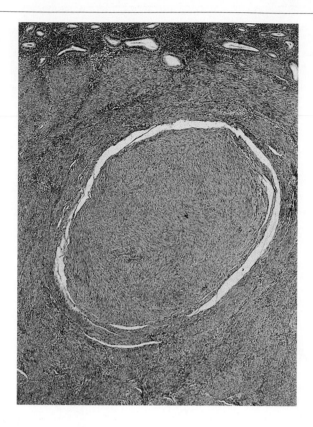

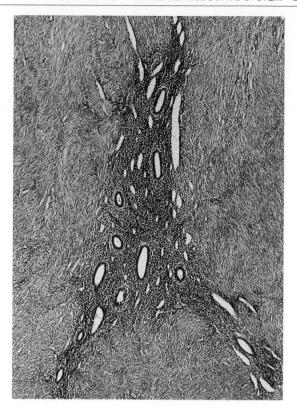

20 A 38-year-old woman underwent hysterectomy for severe pelvic pain. Several nodules were present in the uterus, and a microscopic section of one of these nodules is shown in the figure above. Which of the following most likely would be a complication of the pathology depicted, if left untreated?

☐ A. Amenorrhea

☐ B. Adenomyosis

☐ C. Endometrial hyperplasia

☐ D. Infertility

21 The microscopic section shown in the figure above is from the uterus of a 45-year-old woman who underwent hysterectomy for abdominal pain. Which of the following is the most likely diagnosis?

☐ A. Adenomyosis

☐ B. Endometrial adenocarcinoma

☐ C. Endometritis

☐ D. Leiomyoma

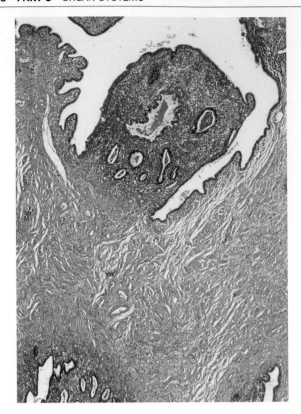

22 A 22-year-old woman underwent exploratory laparotomy for severe abdominal pain. She was found to have lesions in her fallopian tube. A microscopic section of one of these lesions is shown in the figure above. This patient has an increased risk for developing which of the following complications?

☐ A. Endometrial carcinoma
☐ B. Infertility
☐ C. Pelvic inflammatory disease
☐ D. Ovarian failure
☐ E. Uterine prolapse

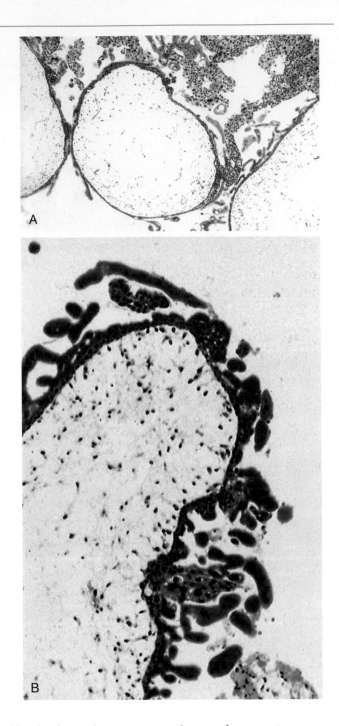

Use the figure above to answer the next four questions.

23 A 28-year-old woman, who is in the 12th week of her pregnancy, presents to the emergency room with vaginal bleeding. On physical examination, her uterus is large for gestational age. A vaginal examination reveals a grapelike mass protruding from the cervical os. The mass was sent to pathology for examination. Based on the microscopic section shown in the images above, which of the following is the most likely diagnosis?

☐ A. Acute cervicitis
☐ B. Complete mole
☐ C. Endometrial polyp
☐ D. Nabothian cyst
☐ E. Uterine prolapse

24 Chromosomal analysis of the tissue depicted in the image would most likely show which of the following karyotypes?
- [ ] A. 45X0
- [ ] B. 46XX
- [ ] C. 47XXY
- [ ] D. 55XY
- [ ] E. 69XXY

25 Serum measurement of which of the following would be most useful in the diagnosis and follow-up of this patient?
- [ ] A. Alpha-fetoprotein
- [ ] B. Carcinoembryonic antigen
- [ ] C. CA 19.5
- [ ] D. CA 125
- [ ] E. Human chorionic gonadotropin

26 This patient has an increased risk for developing which of the following?
- [ ] A. Choriocarcinoma
- [ ] B. Endometrioid adenocarcinoma
- [ ] C. Leiomyosarcoma
- [ ] D. Squamous cell carcinoma of the cervix
- [ ] E. Uterine carcinosarcoma

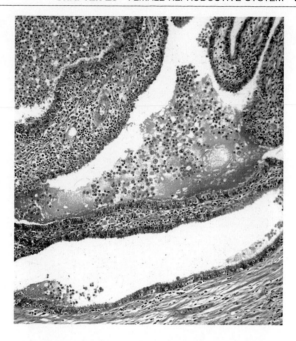

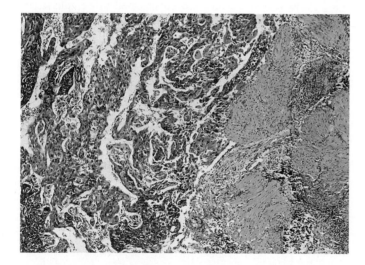

27 A 28-year-old woman underwent total hysterectomy due to profuse vaginal bleeding. She had a history of spontaneous abortion 1 month before presentation. A microscopic examination of her uterus revealed a malignant tumor composed of a proliferation of cytotrophoblasts and syncytiotrophoblast, as shown in the figure above. A CT scan showed multiple nodules in her lung, which were thought to be metastatic in nature. Which of the following most likely would be a presenting sign and symptom resulting from the lung lesions in this patient?
- [ ] A. Fever
- [ ] B. Hemoptysis
- [ ] C. Hoarseness of voice
- [ ] D. Pleuritic chest pain
- [ ] E. Wheezing

28 A 31-year-old woman was referred to a gynecologist for evaluation of right lower quadrant abdominal pain. On physical examination, a right adnexal mass was present. Surgery was performed, and the right fallopian tube and ovary were removed. A microscopic section of the fallopian tube is shown in the figure above. Which of the following is the most common etiologic agent of the pathology shown in the image?
- [ ] A. *Haemophilus ducreyi*
- [ ] B. Herpes simplex virus
- [ ] C. Human papillomavirus
- [ ] D. *Neisseria gonorrhoeae*
- [ ] E. *Trichomonas vaginalis*

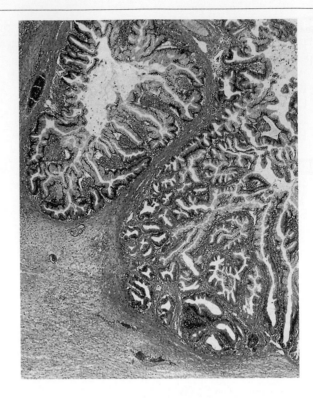

Use the figure above to answer the next two questions.

29 A 26-year-old woman was rushed to the emergency room with severe abdominal pain. Imaging studies showed a distended, fluid-filled left fallopian tube. Exploratory laparotomy was performed with removal of the left fallopian tube. Based on the microscopic section shown in the figure above, which of the following is the most likely cause of her abdominal pain?

☐ A. Ascending vaginal infection
☐ B. Ectopic pregnancy
☐ C. Endometriosis
☐ D. Ruptured cyst
☐ E. Metastatic tumor

30 Which of the following most likely would be present on examination of this patient?

☐ A. Blood pressure 70/50 mm Hg
☐ B. Cardiac murmur
☐ C. Milky vaginal discharge
☐ D. Petechial rash on the abdomen
☐ E. Temperature 103° F

31 A 46-year-old woman was examined by her physician after the onset of irregular menstrual bleeding. A mass with a diameter of about 8 cm could be palpated on the left ovary. A biopsy specimen of the mass is shown in the figure above. What does the histology of this mass indicate?

☐ A. Corpus albicans
☐ B. Enlarged corpus luteum
☐ C. Follicular cyst
☐ D. Hydatidiform mole
☐ E. Mucinous cystadenocarcinoma

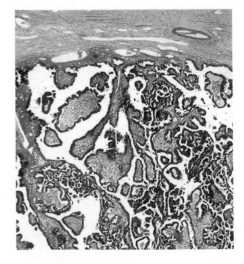

32 A 50-year-old woman complaining of pelvic pain was found to have a cystic mass in her right ovary on ultrasound examination. The mass was surgically removed. Microscopically, the mass showed the findings depicted in the figure on the previous page. This lesion was most likely derived from which of the following structures?

- ☐ A. Embryonic remnants
- ☐ B. Fibrous tissue of broad ligament
- ☐ C. Germ cells
- ☐ D. Ovarian stroma
- ☐ E. Surface epithelium of ovary

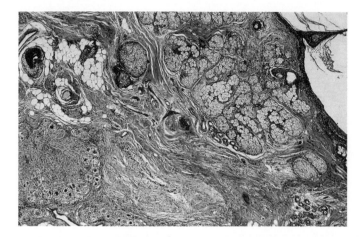

33 A 38-year-old woman underwent surgical removal of an ovarian mass. A microscopic section of the mass is shown in the figure above. This lesion was most likely derived from which of the following structures?

- ☐ A. Embryonic remnants
- ☐ B. Fibrous tissue of broad ligament
- ☐ C. Germ cells
- ☐ D. Ovarian stroma
- ☐ E. Surface epithelium of ovary

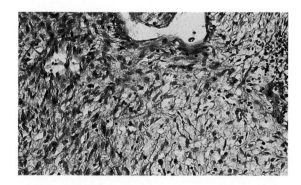

Use the figure above to answer the next two questions.

34 A 52-year-old woman was found to have an ovarian tumor. On examination following surgical removal, the mass was found to be firm and lobulated with a yellow cut surface. A microscopic section of the mass showed the pathologic finding depicted in the figure above. Which of the following is the most likely diagnosis?

- ☐ A. Cystadenocarcinoma
- ☐ B. Endometriosis
- ☐ C. Luteal cyst
- ☐ D. Theca cell tumor
- ☐ E. Teratoma

35 This patient has an increased risk for developing what?

- ☐ A. Adenomyosis
- ☐ B. Endometrial adenocarcinoma
- ☐ C. Endometritis
- ☐ D. Leiomyoma

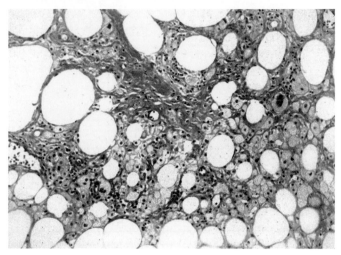

36 A 52-year-old woman presents to her primary care physician after finding a mass in her right breast during her monthly self-examination. She was referred to a surgeon who performed a biopsy of the mass. The microscopic section shown in the figure above is from the mass. Which of the following is the most likely etiology of the pathology depicted?

- ☐ A. Acute infection
- ☐ B. Atrophy
- ☐ C. Excess estrogen
- ☐ D. Genetic mutation
- ☐ E. Trauma

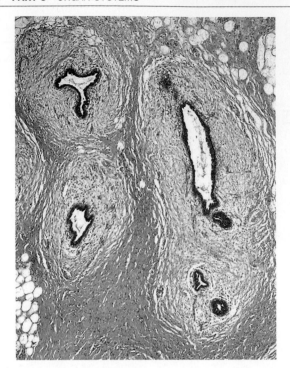

37 Physical examination of a 57-year-old man reveals bilateral breast masses. A biopsy was performed and shows the finding depicted in the figure above. Which of the following conditions would most likely be present in this patient?

☐ A. Gallstones
☐ B. Liver cirrhosis
☐ C. Lung carcinoma
☐ D. Pancreatic insufficiency
☐ E. Prostatic hyperplasia

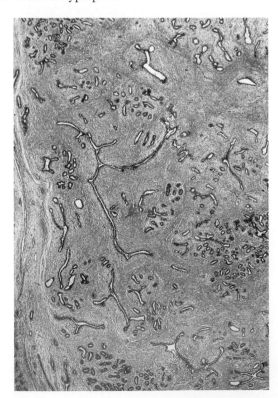

38 A 16-year-old girl was brought to the pediatrician by her mother because of a swelling in her right breast. Physical examination showed a well-defined, rubbery mass, and she was referred to a surgeon. The mass was removed, and a microscopic section is shown in the figure at bottom left. Which of the following is the most likely diagnosis?

☐ A. Ductal carcinoma in situ
☐ B. Fibroadenoma
☐ C. Fibrocystic change
☐ D. Intraductal papilloma
☐ E. Sclerosing adenosis

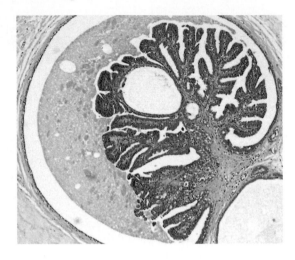

39 A 49-year-old woman with a breast mass had an excisional biopsy shown in the figure above. Which of the following is the most likely clinical presentation of this lesion?

☐ A. Ulcerating lesion on the nipple
☐ B. Bloody nipple discharge
☐ C. Draining abscess
☐ D. Massive edema of the breast

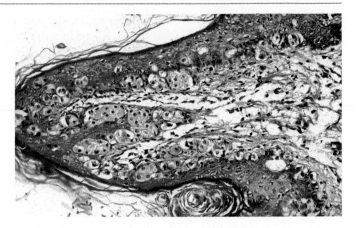

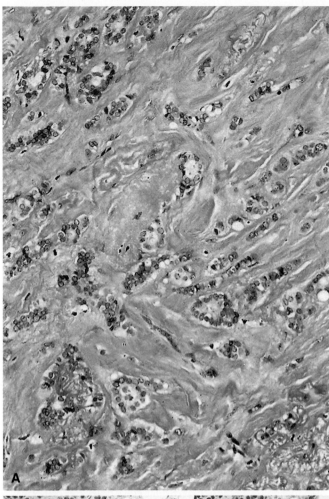

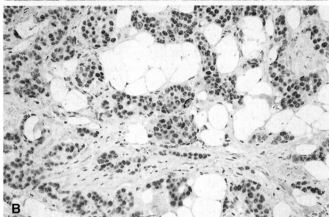

40 A microscopic section taken from a breast mass in a 53-year-old woman is shown in part A of the figure above. This tumor was stained with an antibody directed against estrogen receptors, as shown in part B. Based on these findings, which of the following is most likely regarding this lesion?

- ☐ A. Estrogen receptor positivity imparts a poor prognosis
- ☐ B. It is an intraductal proliferation
- ☐ C. It presents as a circumscribed rubbery mass
- ☐ D. It is likely to respond to hormone therapy

41 A 56-year-old woman was found to have a reddened and thickened nipple and areola. A biopsy of the nipple was performed, and the finding shown in the figure above. Which of the following underlying lesions is the patient most likely to have?

- ☐ A. Fibroadenoma
- ☐ B. Fibrocystic change
- ☐ C. Intraductal papilloma
- ☐ D. Invasive ductal carcinoma
- ☐ E. Sclerosing adenosis

ANSWERS

1. A This is the surface (peritoneal) epithelium of the ovary. These cells are the most common source of ovarian tumors. **FH p. 362, BH p. 229**

2. B This is a primary oocyte. All female germ cells begin meiosis I before birth and are paused during prophase. They are held this way until just before ovulation when meiosis I is completed. Meiosis II is completed at fertilization. **FH p. 362**

3. E The theca interna produces androstenedione, which is then converted to estrogen in granulosa cells. The other labeled cells in the ovary lack the capacity for steroid synthesis. **FH p. 363**

4. C Many ovarian follicles degenerate instead of becoming fully mature. On page 160 are two examples of such atretic follicles, which have a characteristically thickened glassy membrane surrounding clearly degenerating cells or traces of an abnormal oocyte. A corpus luteum would lack an oocyte, which would have been ovulated; in polycystic ovarian disease, large fluid-filled cysts are present. Benign serous adenoma would be characterized by papillary proliferation on the surface of the ovary. The cells surrounding the atretic follicles are clearly well preserved. **FH p. 366**

5. B The simple columnar epithelium with both ciliated and nonciliated cells is characteristic of the fallopian tube. This is the most common site of ectopic implantation. The broad ligament is composed of connective tissue covered by a simple squamous mesothelium; the rectal pouch also is lined by a simple squamous mesothelium, and the uterine cervix has a stratified squamous epithelium. The ovary lacks ciliated simple columnar epithelium. **FH p. 368**

6. C The ampulla of the fallopian tube is the typical site of fertilization. Capacitation and implantation typically occur within the corpus of the uterus; corpora lutea and first polar bodies are formed during ovulation in the ovary. **FH p. 368**

7. E The figure shows a proliferation of endometrial glands with the formation of numerous cysts. This is characteristic of simple endometrial hyperplasia, which is frequently associated with diabetes or with polycystic ovarian syndrome. Because the tissue was taken from the endometrium, these cysts do not represent ectopic endometrial structures, as in endometriosis. There is no proliferation of smooth muscle, as in a leiomyoma. Unlike endometrioid adenocarcinoma, the epithelial cells show no evidence of dysplasia. An endometrial polyp also shows proliferation of glands; however, the outer layer of the polyp is covered by a flattened epithelial layer and the polyp protrudes into the endometrial cavity. **FH p. 372, BH p. 224**

8. A These cells actively synthesize and secrete glycogen, which does not stain well with most histologic stains. The rough endoplasmic reticulum is basophilic, rather than pale-staining, and other membranous organelles would not be so abundant as to account for the widespread pale-staining appearance of these cells. Lipid would appear as discrete pale droplets within the cells. **FH p. 373**

9. E The figure shows a drastic decline in the abundance of endometrial glands, signifying an atrophic, postmenopausal endometrium. This can be provoked by excessive postpartum bleeding that compromises pituitary function (Sheehan syndrome). The lack of hormonal stimulation of the endometrium leads to its atrophy. In hyperplasia, there would be proliferation of glands rather than atrophy. Chronic endometritis is characterized by the presence of numerous plasma cells in the stroma. Nabothian cysts are confined to the uterine cervix. **FH p. 374**

10. B The cytoplasm of vaginal epithelial cells appears pale because of the high content of glycogen in these cells. Proteins like collagen, actin, keratin, and mucin stain pink with hematoxylin and eosin and green with Masson trichrome stain. Lipid would appear as discrete pale droplets within the cells. **FH p. 377**

11. B The glycogen is converted to lactic acid, which inhibits bacterial proliferation. Glycogen production is not linked to mucus secretion or a dry vaginal mucosa, nor to cervical cancer. **FH p. 377**

12. B The early proliferative stage of the endometrium is shown. It is characterized by straight, tubular glands with numerous mitoses in both the glands and the stroma. Glycogen production and implantation occur during the secretory stage of the cycle, in which the endometrial glands have a tortuous rather than straight appearance with numerous secretory vacuoles. During menstruation and endometrial shedding, there is breakdown of the glands and stroma, with evidence of bleeding, and the endometrium is much thinner than in this figure. **FH p. 372**

13. A The immunostained cells are myoepithelial cells that have a high content of actin. Antibodies to collagen or vimentin would label the connective tissue surrounding the ducts, whereas immunoreactivity for casein would be confined to the lumens, and apical cells of the ducts, rather than the basal cells. Antibodies to keratin would stain both the apical cells and the myoepithelial cells. **FH p. 387**

14. D These are the myoepithelial cells. They form the basal layer of epithelium of the ductules and acini. They are stimulated to contract by oxytocin. Connective tissue cells like fat cells or fibroblasts lack oxytocin receptors. **FH p. 387**

15. C A proliferation of duct cells that fills the lumens of the ducts with cells showing evidence of dysplasia is characteristic of ductal carcinoma in situ. Hyperplasia of myoepithelial cells may occur in conjunction with ductal epithelial cell proliferation. However, in these cases, neither the myoepithelial nor the ductal epithelial cells show dysplastic cellular changes. In regressive changes of the breast following the cessation of lactation, the epithelial cells show evidence of apoptosis, that is, dark-stained, irregular cell nuclei and crinophagy (autophagy) of secretory granules. Bacterial infection would be characterized by neutrophils infiltrating the ducts and their surrounding connective tissue. **FH p. 388, BH p. 241**

16. E The figure shows an endocervical polyp composed of a benign proliferation of cystically dilated endocervical glands. The polyp is large, and protrusion through the cervical os generally results in trauma to the polyp. Therefore, the patient would present with vaginal bleeding. Milky vaginal discharge, pain, and fever are symptoms of an infection and would be accompanied by accumulations of inflammatory cells. Patients with primary amenorrhea present with a lack of secondary sexual characteristics and a failure of menstruation, not endocervical polyps. Anorexia and weight loss are nonspecific symptoms, but they are indicators of a long-standing or generalized disorder or neoplastic process rather than a benign localized lesion. **BH p. 217**

17. C The organisms listed are all causes of sexually transmitted diseases. Some of the organisms have a characteristic appearance, whereas in the others, the infected epithelium shows characteristic morphologic changes allowing for a presumptive diagnosis. The cells depicted by the arrows are koilocytes, which are characteristic of human papillomavirus–infected cells. These virally infected cells have enlarged, irregular nuclei and a clear cytoplasm, which forms a halo around the nucleus. The epithelium in herpes simplex virus infection shows multinucleation and glassy intranuclear inclusions. The trophozoites of *Trichomonas vaginalis* are best seen on wet mounts of vaginal discharge or Pap smears, where they exhibit an oval shape with an ill-defined nucleus and the presence of a flagellum. *Neisseria gonorrhoeae* is identified by Gram staining as a gram-negative intracellular diplococcus. Both *N. gonorrhoeae* and *Chlamydia trachomatis* infections are diagnosed using cultures or nucleic acid amplification techniques. **BH p. 220**

18. D The figure shows an invasive squamous cell carcinoma of the cervix. Postcoital bleeding is the most common clinical presentation in patients with this tumor. Other symptoms of cancer of the cervix include vaginal discharge and painful intercourse. The other choices listed are menstrual abnormalities related to disorders of the uterus or hormonal imbalance and do not cause an abnormal Pap test finding. **BH p. 221**

19. B The figure shows invasive endometrioid adenocarcinoma. Complex endometrial hyperplasia is a risk factor for development of this cancer. The other pathologies of the uterus listed are not associated with an increased risk for developing endometrial adenocarcinoma. **BH p. 225**

20. D The nodule, composed of fascicles of smooth muscle cells, is characteristic of leiomyoma. These benign tumors cause pelvic pain and excessive menstruation and may result in infertility due to compression of the endometrial cavity. The other choices listed are not associated with leiomyoma. Amenorrhea results from ovarian failure or hormonal imbalance, and endometrial hyperplasia results from excess stimulation of the endometrium by estrogen. The cause of adenomyosis is not known. **BH p. 225**

21. A The presence of benign endometrial glands and stroma embedded deep within the myometrium is a diagnostic feature of adenomyosis. The glands resemble normal endometrial glands with no evidence of dysplasia, ruling out the possibility of endometrial adenocarcinoma. Endometritis is characterized by an inflammatory infiltrate of the endometrial lining mucosa. Leiomyoma is a nodular proliferation of bundles of smooth muscle from the myometrium without the presence of endometrial glands. **BH p. 223**

22. B The figure shows the presence of endometrial glands and stroma outside of the endometrium, in this case the wall of the fallopian tube. This process is termed *endometriosis*. Infertility is a complication of endometriosis. The precise mechanism of infertility caused by endometriosis is not fully understood. It is partly due to scarring and fibrosis of the fallopian tube, a common site where endometriosis occurs. Endometriosis can occur in the ovaries, but total destruction of both ovaries due to endometriosis is extremely rare; therefore, ovarian failure is unlikely. Endometriosis does not predispose to the development of endometrial carcinoma, pelvic inflammatory disease, or uterine prolapse. **BH p. 223**

23. B The figure shows large, edematous chorionic villi with a large central cavity (cisterna) (A) surrounded by a proliferation of cytotrophoblasts and syncytiotrophoblast (B). The microscopic findings and the clinical presentation are characteristic of a complete hydatidiform mole. A grapelike mass and proliferation of trophoblastic tissue are not seen in any of the other pathologies listed. **BH p. 226**

24. B Almost all complete hydatidiform moles show a 46XX karyotype. All the chromosomes are paternally derived as the condition results from fertilization of an empty egg. In most cases, the empty egg is fertilized by a single haploid sperm with duplication of the sperm DNA, or in a minority of cases, the egg is fertilized by two different haploid sperm. By contrast, in partial moles, the haploid egg is fertilized by either one diploid or two haploid sperm resulting in triploid karyotype (i.e., 69XXY). A 45X0 karyotype occurs in Turner syndrome due to loss of one of the X chromosomes. The mechanism of this loss is not known. In Klinefelter syndrome, meiotic nondisjunction results in an extra X chromosome, thus the karyotype is 47XXY. An abnormal chromosome complement such as 55XY can be seen in tumor cells which acquire extra chromosomes during unregulated cell proliferation. **BH p. 226**

25. E In both complete and partial molar pregnancies, the serum human chorionic gonadotropin levels are markedly elevated. Measurement of this hormone is useful in the diagnosis and monitoring of these patients. The other choices listed are serum markers that are useful in diagnosing or monitoring a variety of tumors: alpha-fetoprotein for hepatocellular carcinoma and yolk sac tumors; carcinoembryonic antigen for colon cancer; CA 19.5 for pancreatic cancer; and CA 125 for ovarian cancer. **BH p. 226**

26. A A small number of complete moles can give rise to choriocarcinomas, which are malignant tumors derived from placental tissue or germ cells. Molar pregnancies are not risk factors for the other tumors listed. **BH p. 226**

27. B This patient has choriocarcinoma, a malignant tumor of trophoblastic cells. These tumors are typically hemorrhagic owing to their propensity to invade blood vessel walls, in both the uterus and metastatic sites. Invasion of lung tissue usually manifests clinically as hemoptysis. Fever and pleuritic chest pain usually indicate an infectious or inflammatory process. Both fever and pleuritic chest pain may be manifestations of some tumors; however, they are not a common presenting symptom in choriocarcinoma. Hoarseness of voice occurs in laryngeal carcinoma. Wheezing is a manifestation of airway diseases of the lung and may be caused by tumor masses that obstruct a major airway, but is not commonly seen in choriocarcinomas. **BH p. 227**

28. D The figure shows acute salpingitis with an inflamed and distended fallopian tube; the lumen is filled with white blood cells. *Neisseria gonorrhoeae* is the most common etiologic agent of acute salpingitis. All the organisms listed are causes of sexually transmitted diseases that show a propensity to preferentially involve different anatomic areas of the genital tract. *Haemophilus ducreyi* causes a painful ulcer of the external genitalia with suppurative lymphadenopathy. Herpes simplex infections cause vesicular lesions of the external genitalia or the uterine cervix. Infections with human papillomavirus cause genital warts, and *Trichomonas* causes inflammation of the uterine cervix. **BH p. 227**

29. B The fallopian tube lumen in the figure is filled with blood and chorionic villi, a characteristic finding in ectopic pregnancy. The other pathologies listed can cause distention of the fallopian tube, with or without the presence of blood. However, chorionic villi are seen only in ectopic pregnancy. **BH p. 228**

30. A Tubal ectopic pregnancies result in hemorrhage into the fallopian tube lumen and peritoneal cavity and subsequent hypovolemic shock. The other symptoms and signs listed are not usually seen in ectopic pregnancy. **BH p. 228**

31. E The figure shows an ovarian tumor derived from the surface epithelium with tall columnar cells showing abundant mucin in the cytoplasm. The proliferation of the epithelium has resulted in complex papillary infoldings and invasion of the tumor cells into the surrounding stroma. This is a characteristic feature of a mucinous cystadenocarcinoma. The corpus luteum is derived from the ovarian follicle and enlarges during the luteal phase of the menstrual cycle. It is recognizable as a collection of large cells with abundant, eosinophilic cytoplasm. A corpus albicans is a regressed, atretic, and fibrotic corpus luteum. A follicular cyst is a fluid-filled cyst lined by low cuboidal cells. A hydatidiform mole is a gestational abnormality in the uterus that results in abnormal placental tissue composed of grapelike vesicles. **BH p. 232**

32. E The figure shows an ovarian tumor composed of complex, branching papillary structures lined by columnar epithelium and with stromal invasion. These features are characteristic of cystadenocarcinomas, which are tumors derived from the surface epithelium. The other tissues listed can give rise to a variety of ovarian tumors, but epithelial tumors are derived only from the surface epithelium. **BH p. 231**

33. C The figure shows features of a mature teratoma composed of tissue derived from the various germ cell layers. Epidermal, neural, and glandular tissue can be seen in the image. The other tissues listed can give rise to a variety of ovarian tumors, but only germ cells give rise to teratomas. **BH p. 234**

34. D The gross features described and the microscopic finding of plump, spindle cells with foamy cytoplasm are characteristic of theca cell tumors. Cystadenocarcinomas are epithelial tumors composed of tall columnar cells, and teratomas are composed of a variety of tissues derived from ectoderm, endoderm and mesoderm. Luteal cysts are lined by large cells

with abundant eosinophilic cytoplasm. In endometriosis, benign endometrial glands and stroma would be present in the ovary. **BH p. 233**

35. B Theca cell tumors secrete excessive amounts of estrogen and may lead to hyperplasia and adenocarcinoma of the endometrium. They do not increase the risk for endometritis, adenomyosis, or leiomyoma **BH p. 233**

36. E The figure shows features of fat necrosis with chronic inflammation, foamy macrophages and necrotic adipose tissue. This pathology is most commonly caused by trauma. Acute infections result in infiltration of the breast by inflammatory cells. If the infection is extensive, it may be accompanied by focal areas of fat necrosis; however, infection is not a common cause of fat necrosis. Excess estrogen leads to hyperplasia of the glandular epithelium, whereas a lack of hormonal stimulation causes atrophy of the glands. Genetic mutations lead to an increased risk for developing malignancies of the breast. **BH p. 236**

37. B Hyperplasia of the male breast, characterized by enlarged and dilated mammary ducts with periductal fibrosis, is characteristic of gynecomastia. This condition may be seen as a physiologic response in males during puberty and, pathologically, in patients with liver cirrhosis. Liver cirrhosis impairs the degradation of estrogen, which leads to hyperplasia of the breast tissue. The other entities listed do not show an increased incidence of developing gynecomastia. **BH p. 239**

38. B Fibroadenomas are common benign tumors in young females. They are well-circumscribed tumors composed of a proliferation of both the glandular and stromal tissue of the breast, as shown in the image. Ductal carcinoma in situ is characterized by malignant epithelial cells filling up the ducts. These tumors are extremely rare in young patients. Fibrocystic changes are benign proliferations of breast tissue, which usually present as ill-defined nodularity and a "lumpy bumpy" breast on physical examination. They are characterized by cystically dilated ducts, epithelial hyperplasia, adenosis, and apocrine metaplasia. Papillomas are proliferations of epithelial cells within a duct with branching fibrovascular cores. These lesions are uncommon in adolescent girls. **BH p. 240**

39. B The figure shows a benign intraductal papilloma composed of a dilated duct with proliferation of epithelial cells within a duct that has branching fibrovascular cores. These tumors present clinically with a blood-stained nipple discharge, but the other symptoms are not commonly associated with intraductal papillomas. Ulcerating lesions on the nipple are seen in mammary Paget disease, which is associated with an underlying malignant breast cancer. Likewise, massive edema of the breast signifies extensive infiltration of the breast by a malignant breast cancer, whereas infections of the breast result in abscess formation. **BH p. 240**

40. D The lesion depicted is an invasive ductal carcinoma characterized by invading nests of epithelial cells that are dissecting through the stroma. The epithelial cells are no longer confined within ducts, and the stroma is very fibrotic. Hence, these tumors would present as poorly defined, hard masses. Estrogen receptor–positive tumors are more likely to respond to hormonal therapy; therefore, estrogen receptor positivity indicates a better (not poor) prognosis. **BH pp. 241-243**

41. D The figure shows features of Paget disease of the nipple, in which the overlying epidermis of the nipple is infiltrated by malignant epithelial cells. These cells are enlarged with hyperchromatic nuclei and pale cytoplasm, imparting a halo around the nucleus. Paget disease of the nipple is characteristic of the spread of ductal carcinoma cells to the nipple along the epithelium of the mammary ducts. All the other lesions listed are benign proliferations of breast tissue that are not associated with Paget disease of the nipple. **BH p. 244**

FH5 Chapter 7: Nervous Tissues
FH5 Chapter 20: Central Nervous System
BH5 Chapter 11: Cardiovascular System
BH5 Chapter 23: Nervous System

20

Central Nervous System

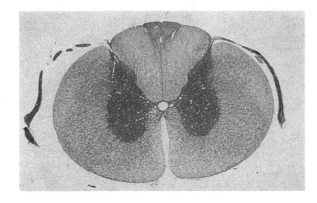

1 Which portion of the spinal cord is illustrated by the figure above?
- ☐ A. Cervical
- ☐ B. Lumbar
- ☐ C. Sacral
- ☐ D. Thoracic

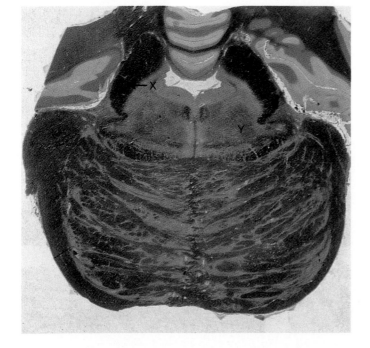

Use the figure at bottom left to answer the next three questions.

2 The figure illustrates a section through which region of the brain?
- ☐ A. Hypothalamus
- ☐ B. Medulla
- ☐ C. Midbrain
- ☐ D. Pons
- ☐ E. Thalamus

3 The large collection of nerve fibers at *X* contains axons that originate in which brain region?
- ☐ A. Cerebellar nuclei
- ☐ B. Globus pallidus
- ☐ C. Lateral geniculate nucleus
- ☐ D. Reticular formation
- ☐ E. Substantia nigra

4 Damage to the structure labeled *Y* would produce what type of neurologic deficit?
- ☐ A. Bilateral loss of pain and heat sensation
- ☐ B. Bilateral spasticity of the lower limbs
- ☐ C. Rest tremor, rigidity, and a masklike facial expression
- ☐ D. Unilateral flaccid paralysis of the limbs
- ☐ E. Unilateral loss of fine touch sensation

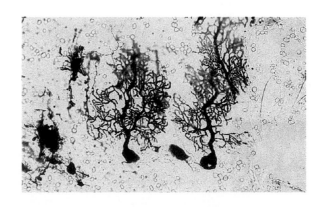

5 In what CNS region are the morphologically distinctive neurons shown on the bottom right of the previous page found?

☐ A. Cerebellar cortex
☐ B. Dorsal horn of the spinal cord
☐ C. Hypothalamus
☐ D. Substantia nigra
☐ E. Visual cortex

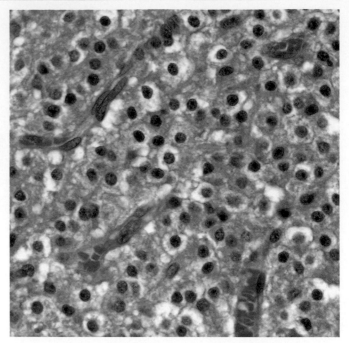

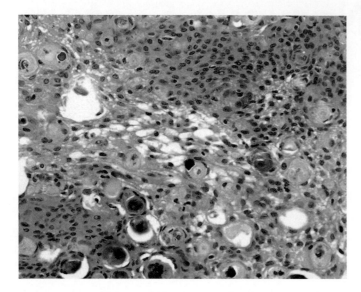

Use the figure above to answer the next two questions.

6 A 45-year-old woman was taken to her neurologist after suffering a seizure while working in her garden. A CT scan of her cranium showed a mass on the surface of the right parietal cortex. A biopsy of the mass is shown in the figure above. What do the histologic features of this biopsy suggest?

☐ A. Astrocytoma
☐ B. Ependymoma
☐ C. Meningioma
☐ D. Oligodendroglioma
☐ E. Schwannoma

7 Which of the following is the most likely location of the mass in this patient?

☐ A. Corpus striatum
☐ B. Inferior olive
☐ C. Surface of the cortex
☐ D. Thalamus
☐ E. Third ventricle

8 A 61-year-old man is referred to a neurologist after complaining of chronic headaches of 2 months' duration. A neurologic examination shows that he has difficulty discerning objects in his left visual field. A CT scan of his cranium reveals a mass within his right occipital cortex. What does histologic analysis of the biopsy specimen of the mass shown in the figure above suggest?

☐ A. Astrocytoma
☐ B. Ependymoma
☐ C. Meningioma
☐ D. Oligodendroglioma
☐ E. Schwannoma

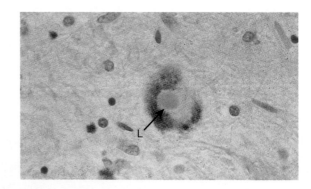

9 The figure above shows brain tissue obtained from a patient suffering from Parkinson disease. In this disease, cells containing pink-staining Lewy bodies (*L*) are seen. These cellular inclusions are aggregations of what?

☐ A. Glycogen
☐ B. Lipid
☐ C. Lipofuscin
☐ D. Neuromelanin
☐ E. Protein

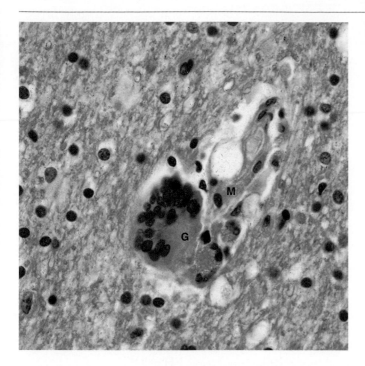

10 The figure above illustrates what pathologic process in the CNS tissue?

☐ A. Demyelination
☐ B. Deposition of amyloid plaques
☐ C. Encephalitis
☐ D. Mast cell degranulation
☐ E. Neuronal apoptosis

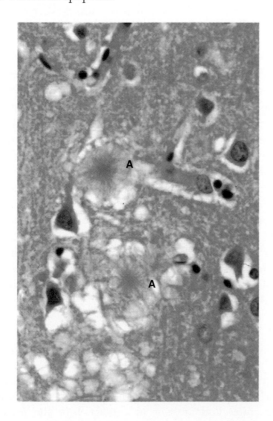

11 The figure at below left shows an autopsy specimen from a patient with Creutzfeldt-Jakob disease. What is the cause of this pathology?

☐ A. Breakdown product of abnormal digestion of extracellular matrix
☐ B. Calcified deposits
☐ C. Degenerating myelin
☐ D. Normal cellular protein that has misfolded
☐ E. Secretory material from a pathogenic organism

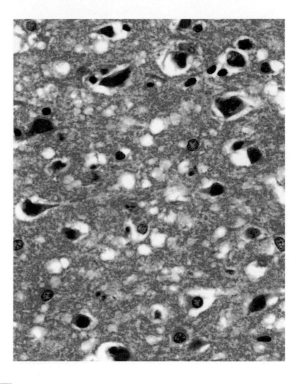

12 The figure above illustrates which pathologic condition?

☐ A. Cerebral infarct
☐ B. Deposition of amyloid plaques of Alzheimer disease
☐ C. HIV encephalopathy
☐ D. Lewy bodies of Parkinson disease
☐ E. Spongiform encephalopathy of the cortex

13 A 25-year-old woman was brought to the emergency room with a loss of consciousness. She has a history of berry aneurysm in the vessels of her brain. As a result of her condition, which cell type would be expected to be elevated in her CSF?

☐ A. Ependymal cells
☐ B. Malignant cells
☐ C. Monocytes
☐ D. Neutrophils
☐ E. Red blood cells

14 A 22-year-old man presents with headache, nausea, and vomiting. He was found to have an elevated blood pressure of 150/95 mm Hg. Imaging studies showed a mass arising from the choroid plexus. The mass would most likely be located in which of the following sites?

☐ A. Gray matter
☐ B. Pons
☐ C. Thalamus
☐ D. Ventricles
☐ E. White matter

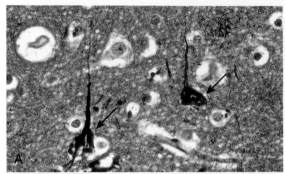

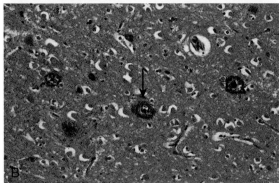

15 A 65-year-old man died from complications of a severe neurologic disease. Autopsy examination of the brain showed significant atrophy of the frontal and temporal lobes. Silver-stained histologic sections of his hippocampus are shown in the figure above. Based on the findings in the image, which of the following clinical signs and symptoms were most likely present in this patient?
☐ A. Hyperreflexia and positive Babinski sign
☐ B. Loss of sensation of temperature and vibration in the left leg
☐ C. Lower extremity weakness
☐ D. Memory loss and disorientation as to time and place
☐ E. Motor rigidity and shuffling gait

ANSWERS

1. A The presence of both the cuneate and gracile fasciculi in the dorsal funiculus indicates that sensory fibers from both the arms and the legs are present. This is only possible in the cervical region of the cord. **FH p. 393**

2. D The prominent crossing tracts seen in the ventral half of this section communicate between portions of the pontine nuclei. Also, the characteristic flattened profile of the fourth ventricle identifies this region as the pons. In the medulla, the

fourth ventricle is open dorsally, whereas in the regions of the hypothalamus and thalamus, the third ventricle is present as a slitlike space. **FH p. 395**

3. A The structure labeled X in the figure is the superior cerebellar peduncle, which is composed mainly of fibers ascending to the cortex from the cerebellar nuclei. A major tract leaving the globus pallidus is the anterior commissure, a more rostral structure. Similarly, the lateral geniculate nucleus and substantia nigra are located more rostrally in the brain. The reticular formation is ventromedial to the labeled structure. **FH p. 395**

4. E The indicated structure is the medial lemniscus, which carries sensations of fine touch from the contralateral side of the body. Sensations of pain are carried through the spinothalamic tracts, which are located more laterally than the structures indicated. Spastic or flaccid paralysis results from injury to different components of the corticospinal motor system, located on the ventral aspects of the pons and spinal cord. A rest tremor is usually a sign of damage to the substantia nigra, as occurs in Parkinson disease. **FH p. 395**

5. A The highly branched dendritic tree of these cells is a unique feature of Purkinje neurons of the cerebellar cortex. **FH p. 396**

6. C Meningiomas are benign tumors derived from meningothelial cells of the arachnoid. They are characterized by proliferation of epithelial cells and spindle cells arranged in whorls. At the center of these whorls, there may be eosinophilic, calcified masses called *psammoma bodies*. All the choices listed are tumors derived from various components of nervous tissue and are distinguished based on their cell of origin, histologic finding, and location. Astrocytomas are intracerebral glial tumors derived from astrocytes. Microscopically, they are characterized by a proliferation of astrocytes, which are recognized by their pale-staining oval nuclei. Oligodendrogliomas are also intracerebral glial tumors. They are derived from oligodendrocytes and are characterized by a proliferation of cells that show nuclear halos. Ependymomas are derived from the ependymal lining cells and show a proliferation of cells with a dense, fibrillary background and perivascular pseudorosette formation. Schwannomas are derived from Schwann cells and histologically appear as a proliferation of compact spindle cells with a palisading pattern. They arise more commonly from peripheral nerve. In the brain, they most often arise from the eighth cranial nerve. **BH p. 310**

7. C The microscopic finding of spindle cells arranged in whorls with psammoma bodies is characteristic of meningiomas. These are benign tumors that arise from the arachnoidal epithelial cells of the meninges and are usually located at the surface of the cortex. The other choices listed are internal structures and are not in contact with the meninges. **BH p. 310**

8. D Oligodendrogliomas are glial tumors characterized by a proliferation of sheets of uniform cells with vacuolated cytoplasms that form halos around the nuclei. Astrocytomas are characterized by a proliferation of astrocytes, which are recognized by their pale-staining oval nuclei. Ependymomas are derived from the ependymal lining cells and show a proliferation of cells with a dense, fibrillary background and perivascular pseudorosette formation. Schwannomas are derived from Schwann cells, and histologically, there is a proliferation of compact spindle cells with a palisading pattern. They arise more commonly from peripheral nerves. In the brain, they most often arise from the eighth cranial nerve. **BH. p. 309**

9. E Aggregations of protein are commonly eosinophilic; Lewy bodies contain aggregations of a protein called *alpha-synuclein*. Glycogen and lipid are almost never found within CNS neurons. Neuromelanin is derived from metabolism of dopamine and forms the brown granules seen in this figure. Lipofuscin is likewise a brown cellular inclusion. **FH p. 126, BH p. 302**

10. C In HIV infections of the CNS (viral encephalitis), multinucleate giant cells (G) derived from monocytes (M) are loaded with viral particles and are commonly found adjacent to blood vessels. Such a multinucleated cell can be seen in this image. Mast cells are not present in this image and are normally rare in the brain. The large, amorphous masses that form amyloid plaques are not visible here, nor are the large dark-staining nuclei that would result from neuronal apoptosis. In demyelinating diseases, large pale plaques would be visible. **FH p. 126, BH p. 305**

11. D Creutzfeldt-Jakob disease typically is caused by prion proteins, which are normal cellular proteins, but in an abnormal configuration. The abnormally folded proteins can form large aggregates (A), leading to neurologic damage. The extracellular matrix of the CNS is far too sparse to account for these aggregations. Demyelinated areas of the brain typically stain pale rather than pink, owing to loss of myelin-associated protein. Calcified deposits are rare in the brain except for the pineal gland. **FH p. 127, BH p. 303**

12. E The pyramidal-shaped cells in this illustration are neurons; the pale spaces in the neuropil are areas of degeneration typical of spongiform encephalopathy. This disorder is caused by the toxic effects of abnormal prion proteins that are not visible in this brain section. Amyloid plaques or Lewy bodies are easily visible aggregations of proteins and would stain pink rather than white. A cerebral infarct would appear as a large area of damage rather than the discrete vacuoles seen in this image. HIV encephalopathy is perivascular. **FH p. 140, BH p. 303**

13. E Aneurysms in the brain lead to rupture of blood vessels and leakage of red blood cells into the CSF. Hence, examination of the CSF would show an increase in red blood cells. The presence of neutrophils in the CSF indicates a bacterial infection such as meningitis. The presence of monocytes in the CSF may be seen in chronic inflammation. Malignant cells in the CSF indicate a metastatic tumor. Ependymal cells form the lining of the ventricles and normally may be seen in the CSF. **FH p.146 , BH p. 115, 299**

14. D The choroid plexus is a vascular structure arising from the walls of the lateral and fourth ventricles. Tumors that develop from the choroid plexus would be located close to the ventricles. Because of their location, these tumors may obstruct CSF flow, with a subsequent increase in intracranial pressure, which accounts for the signs and symptoms observed in this patient. The choroid plexus is not intimately associated with any of the other structures listed. **FH p. 145, BH p. 310**

15. D The images show neurofibrillary tangles in neurons (arrows in A) and amyloid plaques in the neuropil (arrow in B). These structures are found in Alzheimer disease. These plaques and tangles are most numerous in the hippocampus and the frontal cortex. Hence, patients with Alzheimer disease have progressive dementia characterized by loss of cognitive function with memory loss, disorientation, and disrupted thinking and reasoning. Motor rigidity and a shuffling gait are symptoms of Parkinson disease, which results from damage to the substantia nigra and not to the cortex. Symptoms of motor or sensory impairment would arise from damage to the postcentral or precentral gyri and not from damage to the frontal or temporal lobes. **BH p. 301**

21

Special Sense Organs

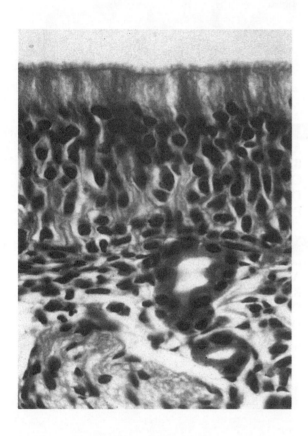

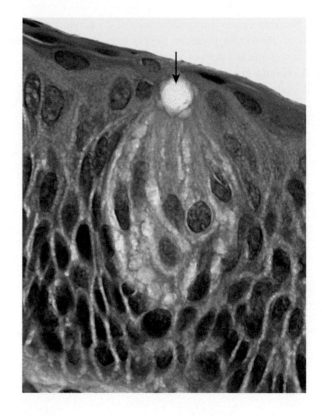

1 Which sensory epithelium is illustrated in the figure above?
- ☐ A. Epithelium of the organ of Corti
- ☐ B. Epithelium of the utricular macula
- ☐ C. Olfactory epithelium
- ☐ D. Stria vascularis of the inner ear
- ☐ E. Taste buds of circumvallate papillae

2 A biopsy taken from the oral cavity is shown in the figure above right. What does the *arrow* indicate?
- ☐ A. Carcinoma in situ
- ☐ B. Epithelial metaplasia
- ☐ C. Necrosis due to ischemia
- ☐ D. Small mucous gland
- ☐ E. Taste bud

3 Cilia do not play a role in the development or function of what?
- ☐ A. Hair cells of the ear
- ☐ B. Olfactory receptor cells
- ☐ C. Rods or cones
- ☐ D. Taste bud gustatory cells

4 A 45-year-old man complains that he has trouble seeing close objects clearly. What is the mostly likely cause of his problem?
- ☐ A. Abnormal growth of the ciliary processes
- ☐ B. Loss of lens fibers
- ☐ C. Loss of elasticity in the lens
- ☐ D. Loss of elasticity in the suspensory ligament of the lens
- ☐ E. Weakness in the ciliary muscles

5 A young man with severe myopia comes to the hospital complaining of a distortion in his vision. He stated that he sees a shadow and has a blind area in his left eye. He further stated that he had been in an auto accident several days previously. An assessment with an ophthalmoscope indicates a tear and detachment of a portion of the retina. What is the most likely location for this detachment?

☐ A. Between Bruch membrane and the retinal pigment epithelium
☐ B. Between choroid and retina
☐ C. Between photoreceptors and bipolar cells
☐ D. Between retinal pigment epithelium and photoreceptors
☐ E. Between vitreous and retina

6 Routine eye examinations normally include a measurement of intraocular pressure. This is because increased intraocular pressure is a sign of what?

☐ A. Cataracts
☐ B. Glaucoma
☐ C. Keratoconus
☐ D. Macular degeneration
☐ E. Presbyopia

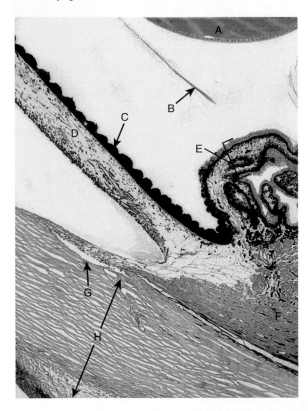

Use the figure above to answer the next four questions.

7 Which region varies with different eye colors?

8 Which structure will stain well with antibodies to the protein fibrillin?

9 Which labeled structure in the figure above produces the aqueous humor?

10 A diabetic 53-year-old African American woman comes in for her yearly eye examination and is told that her intraocular pressure is high (>21 mm Hg), but production of aqueous humor is normal. Which labeled structure is the likely cause of the high intraocular pressure recorded?

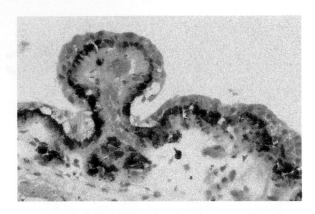

11 Which ocular structure is shown in the figure above?

☐ A. Ciliary epithelium
☐ B. Corneal endothelium
☐ C. Corneal epithelium
☐ D. Epithelium of the posterior surface of the iris
☐ E. Pigment epithelium of the retina

12 What usually causes swelling and cloudiness in the cornea?

☐ A. Abnormal ion content in the aqueous humor
☐ B. Abnormal ion content in lacrimal gland secretions
☐ C. Aging changes in corneal fibroblasts
☐ D. Damage to the anterior epithelium of the cornea
☐ E. Loss of cells in the corneal endothelium

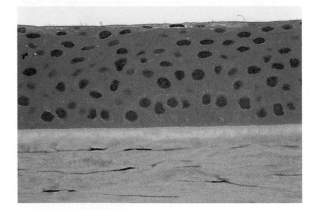

13 The figure above illustrates what structure?

☐ A. Corneal epithelium
☐ B. Corneal endothelium
☐ C. Olfactory epithelium
☐ D. Tympanic membrane
☐ E. Utricular macula

14 A 53-year-old woman complains of tinnitus, dizziness, and an occasional hearing loss in her left ear. From what is the patient most likely suffering?
☐ A. Bacterial meningitis
☐ B. Influenza
☐ C. Lyme disease
☐ D. Ménière disease
☐ E. Viral meningitis

15 What treatment might be helpful for the above patient?
☐ A. ACE inhibitors
☐ B. Antiarrhythmics
☐ C. Antibiotics
☐ D. Diuretics
☐ E. Protease inhibitors

16 What will repeated inflammation of the endolymphatic sac directly affect?
☐ A. Addition of potassium to endolymph
☐ B. Detection of linear acceleration
☐ C. Resorption of endolymph
☐ D. Synthesis of perilymph

17 Connexin mutations appear to be a major cause of what?
☐ A. Anosmia
☐ B. Deafness
☐ C. Presbyopia
☐ D. Taste deficiencies

18 Which feature is unique to the organs which sense angular acceleration?
☐ A. Basilar membrane
☐ B. Cupula
☐ C. Hair cells
☐ D. Otolithic membrane
☐ E. Tectorial membrane

19 A 45-year-old man presents to his physician with complaints of sudden and severe nausea, vomiting, and dizziness. The patient has difficulty standing because he states that the room is spinning. On physical examination, the patient is noted to have abnormal eye movement. From what is he most likely suffering?
☐ A. A cerebrovascular accident
☐ B. A gastrointestinal bacterial infection
☐ C. An inner-ear viral infection
☐ D. Bell palsy
☐ E. Viral meningitis

20 Auditory hair cells rest directly on what structure?
☐ A. Basilar membrane
☐ B. Phalangeal cells
☐ C. Pillar cells
☐ D. Spiral ligament
☐ E. Spiral limbus

ANSWERS

1. C The very thick, ciliated, pseudostratified columnar epithelium shown here is characteristic of the respiratory system. The presence of cilia can be recognized by the dark row of basal bodies right under the apical membranes of the epithelial cells. Also, the presence of Bowman glands beneath the epithelium, which produce a watery secretion that dissolves odorants, is diagnostic for the olfactory sensory region. The organ of Corti and the utricular macula have stereocilia (microvilli) rather than true cilia. The stria vascularis shows only two layers of nuclei in the epithelium and is not sensory. Taste buds are surrounded by a stratified squamous epithelium. **FH. p. 401**

2. E The arrow indicates a taste bud, which is embedded within the stratified squamous oral mucosal epithelium. Taste buds are characteristically barrel shaped with elongated spindle-shaped cells, and they communicate to the surface through the taste pores (circular holes). Such structures are common on the back of the tongue. Mucous glands would have much larger cells, filled with large mucous secretion granules. The orderly nature of these structures and their association with the taste pore rule out epithelial metaplasia and carcinoma in situ. Necrosis due to ischemia would be characterized by cells with a dense eosinophilic cytoplasm and loss of nuclei. **FH p. 400**

3. D Taste buds have their receptors on long microvilli, not cilia. The olfactory receptors and rods and cones include a modified cilium in their structure. In the ear, the organization of the microvilli on the apical surface of the hair cells reflects an initial location of a cilium. This cilium is lost from cells in the organ of Corti but is retained in the vestibular sensory cells. **FH p. 400**

4. C With age, the lens loses its ability to round up when tension in the suspensory ligament is reduced, leading to an inability to focus on close objects. This presbyopia is common after the age of 40 to 45 years and is caused by changes in the structure of the lens fibers. The number of lens fibers increases with age. The suspensory ligament and the ciliary body are relatively unaffected by aging changes. **FH pp. 403, 409**

5. D The retinal pigmented epithelial cells are not anchored tightly to the rod and cone photoreceptors that they support metabolically and may separate from them under mechanical stress. Other layers of the eye have more robust adhesion mechanisms and are unlikely to separate. **FH p. 406**

6. B Glaucoma is characterized by increased intraocular pressure and, if left untreated, may lead to retinal damage. The other conditions listed do not affect intraocular pressure. In cataracts, denaturation of the proteins in the lens leads to increased opacity and loss of vision. Keratoconus is an abnormal curvature of the cornea, and macular degeneration is a disorder that specifically affects the center of the visual field in the retina. Presbyopia is due to loss of elasticity in the lens. **FH p. 409**

7. D This area is the iris stroma, recognizable as a layer of loose connective tissue bounded on one side by the heavily pigmented iris epithelium (C) and anchored at one end to the ciliary body (E). The iris epithelium preferentially absorbs yellow light, so that in individuals with little pigment in the iris stroma, the eyes appear blue. Individuals with more iris stromal pigment have brown or black eyes. **FH pp. 409-410**

8. B This is the suspensory ligament, which runs between the lens and the ciliary body. It is composed of the elastic protein fibrillin and holds the lens in place. **FH p. 409**

9. E The epithelium of the ciliary processes produces the aqueous humor. The ciliary epithelium has two layers of cells and forms a highly folded structure posterior to the iris. **FH p. 409**

10. G Because fluid production is normal, removal of fluid, beginning with the trabecular meshwork and the canal of Schlemm, is suspected of being impaired. This is a common cause of glaucoma, particularly among African Americans. The canal of Schlemm (G) can be recognized as a channel that is found in the deeper regions of the limbus (H), just lateral to the cornea. The trabecular meshwork is between the canal of Schlemm and the lateral edge of the anterior chamber, close to where the iris attaches to the ciliary body. **FH p. 409**

11. A The ciliary epithelium is distinctive because, unlike the epithelia of the cornea or iris, it possesses an inner unpigmented layer above an outer pigmented layer. The pigmented epithelium of the retina is a single layer of cells with the choroid on one side and the neural retina on the other. The iris epithelium consists of two layers of heavily pigmented cells. The corneal epithelium and endothelium are unpigmented. **FH p. 409**

12. E Corneal endothelial cells pump ions out of the corneal stroma, keeping it partially dehydrated. As these endothelial cells are gradually lost through aging or damage, their ion-pumping activity is compromised, and the cornea swells and becomes cloudy. Corneal transplantation is used to replace such damaged corneas. **FH p. 412**

13. A The corneal epithelium is a stratified squamous epithelium that can be recognized by its very regular, smooth surfaces. Also, an unusually thick basement membrane, Bowman membrane, is a prominent feature of this epithelium. The corneal endothelium is a simple squamous epithelium, whereas the olfactory and utricular macular epithelia are pseudostratified columnar epithelia. The epithelium of the tympanic membrane is exposed to air and is keratinized stratified squamous. **FH pp. 401, 412, 423**

14. D The patient's symptoms are indicative of a disturbance of the inner ear. Ménière disease is a disorder of the labyrinth of the inner ear. The other diseases listed do not ordinarily involve hearing loss. Symptoms of both viral and bacterial meningitis include fever, headache, and neck stiffness. In influenza, the patient usually complains of fever, muscle, and joint pain. Patients with Lyme disease have a characteristic targetoid skin rash and may complain of influenza-like symptoms and joint pain. **FH p. 423**

15. D Ménière disease is believed to be caused by increased fluid pressure in the membranous labyrinth of the inner ear. Mild symptoms are helped by decreasing fluid retention in the body with diuretics and a low-salt diet. The exact cause of Ménière disease is not known. Infections of the middle ear have been implicated as a cause. However, because the symptoms are caused by an increase in the fluid pressure rather than an active infection, antibiotics are not indicated as a treatment modality. ACE inhibitors are used to treat hypertension and congestive heart failure, whereas antiarrhythmics are used to treat disturbances of heart rhythm. Protease inhibitors are used to treat HIV. **FH p. 423**

16. C The endolymphatic sac is composed of a columnar epithelium specialized for resorption of the endolymph. Repeated inflammation at the endolymphatic sac will lead to impaired resorption of the endolymph. This in turn may lead to Ménière disease. Infections in the endolymphatic sac will not affect formation of endolymph or perilymph because they are not formed here. Long-standing disruption of endolymph absorption indirectly may cause problems with the detection of linear acceleration. **FH p. 423**

17. B Mutations in the gap junction protein connexin 26 are a leading cause of deafness in Americans, but the role of connexin 26 in hearing is not understood. The other conditions are not correlated with connexin mutations. **FH p. 421**

18. B The cristae ampullares located in the semicircular canals are the sensors of angular acceleration and are covered by a gelatinous mass, the cupula. Hair cells are the sensory receptors of both the vestibular and cochlear systems and therefore are found in all inner-ear sensory areas. Otolithic membranes are found in the maculae of the utricle and saccule and sense linear acceleration. The tectorial and basilar membranes are part of the organ of Corti and detect sound. **FH pp. 424-425**

19. C Nausea, vomiting, and dizziness can be caused by a variety of diseases, including a gastrointestinal bacterial infection as well as viral meningitis. However, the patient's vertigo (spinning room) and the abnormal movement of the eye (nystagmus) indicate a disorder of the vestibular system. This may be caused by labyrinthitis, a viral or bacterial infection in the inner ear. Dizziness, vertigo, and nystagmus may also be symptoms of a cerebrovascular accident (stroke); however, the sudden onset of severe nausea and vomiting is not a common presentation. Bell palsy is a unilateral paralysis of the facial nerve resulting in a loss of control of facial muscles on the affected side. The other symptoms are usually not seen in this disorder. **FH p. 423**

20. B The auditory hair cells sit on the phalangeal cells, which in turn rest on the basilar membrane. Pillar cells are between the inner and outer hair cells. The spiral ligament forms the lateral attachment of the organ of Corti, and the spiral limbus forms the medial attachment. **FH pp. 420-421**

Final Examination

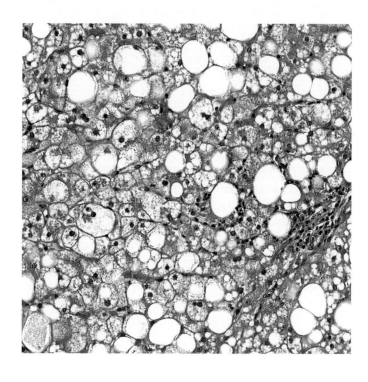

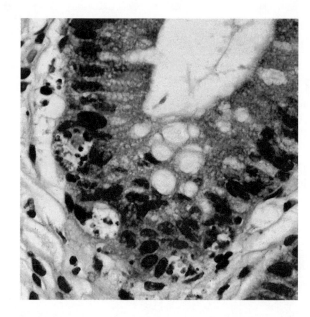

1 The pathology in the microscopic image of the liver shown in the figure above would most likely be seen in which of the following patients?
- ☐ A. A 20-year-old man with sickle cell disease
- ☐ B. A 25-year-old woman with acetaminophen overdose
- ☐ C. A 40-year-old man with ulcerative colitis
- ☐ D. A 45-year-old woman with morbid obesity
- ☐ E. A 65-year-old man with right heart failure

2 A 47-year-old hospitalized man underwent bone marrow transplantation for acute leukemia. He subsequently developed bloody diarrhea, a skin rash, and jaundice. A microscopic section of a biopsy of his colon is depicted in the image above. Which of the following is the most likely cause of the pathology shown?
- ☐ A. Chemotherapy-induced colitis
- ☐ B. Graft-versus-host disease
- ☐ C. Normal turnover of colonic epithelium
- ☐ D. Rejection of the transplant
- ☐ E. Viral infection due to immunosuppression

3 Which of the following changes in organelles is the earliest evidence of a response to cellular injury?
- ☐ A. Endoplasmic reticulum swelling
- ☐ B. Golgi complex dispersal
- ☐ C. Lysosomal disruption
- ☐ D. Nuclear condensation
- ☐ E. Ribosome clustering

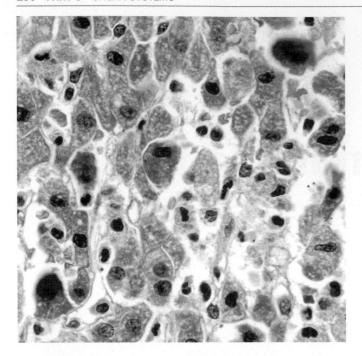

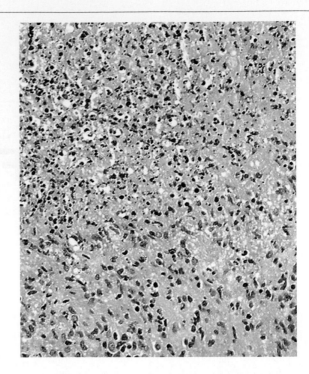

4 Which feature, visible in the image of the liver above, indicates a necrotic cell?

☐ A. A large pale nucleus
☐ B. A lobulated nucleus
☐ C. Highly eosinophilic cytoplasm
☐ D. Poorly stained cytoplasm
☐ E. Vacuolated cytoplasm

6 A 21-year-old woman is being followed by her physician for a workup of fever, weight loss, recurrent pneumonia, and cervical lymphadenopathy. The patient had been in good health previous to her current symptoms, which started about 3 months before her presentation. A cervical lymph node biopsy is performed, and a microscopic image is shown above. Which of the following is the most likely cause of the pathology?

☐ A. Acquired immunodeficiency syndrome
☐ B. Diffuse large cell lymphoma
☐ C. Infectious mononucleosis
☐ D. Kaposi sarcoma
☐ E. Sarcoidosis

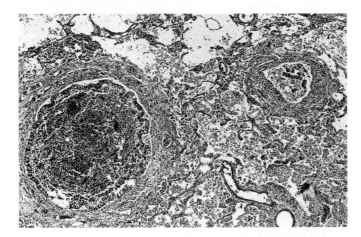

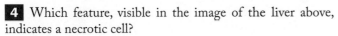

5 A 17-year-old boy who had a long-standing history of chronic cough, nasal polyps, and diarrhea died of respiratory complications. An autopsy was performed, and a microscopic section of his lung is shown in the image above. Which of the following pathologies also would be present in this patient?

☐ A. Aortic dissection
☐ B. Chronic pancreatitis
☐ C. Multiple gallbladder stones
☐ D. Numerous colonic adenomas
☐ E. Tracheoesophageal fistula

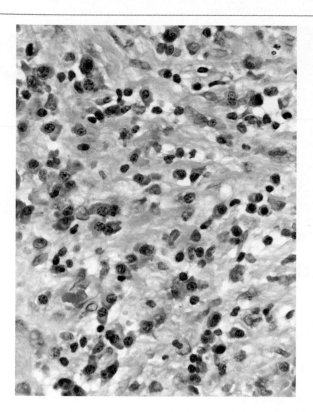

8 A 25-year-old man who has been HIV positive for 2 years comes to his physician complaining of shortness of breath and a mild fever. He is diagnosed with mild respiratory difficulty, and a lung biopsy (shown below left) is taken. Based on the appearance of cells in the biopsy indicated by the arrows, what type of infection most likely caused his symptoms?

☐ A. *Aspergillus fungus*
☐ B. Cytomegalovirus
☐ C. Herpesvirus
☐ D. *Pneumocystis carinii*
☐ E. *Streptococcus pneumoniae*

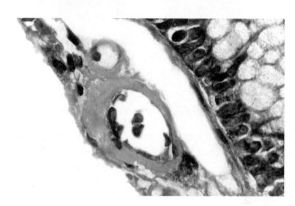

7 A 47-year-old man is admitted to the hospital after complaining of chronic stomach pain. He is diagnosed with peptic ulcer, and a biopsy of the stomach lining is obtained (shown above). What signs are seen in the lamina propria of his stomach?

☐ A. Abscess formation
☐ B. Apoptosis
☐ C. Chronic inflammation
☐ D. Edema
☐ E. Necrosis

9 A 62-year-old woman was referred to a gastroenterologist by her primary care physician for investigation of unexplained anemia. The patient underwent a colonoscopy with biopsy of her colon and rectum. A microscopic section of her rectal biopsy is shown in the image above. A Congo red stain of the same biopsy showed apple-green birefringence under polarized light. What would a bone marrow examination most likely show?

☐ A. Extensive fibrosis
☐ B. Markedly increased iron
☐ C. Numerous plasma cells
☐ D. Replacement by fat
☐ E. Sheets of myeloblasts

10 Which of the following laboratory tests would be useful in arriving at a diagnosis for the above patient?

☐ A. Chromosome analysis
☐ B. Liver function tests
☐ C. Measurement of hemoglobin
☐ D. Serum protein electrophoresis
☐ E. Thyroid hormone measurement

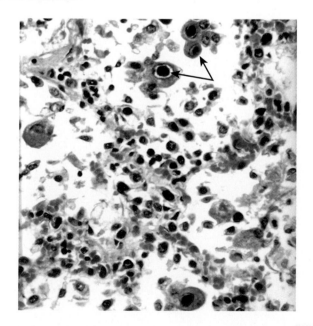

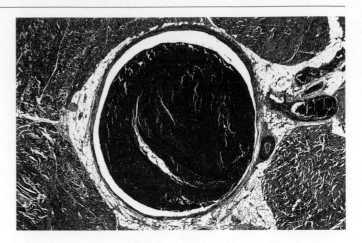

In reviewing a slide made from a biopsy of the uterus of a 30-year-old woman, a pathologist notes numerous light areas in the tissue, shown by the *arrows* in the image above. Use for questions 11 to 13.

11 What process has the cells indicated by the *arrows* undergone?
☐ A. Apoptosis
☐ B. Cytokinesis
☐ C. Fatty change
☐ D. Mitosis

12 Which intracellular molecules cause the nuclear and cytoplasmic changes that the cells in the light areas have undergone?
☐ A. Caspase
☐ B. Cyclic AMP
☐ C. Cyclins and cyclin-dependent kinases
☐ D. Cytokines
☐ E. Tyrosine kinases

13 This image shows the normal appearance of uterine glands in which condition?
☐ A. Luteal phase
☐ B. Menopause
☐ C. Menstrual phase
☐ D. Proliferative phase
☐ E. Secretory phase

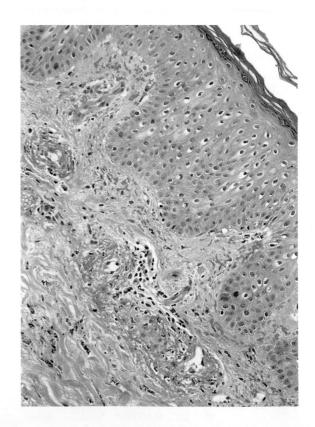

14 A 32-year-old woman collapsed and died after experiencing a sudden onset of chest pain while at work. The woman was in apparently good health with no prior medical history. An autopsy was performed to determine the cause of death. A cross section of her popliteal vein is shown in the image above. A similar finding was also present in the left pulmonary vein. A mutation in a gene encoding for which of the following was most likely responsible for her condition?
☐ A. Factor V
☐ B. Hemoglobin
☐ C. Myosin heavy chain
☐ D. Type I collagen
☐ E. von Willebrand factor

15 A 53-year-old woman was seen by her physician for complaints of fever, fatigue, and malaise. On physical examination, there were scattered, palpable purpura over her upper and lower extremities. A skin biopsy of one of these lesions was taken, and a microscopic section is shown in the image at the bottom of the previous page. The physician ordered a urinalysis, which showed numerous red blood cells. What is the most likely cause of this latter finding?

- ☐ A. Acute tubular necrosis
- ☐ B. Chronic pyelonephritis
- ☐ C. Glomerulonephritis
- ☐ D. Renal cell carcinoma
- ☐ E. Renal papillary necrosis

16 Which organelle is most important in determining whether an injury is reversible?

- ☐ A. Endoplasmic reticulum
- ☐ B. Golgi complex
- ☐ C. Lysosome
- ☐ D. Mitochondrion
- ☐ E. Nucleus

17 Large numbers of apoptotic cells are common and are not a sign of pathology in which structure?

- ☐ A. Bone marrow
- ☐ B. Epidermis
- ☐ C. Hyaline cartilage
- ☐ D. Seminiferous tubule
- ☐ E. Thymic cortex

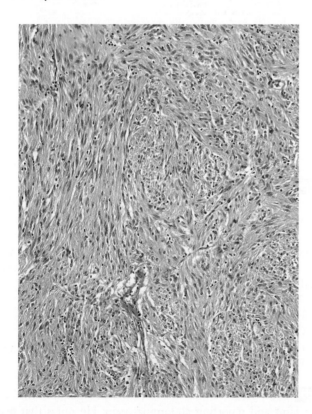

18 A 49-year-old man who complained of abdominal pain and weight loss was found to have a gastric mass. A partial gastrectomy was performed, and a microscopic section of the mass is shown in the image below left. Which of the following is most likely regarding the tumor shown?

- ☐ A. It arises from the glandular epithelium
- ☐ B. It can be treated with a tyrosine kinase inhibitor
- ☐ C. It expresses chromogranin A
- ☐ D. It is associated with *Helicobacter pylori* infection
- ☐ E. It produces mucin

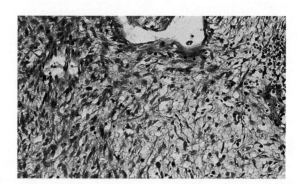

19 A 50-year-old woman was seen by a gynecologist for lower abdominal pain and vaginal bleeding. On physical examination, a right adnexal mass was palpated. Imaging studies showed that the mass was in the right ovary. A hysterectomy and bilateral salpingo-oophorectomy were performed. A microscopic section of the ovarian mass is shown in the image above. Which of the following also would be present on morphologic examination of the uterus?

- ☐ A. Adenomyosis
- ☐ B. Chronic endometritis
- ☐ C. Complex endometrial hyperplasia
- ☐ D. Leiomyoma
- ☐ E. Serous cystadenoma

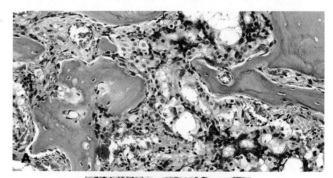
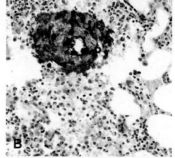

20 A 65-year-old man has come to his physician complaining of back pain. A computed tomography scan of his lumbar vertebrae showed a localized osteosclerosis at the third lumbar vertebra. A biopsy of the affected region is taken and is shown at bottom right on the previous page. Some of the cells in the marrow cavity stain positively for prostate-specific antigen (brown stain seen in part B). What is the cause of this pathology?

☐ A. Ectopic endochondral ossification
☐ B. Excessive numbers of megakaryocytes that stimulate bone remodeling
☐ C. Osteoclast hyperactivity
☐ D. Reaction of marrow cells to multiple fractures in surrounding bone
☐ E. Tumor-induced bone formation

21 A 40-year-old woman presents to her physician with an unusual array of symptoms. She has had chronic yeast infections in her mouth (candidiasis, or thrush); scaly, dry skin with signs of hyperpigmentation; unusually low blood pressure upon standing; and muscle spasms in her hands. She ceased menstruating 3 years previously. What is at the root of her complaints?

☐ A. Diabetes mellitus, adult onset (type 2)
☐ B. Hyperparathyroidism
☐ C. Hyperthyroidism
☐ D. Pituitary insufficiency (Sheehan syndrome)
☐ E. Thymic abnormality provoking autoimmune processes

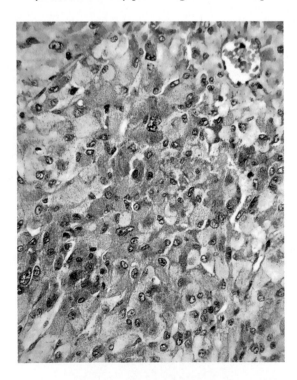

22 A 30-year-old man was seen by his physician for complaints of palpitation, excessive sweating, and generalized anxiety. On physical examination, the patient was found to have an elevated blood pressure, multiple skin nodules, and an enlarged thyroid gland. The patient states that his father

and sister have similar problems. Imaging studies show a mass in the right adrenal gland, which was surgically resected. A microscopic section of the mass is shown in the image at bottom left. The thyroid gland also was removed. Which of the following morphologic findings would most likely be present in the thyroid gland?

☐ A. Hemorrhage, calcification, and fibrosis
☐ B. Hyperplastic acini with tall columnar cells
☐ C. Lymphoid infiltration with germinal centers
☐ D. Nests of polygonal cells with amyloid deposition
☐ E. Epithelial cells with nuclear inclusions and grooves

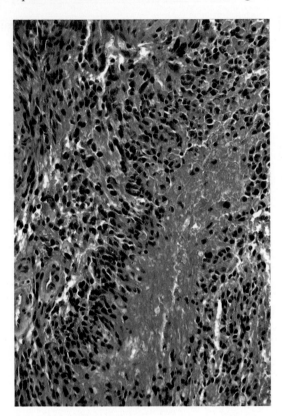

23 A 50-year-old man had a seizure while at work. He was taken to the emergency room, where a neurologic examination showed weakness of the right upper and lower extremities. Magnetic resonance imaging examination of the head shows a large, ring-enhancing lesion in the temporal lobe. A biopsy of the mass was performed, and a microscopic section is shown in the above image. What can be said about this tumor?

☐ A. It arises from cranial nerves
☐ B. It has numerous mitoses and a poor prognosis
☐ C. It is associated with a mutation in the *NF-1* gene
☐ D. It is cystic and more commonly seen in the cerebellum
☐ E. It is easily resectable

24 A 50-year-old man comes to the emergency room feeling faint and reporting abdominal pain. He notes that over the past few days, he has felt uncomfortable after meals. An endoscopy showed an ulcer, which was excised. A section of the ulcer is shown in the image on the following page. Where was this ulcer located?

☐ A. Esophagus
☐ B. Stomach
☐ C. Small intestine
☐ D. Large intestine

☐ A. Bacterial infection
☐ B. Excessive estrogen stimulation
☐ C. Reaction to suture
☐ D. Recurrence of the tumor
☐ E. Trauma to the breast

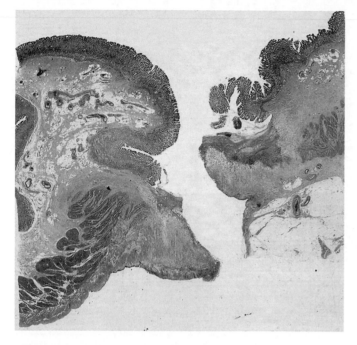

25 Which of the following laboratory tests would be abnormal in the above patient?
☐ A. Bilirubin
☐ B. Blood glucose
☐ C. Blood urea nitrogen
☐ D. Hemoglobin
☐ E. Triglyceride

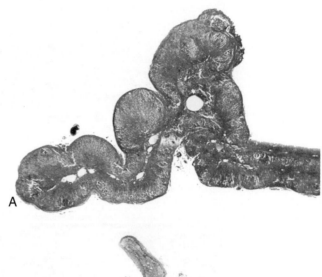

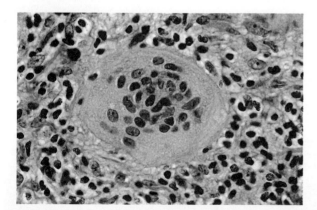

26 Two months after undergoing surgical removal of a breast mass, a 40-year-old woman returned to her physician with complaints of a lump at the site of her previous surgery. The mass that was previously removed was examined by a pathologist who reported the presence of a microscopic focus of ductal carcinoma in situ. At that time, the patient was told that additional surgery would not be required because the tumor was completely removed. The new lump, which felt firm on palpation, was removed, and a microscopic section is depicted in the image above. Which of the following is the most likely cause of the mass?

27 The photomicrograph in the above image shows a normal adrenal gland (part A) compared with the right adrenal gland from a patient (part B). The left adrenal gland was similar in appearance to the right adrenal gland. This pathology would be seen in which of the following patients?
☐ A. A 30-year-old woman with headache and bilateral hemianopia
☐ B. A 32-year old woman with severe joint pain and a malar rash
☐ C. A 35-year old man with palpitation and episodic hypertension
☐ D. A 40-year-old man with hypertension, hyperkalemia, and hyponatremia
☐ E. A 55-year-old male smoker with shortness of breath and marked weight loss

28 Which of the listed cells undergo hypertrophy, but not hyperplasia?
☐ A. Cardiac muscle cell
☐ B. Central nervous system neuron
☐ C. Hepatocyte
☐ D. Mammary epithelial cell
☐ E. Postganglionic parasympathetic neuron

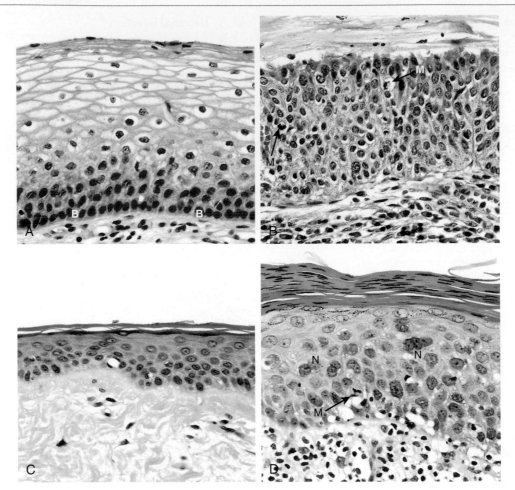

29 In the figure above, the cervix is shown in part A and B, and the skin is shown in parts C and D. The two images on the left show normal tissues. The two on the right illustrate which process?

☐ A. Dysplasia
☐ B. Hypertrophy
☐ C. Metaplasia
☐ D. Hyperplasia

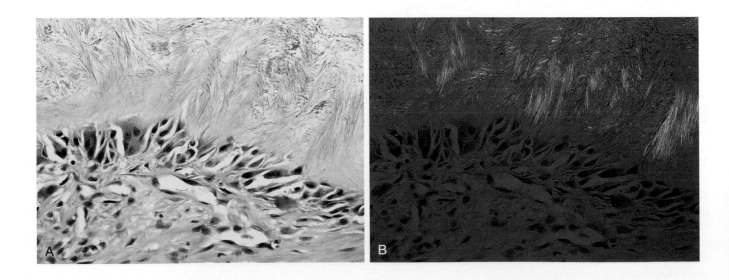

30 A 55-year-old man was found to have small subcutaneous nodules around his heel and knee. A laboratory examination shows an elevated blood urea nitrogen and creatinine. A biopsy of one of the nodules was performed, and the image on the previous page shows a histologic section (part A) and examination of the tissue under polarized light (part B), which shows negative birefringence, that is, the needles appear blue when the angle of light is perpendicular to the crystal and yellow when it is parallel. Which of the following was the most likely cause of the patient's abnormal renal function tests?
- A. Acute glomerulonephritis
- B. Renal stones
- C. Rhabdomyolysis
- D. Severe hypotension
- E. Urinary tract infection

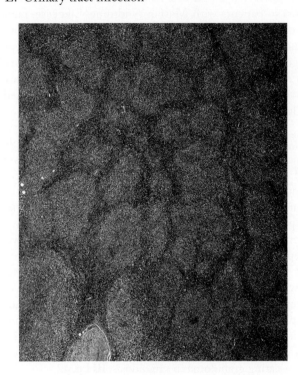

31 A 56-year-old man went to his physician with complaints of fever, night sweats, and weight loss. Physical examination showed cervical, axillary, and inguinal lymphadenopathy. A biopsy of one of the enlarged cervical lymph nodes was performed, and a section is shown in the figure above. Cytogenetic analysis performed on the lymph node showed a translocation involving chromosomes 14 and 18 [t(14;18)]. The patient's signs and symptoms were due to a dysregulation of what process?
- A. Apoptotic cell death
- B. DNA repair
- C. Growth signal reception
- D. Progression into the cell cycle
- E. Signal transduction

32 A 23-year-old woman is being examined by her physician after complaining of chronic respiratory infections. Stethoscope examination reveals that her lungs are clear, but her heart is on the right side of her thorax. A disturbed function of which cellular organelle is responsible for this condition?
- A. Actin filaments
- B. Cilia
- C. Golgi vesicles
- D. Lysosomes
- E. Mitochondria

33 A 35-year-old woman has come to her physician because of a recent weight gain and a failure to conceive a child after 3 years. She has some signs of increased facial hair. What diagnostic test should be ordered to confirm a diagnosis?
- A. Blood assay for decreased levels of prolactin
- B. Computed tomography of the head for pituitary involution
- C. Mammogram for breast tumors
- D. Papanicolaou staining of a cervical smear
- E. Ultrasound of pelvic organs

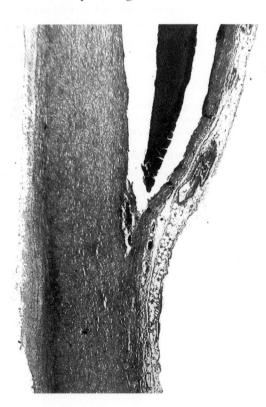

34 Autopsy examination of the aorta in a case of a sudden death revealed the pathology shown in the image above. This pathology would most likely have been seen in which of the following patients?
- A. A 23-year-old with lax joints and dislocated eye lens
- B. A 30-year-old with long-standing shortness of breath and heart murmur
- C. A 32-year-old intravenous drug abuser with fever and shortness of breath
- D. A 49-year-old alcoholic with severe vomiting
- E. A 55-year-old smoker with hypercholesterolemia

ANSWERS

1. D The image shows large vacuoles in the cytoplasm of hepatocytes that displace the nucleus. This is due to an accumulation of lipids, which is characteristic of fatty change, also known as *steatosis*. The most common causes of fatty change in the liver are toxins such as alcohol. In the absence of a history of alcohol intake or exposure to toxins, steatosis is most frequently associated with obesity, diabetes, or dyslipidemia and is known as *nonalcoholic steatohepatitis* (NASH). The other conditions listed are all associated with various pathologic changes in the liver but do not cause fatty change. In patients with sickle cell disease or other hemoglobinopathies, hemolysis of red blood cells and frequent blood transfusions result in excessive iron accumulation in the liver and other organs, giving rise to secondary hemosiderosis. Acetaminophen overdose causes extensive hepatocyte necrosis. Patients with ulcerative colitis can have an inflammatory disorder that leads to destruction and fibrosis of intrahepatic and extrahepatic bile ducts known as *primary sclerosing cholangitis*. The backup of blood into the liver in right-sided heart failure results in ischemia and necrosis of hepatocytes around the central veins. **BH p. 166**

2. B The micrograph shows colonic glands with numerous apoptotic bodies. A patient who has undergone transplantation is at risk for developing graft-versus-host disease, in which the cytotoxic T cells present in the donor's tissue attack various cells in the patient, resulting in apoptosis-induced cell death. The most common target tissues are the epithelial cells of the colon, epidermis, and bile ducts, and this is clinically manifested by a bloody diarrhea, skin rash, and jaundice. Although apoptosis is a normal physiologic process in the colonic epithelium, it does not lead to bloody diarrhea or any of the other symptoms noted. Transplant rejection occurs as a result of the recipient's T cells rejecting the transplanted tissue, which leads to failure of engraftment. In this case, the patient would present with symptoms of marrow failure. Apoptosis may be seen in chemotherapy-induced colitis or viral infections, but it would be accompanied with necrosis, inflammation, and, in the latter case, viral cytopathic changes. These patients may have diarrhea, but the triad of skin rash and jaundice are not seen. **BH p. 10**

3. A Injury, such as that caused by hypoxia, causes ionic imbalances leading to swelling of cellular organelles, particularly the endoplasmic reticulum. While there may be swelling of the Golgi complex, it does not disperse. Lysosomal disruption is a late injury response. Nuclear condensation occurs during apoptosis, which also is a late injury response. Ribosomes disappear from the cytoplasm in cellular injury. **BH pp. 3-6**

4. C As proteins in the necrotic cells degenerate, they form an eosinophilic mass in the cytoplasm causing the necrotic cells to stand out from the surrounding cells. A large pale nucleus is characteristic of cells actively undergoing transcription. Lobulated nuclei are normal features of polymorphonuclear neutrophils, as seen here. A poorly stained cytoplasm and a vacuolated cytoplasm may be early signs of cellular injury, but are not signs of necrosis. **BH pp. 6-7**

5. B The patient's symptoms are characteristic of cystic fibrosis, which causes mucus plugging of various ducts in the body. Thus, mucus blockage of the bronchi results in inflammation and permanent destruction of the walls (bronchiectasis), as shown in the image above. Similarly, blockage of the pancreatic ducts results in chronic pancreatitis with subsequent malabsorption and diarrhea. The other pathologies listed may occur in this age group in association with other diseases but are not typically seen in cystic fibrosis. Thus, multiple gallstones may occur in association with sickle cell disease due to excessive red blood cell hemolysis, and aortic dissection occurs in patients with Marfan syndrome. Likewise, numerous colonic adenomas are seen in young patients with familial adenomatous polyposis due to mutations in a tumor suppressor gene. Tracheoesophageal fistula is a congenital abnormality that manifests in the newborn as cough and difficulty breathing associated with feeding and the symptoms are limited to the lung. Mild cases may present later in life. **BH p. 30**

6. A The image shows replacement of the normal lymphoid tissue by confluent sheets of epithelioid macrophages associated with a suppurative necrosis. This pathology may be seen in immunocompromised patients infected with the opportunistic organism *Mycobacterium avium-intracellulare*. The patient's symptoms are also suggestive of an immune deficiency. The other choices listed can all lead to lymphadenopathy; however, except for Kaposi sarcoma, they are not associated with recurrent infections. In addition, the lymph node biopsy would show different pathologic changes, that is, sheets of large lymphocytes with large nuclei and prominent nucleoli in large cell lymphoma, follicular hyperplasia and proliferation of immunoblasts in infectious mononucleosis, a spindle cell proliferation with extravasated red blood cell in Kaposi sarcoma, and noncaseating granuloma in sarcoidosis. **BH p. 42**

7. C Cells that are characteristic of chronic inflammation (plasma cells, lymphocytes, and macrophages) are seen here. In abscess formation, neutrophils are the predominant cell type that accumulates in the connective tissue. If apoptosis were ongoing, cellular debris, such as fragments of nuclei, would be visible. In edema, large fluid-filled spaces would be present between cells. Necrotic cells are very eosinophilic. **BH p. 28, FH p. 207**

8. B Infection with cytomegalovirus, common in HIV patients, produces markedly enlarged cells with characteristic cellular features such as a dark-staining intranuclear inclusion body surrounded by a pale "halo," as seen in the image (*arrows*). Inclusion bodies may also be seen with herpes infections, but the virally infected cells are usually multinucleate. *Aspergillus* infections commonly form a "fungus ball" within the lung cavities, and fungal hyphae would be visible. In pneumocystis infections, the organisms are too small to be easily visible in hematoxylin and eosin–stained sections and may require Giemsa or silver stains to be seen. **BH pp. 44-46**

9. C The image shows a thickened wall in a mucosal vessel due to deposition of a pink, homogeneous material. The histologic findings and the characteristic birefringence with Congo red are confirmatory of amyloidosis. In the amyloid light-chain (AL) type of amyloidosis, immunoglobulin light chains are deposited in various tissues, some of which occur in association with multiple myeloma. In such cases, examination of the bone marrow would show sheets of plasma cells infiltrating the bone marrow. All the other marrow pathologies listed occur in a variety of disorders but are not characteristic of amyloidosis. Extensive fibrosis occurs in chronic myeloproliferative disorders (myelofibrosis), lymphomas, and metastatic tumors of the marrow. Markedly increased iron is seen in chronic hemolysis, recurrent transfusion, and disorders of iron metabolism. In aplastic anemia and acute myeloid leukemia, the marrow is replaced by fat and myeloblasts, respectively. **BH pp. 55-57**

10. D Since the AL type of amyloidosis is associated with multiple myeloma, measurement of serum proteins by electrophoresis is a useful laboratory test to arrive at a diagnosis. This test would show a monoclonal protein (M-spike) due to overproduction of an immunoglobulin by the neoplastic plasma cells. Measurement of hemoglobin is useful to assess the degree of bone marrow compromise but does not provide specific diagnostic information. Amyloid deposition in the brain may be seen in association with Down syndrome, in which chromosome analysis would show trisomy 21. However, the condition becomes evident early in life owing to the characteristic physical findings. Amyloid deposition may also occur in medullary carcinoma of the thyroid; however, thyroid hormones are usually normal. Similarly, amyloid may be deposited in the liver, but the liver function tests are usually normal. **BH pp. 55-57, 211**

11. A The condensed fragmented chromatin is characteristic of cells undergoing apoptosis. Cytokinesis and mitoses involve whole cells with normal cytoplasm. Here the space around the chromatin appears empty. Although fatty change may show large vacuolar areas, they will not contain chromatin. **FH p. 43**

12. A A characteristic of apoptosis is that caspase causes breakdown of the nucleus and cytoplasm. Cyclic AMP functions as an intracellular messenger which coordinates other cellular processes. Cyclins and cyclin-dependent kinases regulate the cell cycle. Cytokines are intercellular messenger molecules used by cells to coordinate the immune response. Tyrosine kinases are involved in signal transduction. **FH p. 43**

13. C This image shows numerous apoptotic bodies characteristic of the onset of menstruation. Later in the process, the endometrial glands will be absent, except for remnants near the myometrium. The proliferative phase will show numerous

mitotic figures, whereas the secretory stage glands will have a tortuous appearance. There are few glands in the endometrium after menopause. **FH p. 43**

14. A The image illustrates a thrombus filling the lumen of the vein. The thrombus dislodged and resulted in pulmonary embolism, which was the cause of her sudden death. In a young patient with no known risk factors for deep vein thrombosis, an inherited cause should be suspected. A mutation in the clotting factor V gene, also known as factor V Leiden, is most likely because it is the most common cause of inherited clotting disorder. Mutations in the other molecules listed result in various diseases, but an increased risk for thrombosis is not seen except in sickle cell disease, which is caused by a mutation in the hemoglobin gene. In the latter case, the patient would have been symptomatic from early childhood. A mutation in the myosin heavy chain is associated with hypertrophic cardiomyopathy, which is a cause of sudden death in young patients. A mutation in type I collagen results in osteogenesis imperfecta or brittle bone disease. Mutations in von Willebrand factor cause a bleeding disorder, not thrombosis. **BH pp. 95-97**

15. C The microscopic section of the skin shows a small vessel vasculitis with fibrinoid necrosis and neutrophilic infiltration of the vessel walls. This is characteristic of microscopic polyangiitis, which can involve many different organs, including the kidneys. The vasculitis affects the small vessels of the glomeruli leading to glomerulonephritis with hematuria and proteinuria. The other renal pathologies listed may present with hematuria, but are not associated with microscopic polyangiitis. Acute tubular necrosis is caused by ischemia or exposure to a toxin. Chronic pyelonephritis is caused by recurrent infections of the renal tubules. Renal papillary necrosis is most commonly seen in association with diabetes, sickle cell disease, or infections. Patients with microscopic polyangiitis do not have an increased incidence of renal cell carcinoma. **BH p. 117**

16. D Mitochondria are critical in determining whether a cellular injury is reversible. Mitochondria release cytochrome C to trigger apoptosis or, in the case of severe injury, stop producing ATP, which in turn affects all other organelles. Damage to other organelles may be reversible or may be secondary to mitochondrial injury. **BH p. 5**

17. E Nearly all the maturing T cells in the thymic cortex die by apoptosis. Many of these are self-reactive, and their removal prevents autoimmune reactions. Thus, apoptosis is frequently seen in the normal thymus. Bone marrow is the site of new blood cell formation, and little apoptosis would be expected in this location. Epidermal cells constantly turn over, but they are shed and lost to the environment rather than undergoing apoptosis. Chondrocytes of hyaline cartilage are long-lived cells that do not turn over. In osteoarthritis, chondrocytes are lost by apoptosis, and there is a loss of cartilage tissue. In the seminiferous tubules, spermatozoa are constantly produced after the age of puberty. Like the bone marrow, the function of the seminiferous tubules is to produce new cells, and little apoptosis would be expected here. **FH pp. 58-59, 169-171, 186-187, 215, 349**

18. B The microscopic section shows a proliferation of epithelioid and spindle cells arranged in fascicles. This is a characteristic morphologic finding in gastrointestinal stromal tumors (GIST), which are thought to be derived from the interstitial cells of Cajal. Because these tumors express CD117 (Kit), immunohistochemical stains are used to confirm the diagnosis of a GIST. Because of the expression of Kit, these tumors can be treated with imatinib, a tyrosine kinase inhibitor. The tumors are neither derived from the glandular epithelium nor associated with *Helicobacter pylori* infection. Tumors derived from the glandular epithelium would show evidence of gland formation or mucin production, and chronic *H. pylori* infection is a predisposing factor for the development of adenocarcinomas. Chromogranin A, a protein associated with secretory granules, is expressed by neuroendocrine tumors such as carcinoid tumors. **BH p. 150**

19. C The image shows an ovarian mass composed of plump spindle cells with foamy cytoplasm due to lipid droplets. This is characteristic of thecomas, which are stromal tumors of the ovary. These tumors usually secrete estrogen, which leads to excessive stimulation of the endometrium. This in turn results in endometrial hyperplasia, which progresses from simple to complex, and subsequent development of adenocarcinoma. All the other choices listed are common disorders of the uterus, but are not directly associated with thecomas. **BH p. 233**

20. E Metastases of cancerous prostate cells, which stain positively for prostate-specific antigen, commonly occur within the marrow cavities of bones. Signals released from these cells stimulate increased bone formation, resulting in osteosclerosis. Endochondral ossification refers to bone formation around a model made of cartilage, which is absent from this figure; also, excessive numbers of megakaryocytes with folded nuclei are not detectable in this image. Osteoclast hyperactivity would produce signs of bone resorption and destruction, not seen here. **BH p. 210**

21. E This patient is suffering from autoimmune polyendocrine syndrome, which arises when a protein called *Aire* fails to function in the thymus. This prevents the display of autoantigens for the process of deleting T cells that are reactive to self-antigens. The immune system, for uncertain reasons, primarily attacks endocrine organs like the parathyroid and adrenal glands, leading to symptoms of hypoparathyroidism (muscle spasms), hypothyroidism (dry, scaly skin), and Addison disease. Symptoms of Addison disease include hyperpigmentation due to increased adrenocorticotropic hormone (ACTH) production and low blood pressure due to decreased mineralocorticoid secretion. The increased ACTH secretion results from a diminished negative feedback effect of corticosteroids on the pituitary gland, which is otherwise normal. Elevated ACTH levels rule out Sheehan syndrome of a generalized pituitary insufficiency. Additionally, in patients with

this syndrome, immune cells fail to attack certain microorganisms such as yeast cells, resulting in frequent yeast infections. **FH p. 217**

22. D The microscopic section of the adrenal mass shows nests of plump cells with abundant, granular cytoplasm. The patient's clinical presentation and the morphologic findings of the adrenal gland mass are characteristic of pheochromocytoma. In addition, the young age of the patient, the occurrence of multiple tumors, the positive family history, and the thyroid mass all point to a genetic component leading to a diagnosis of multiple endocrine neoplasia (MEN). In such cases, the thyroid mass would be due to a medullary carcinoma, which characteristically shows nests of polygonal cells with amyloid deposition. All the other morphologic changes listed can be seen in the thyroid, but are not associated with MEN. Hemorrhage, calcification, and fibrosis usually are seen in multinodular goiter. Hyperplastic acini with tall columnar cells are present in hyperthyroidism, such as Graves disease, whereas lymphoid infiltration with germinal centers is seen in Hashimoto thyroiditis. Epithelial cells with nuclear inclusions and grooves are characteristic of papillary carcinoma of the thyroid. **BH pp. 263-265**

23. B The image shows a cellular tumor composed of pleomorphic glial cells that palisade around areas of necrosis. This is a characteristic feature of glioblastoma multiforme, which is a high-grade astrocytoma. This tumor has a high proliferation rate, with numerous mitoses, grows rapidly and has a poor prognosis. It is most often located in the cerebrum and has an infiltrating pattern, making it difficult to resect. It is not associated with *NF-1* gene mutations, nor does the tumor arise from cranial nerves. Cyst formation and common occurrence in the cerebellum are more characteristic of the low-grade pilocytic astrocytoma commonly seen in children. **BH p. 308**

24. B The stomach mucosa has a typical layered appearance. The upper portion stains pink, whereas the lower portion stains purple because of the chief cells in the lower half of the gastric glands. The thick stratified squamous esophageal epithelium would appear much lighter. The mucosa of the small intestine has villi and lacks the layered appearance. The large intestine also lacks the layered appearance, and the epithelium has many light-stained goblet cells. **BH p. 147**

25. D The patient's symptoms and the microscopic image are diagnostic for a peptic ulcer. Erosion of blood vessels at the ulcer site will result in bleeding, leading to a low level of hemoglobin (anemia). The bleeding can present as tarry stool (melena). Measuring blood glucose tests for diabetes. A blood urea nitrogen test is carried out to look at kidney function. A test for bilirubin is used to identify the source of jaundice. Triglycerides are used to screen for hypercholesterolemia. **BH p. 147**

26. C The image shows a multinucleated foreign-body type of giant cell, which is formed by the fusion of tissue macrophages. These cells form in response to implanted foreign material, such as the remnant of a surgical suture. On physical examination, a foreign-body granulomatous inflammation at the site of a previous surgery can feel firm, mimicking a tumor. There are no atypical glandular cells to indicate the recurrence of her tumor. In a bacterial infection, numerous neutrophils would be present, and trauma would result in fat necrosis. **BH p. 33**

27. B The microscopic section of the adrenal gland shows atrophy of the gland as evidenced by a marked reduction in the size of the cortex. This was present in both adrenal glands, hence there is bilateral adrenocortical atrophy, which is caused by a lack of ACTH stimulation. Joint pain and a malar rash are typically present in systemic lupus erythematosus, and severe cases usually require corticosteroid therapy. In patients on long-term administration of corticosteroids, ACTH suppression by a negative feedback mechanism results in bilateral adrenocortical atrophy. Headache and bilateral hemianopia are symptoms of a pituitary adenoma, which may secrete excessive ACTH. Shortness of breath and weight loss in a smoker are highly suggestive of a lung carcinoma. The small cell variant of the latter is known to produce ectopic ACTH. An increase in ACTH would result in bilateral, diffuse, cortical hyperplasia, not atrophy. Palpitation and episodic hypertension are symptoms of catecholamine excess due to an adrenal medullary tumor (pheochromocytoma). Hypertension associated with hyperkalemia and hyponatremia is suggestive of an aldosterone-secreting adenoma (Conn syndrome). **BH pp. 254-265**

28. A Under increased load, cardiac muscle cells will hypertrophy but are postmitotic and will not undergo hyperplasia. Neurons do not undergo either hypertrophy or hyperplasia. Hepatocytes undergo both hypertrophy and hyperplasia. Mammary epithelial cells undergo hyperplasia, particularly during pregnancy. **BH p. 61**

29. A The images on the right illustrate dysplasia, which is characterized by a failure of the cells to undergo their normal pattern of differentiation. In the cervix, the cells in the upper layers of the epithelium have large, rounded nuclei rather than condensed flattened nuclei, and the surface cells have not flattened either. In the skin, the surface cells have retained their nuclei, and the nuclei of the cells in the lower layers are enlarged. In both organs, mitotic figures may be seen in the upper layers of the epithelium rather than being confined to the basal layer. Hypertrophy is characterized by cellular enlargement, which is not present in most of the atypical cells here. Metaplasia is the development of a different type of tissue (usually epithelium). Hyperplasia is an increase in the number of cells in the tissue, but with the normal characteristics retained. **BH pp. 59-61, 63, 65-66**

30. B The image shows a granulomatous reaction with a proliferation of macrophages surrounding needle-shaped crystals that have precipitated in the tissue. The negative birefringence is characteristic of urate crystals, which occur in gout. The same crystals can precipitate in the renal tubules and form stones, which can, in turn, lead to renal failure, which is evidenced by an elevated blood urea nitrogen and creatinine in this patient. All the other choices listed can cause renal failure, but are not directly associated with gout. **BH p. 269**

31. A Generalized lymphadenopathy with a proliferation of numerous follicles in the lymph node, as shown in the image, with a genetic translocation involving chromosome 14 and 18 is characteristic of follicular lymphoma. In this type of lymphoma, the translocation, involving the antiapoptotic *BCL-2* gene on chromosome 18 and the immunoglobulin heavy-chain gene on chromosome 14, results in overexpression of the *BCL-2* gene. This leads to inhibition of apoptosis and accumulation of the lymphocytes, resulting in generalized lymphadenopathy. Dysregulation of the other cell processes are caused by other genetic mechanisms. **BH p. 203**

32. B This woman is exhibiting symptoms of Kartagener syndrome, which arises from a defect in ciliary dynein. Dysfunctional cilia provoke impaired clearance of mucus in the respiratory system, leading to recurrent infections. Cilia are important in setting up left-right asymmetries in the body. People with this syndrome sometimes have a reversed left-right asymmetry. Immotile cilia fail to form gradients of morphogen in the developing embryo, which are required for the development of the normal left-right asymmetries. **FH p. 92**.

33. E The obesity, infertility, and increased facial hair are suggestive of polycystic ovarian syndrome, which can be diagnosed by the ultrasound detection of many small cysts within an ovary. In this disease, ovarian follicles are stimulated to produce excessive androgens (perhaps by an obesity-associated increase in circulating insulin) and thus cause signs of virilization. Increased, but not decreased, levels of prolactin may also accompany other syndromes of infertility. In pituitary involution, ovarian atrophy rather than ovarian cysts would be seen. **FH p. 366**

34. A The image shows an aortic dissection with blood tracking into the tunica media caused by a laceration in the intima. Patients with Marfan syndrome are at a risk for developing an aortic dissection because of weakening of the vessel wall caused by abnormal elastic fibers. In addition, these patients have lax joint ligaments, skeletal deformities, and dislocation of the eye lens, referred as *ectopia lentis*. The other signs and symptoms are suggestive of other diseases, which are not directly associated with aortic dissection. Thus, a patient with long-standing shortness of breath and heart murmur would most likely have rheumatic or congenital valvular heart disease. Fever and shortness of breath in an intravenous drug abuser are suggestive of endocarditis, and patients with severe vomiting can develop esophageal lacerations, which is most commonly seen in alcoholics. **BH p. 114**

Index

Liver *(Continued)*
   sinusoids of, 124–126
   supporting framework of, 24, 27
   tumor in, 124, 124f, 127
Loop of Henle, 136–137
Low-density lipoprotein (LDL), 5, 5f, 9
Lung. *See also* Alveoli; Asbestos, in lung;
      Pulmonary entries.
   adenocarcinoma of, 97–98
   autopsy specimen from, in adolescent, 190,
      190f
   biopsy of, in HIV-infected patient, 191, 191f,
      198–199
   squamous cell carcinoma of, 97
Lung nodule(s)
   with fever and night sweats, 94, 94f, 98
   in HIV-positive patient, 94f, 95
   as metastatic tumors, 95, 95f, 98
      from uterus, 167, 173
   with shortness of breath, 92, 92f, 97
Lymph nodes
   afferent lymphatic vessels and, 84
   antigen-presenting cells in, 83
   cervical biopsy of, 190, 190f, 198
   dendritic cells in, 84
   follicles of, 84
   malignant cells in, 84
   mediastinal, granulomas in, 97
Lymphadenopathy
   generalized, with chromosomal translocation,
      197, 197f, 201
   mediastinal, 92, 92f, 97
Lymphatic vessels, afferent, 84
Lymphocytes. *See also* B cells; T cells.
   bone marrow replacement by, 85
   in chronic inflammation, 198
   circulation between tissue and blood, 21
   elevated count of, 21
   epidermal infiltration by, 68
   in granulomas, 98
   in intestinal mucosa, in celiac disease, 116–117
   in intestines, 84
   in leprosy, nerve destruction and, 47
   in lymph node, 83
   in lymphoepithelial lesions, 117–118
   proliferation in tissues and organs, 21
   in rheumatoid arthritis, 75
   in salivary gland, 104
   thyroid infiltration by, 148
Lymphocytic sialadenitis, 101, 104
Lymphoepithelial lesions, gastric, 117–118
Lymphoid follicles
   in Hashimoto thyroiditis, 148
   in lymph nodes, 84
Lymphoid nodules, in intestinal epithelium, 117
Lymphoma
   cutaneous
      MALT, 84–85
      T-cell, 68
   flow cytometry studies in, 79
   follicular, 201
   gastric, 81, 84–85, 113, 113f, 117–118
   Hodgkin, 85
   non-Hodgkin, HIV infection with, 85
Lysosomal storage disorders, 26, 28. *See also*
      Hurler syndrome.
Lysosomes, incomplete digestion in, 9
Lysozyme, from Paneth cells, 117

M
M cells, 117
Macrophages
   alveolar, 21, 28, 95
      asbestos and, 97
   in chronic inflammation, 198
   giant cells formed by, 28, 200–201. *See also*
      Giant cells.
   in gout, 201
   in granulomas, 98
   lysosomal storage disorders and, 28
   monocyte precursors of, 28
   in *Mycobacterium avium-intracellulare* infection,
      198
   after myocardial infarction, 28
   splenic
      in lysosomal storage disorders, 28
      phagocytosis of RBCs by, 20
Macula densa, 129, 136–137
Male reproductive system, 151
Malignant tumor cells. *See also* Carcinoma.
   abnormal mitosis in, 13–14
   cell of origin of, 8, 10
Marantic endocarditis, 58
Marfan syndrome, 23–24, 27, 201
Mast cells
   CD117 expressed on, 84
   metachromatic staining of, with toluidine blue,
      28
Maternally derived genetic defects, 12–13
Media, arterial
   of aorta, 58
   essential hypertension and, 59
Media, venous, 60
Medial lemniscus, 180
Mediastinal lymphadenopathy, 92, 92f, 97
Mediastinal mass, 78, 81, 81f
Medullary carcinoma, thyroid, 200
Megakaryocytes, 20–21
Meiosis, 12–14, 171
Meissner corpuscles, 47
Melanin, tyrosinase in formation of, 67
Melanocytes, 63, 67
   of junctional nevi, 68
Melanoma, 67
Membranous glomerulonephritis, 137
MEN (multiple endocrine neoplasia), 200
Ménière disease, 186
Meningioma, 180
Menstrual cycle
   apoptosis in, 199
   endometrial changes in, 162, 162f, 172
   excessive bleeding in, with nodules, 173
   irregular bleeding in, with mass, 168
Merkel cells, 47
   tumor derived from, 45, 47
Mesangial cells, 136
Mesangium
   hypercellular, in postinfectious
      glomerulonephritis, 137
   IgA deposition in, 137
Mesothelioma, 97
Metachromatic staining, with toluidine blue, 26, 28
Metastatic tumors
   in bone marrow, 85, 200
   in liver, 127
   in lung, 95, 95f, 98
MHC I proteins, 83

Microcirculation, control of, 56f, 57, 59
Microscopic polyangiitis, 199
Microtubules, 10
   of cilia, 32
   of flagella, 156
   in mitosis, 11, 13
   of nerve fibers, 46
Microvilli
   actin cores of, 33
   lactase associated with, 117
   of taste buds, 185
   terminal web supporting, 33
Mitochondria
   beta-oxidation of fatty acids by, 126
   of cardiac muscle, 40
   cellular injury and, 199
   cristae of, 9, 40
      tubular, 148
   energy requirements of cell and, 6, 6f, 9
   highest concentration of, 37, 40
   of ion-transporting cells, 9, 136
   in parathyroid oxyphil cells, 147
   in parietal cell, 116
   in renal oncocytoma, 138
   of skeletal muscle, 40
   of spermatozoa, 156
Mitochondrial DNA, 13
Mitosis
   in brain tumor, rapidly-growing, 200
   chromosome staining in, 13
   cytokinesis and, 13
   in endometrial proliferation, 172
   microtubules in, 11, 13
   tripolar spindle in, 13
   without cytokinesis, 20–21, 127
Mitotic figures, 11, 11f, 13
   in malignant cells, 13–14
   ring-form, 14
Mitral valve, 53, 53f, 58
Monocytes, 21, 28
   osteoclasts derived from, 73
M-spike, 199
Mucinous cystadenocarcinoma, ovarian, 174
Mucosa
   bronchial, squamous metaplasia of, 96
   gastric, 200
   lymphoid tissue of, 104
   nasal, 95
Mucosa-associated lymphoid tissue (MALT)
      lymphoma
   cutaneous, 84–85
   gastric, 84–85, 117–118
   Hashimoto thyroiditis and risk of, 148
Mucous acini, salivary gland, 104
Mucous glands, bronchial
   hypertrophy of, 96
   inflammation of, 96
Mucus
   in airways, 32
   dysfunctional cilia and, 201
   generalized plugging of ducts with, 198
Multiple endocrine neoplasia (MEN), 200
Multiple myeloma, 77, 77f, 83
   amyloidosis in, 199
Multiple sclerosis, 46
Muscle, 35. *See also* Cardiac muscle; Skeletal
      muscle; Smooth muscle.
   desmin staining of, 10

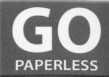
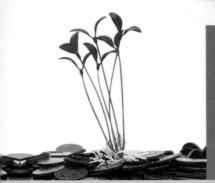
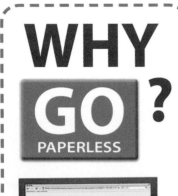
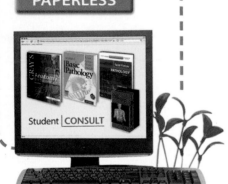
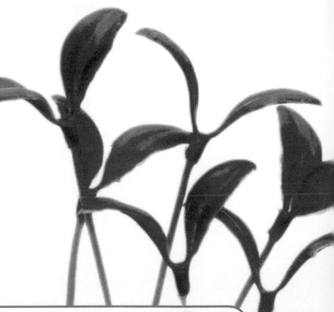